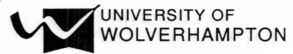
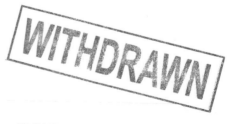

Molecular Diagnostics

Pathology and Laboratory Medicine

Clinical Pathology of Pancreatic Disease, edited by **John A. Lott,** 1997

Molecular Diagnostics: For the Clinical Laboratorian, edited by **William B. Coleman** and **Gregory J. Tsongalis,** 1997

Molecular Diagnostics

For the Clinical Laboratorian

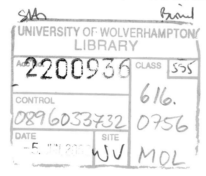
Edited by

William B. Coleman

University of North Carolina, Chapel Hill, NC

and

Gregory J. Tsongalis

Hartford Hospital, Hartford, CT

Humana Press ✳ Totowa, New Jersey

© 1997 Humana Press Inc.
999 Riverview Drive, Suite 208
Totowa, New Jersey 07512

For additional copies, pricing for bulk purchases, and/or information about other Humana titles, contact Humana at the above address or at any of the following numbers: Tel.: 201-256-1699; Fax: 201-256-8341; E-mail: humana@mindspring.com

This publication is printed on acid-free paper. ∞
ANSI Z39.48-1984 (American Standards Institute) Permanence of Paper for Printed Library Materials.

Cover illustration: From Fig. 6 in Chapter 2 "An Overview of Nucleic Acid Chemistry, Structure, and Function: *The Foundations of Molecular Biology,*" by William B. Coleman.

Cover design by Patricia F. Cleary.

Printed in the United States of America. 10 9 8 7 6 5 4 3 2

Library of Congress Cataloging-in-Publication Data

Molecular diagnostics : for the clinical laboratorian / edited by
    William B. Colaman and Gregory J. Tsongalis.
        p.   cm.
    Includes index.
    ISBN 0-89603-373-2 (alk. paper)
    1. Molecular diagnosis.   2. Pathology, Molecular.   I. Coleman.
    William B.   II. Tsongalis, Gregory J.
    [DNLM: 1. Technology, Medical.   2. Genetic Techniques.
    3. Diagnosis, Laboratory—methods.   4. Molecular Biology—methods.
    5. Chemistry, Clinical—methods.   WB 365 M718 1997]
    RB43/7.M65   1997
    616.07'56—dc21
    DNLM/DLC
    for Library of Congress   96-37505
                                                                   CIP

Preface

The clinical laboratory has long functioned as a dynamic environment in which new technologies constantly challenge us by their implementation in new diagnostic tests. With the goal of providing the most sensitive and specific tests for monitoring disease, the clinical laboratory is now challenged by yet another technological advancement, that occasioned by the development and applications of molecular biology to the analysis of nucleic acids. It is already clear that this will have a most significant impact on the clinical laboratory with respect to the sensitivity/specificity of tests as well as their broad application to all areas of laboratory medicine. The information provided by molecular diagnostic testing will change the way laboratory medicine is practiced in an unprecedented manner.

The success of this molecular diagnostic approach in a clinical setting is highly dependent on the training of well-qualified technologists, residents, and clinicians alike, who will not only have to perform these tests and interpret their results, but also understand the limitations of both the technology and the results. We address these issues in chapters specifically dealing with each technique, and in subsequent chapters include applications to the diagnosis of various forms of disease. This book is intended for use by medical technologists, residents, fellows, and clinicians of all medical disciplines who will be affected by one or more applications of this technology to any given subspecialty.

It has been a mere ten years since this technology shifted from the research arena to the clinical arena. In part because of the success of the Human Genome Project, both the technology and its applications are being introduced to the medical community at record-setting speeds. Our goal is to present this revolutionary technology to these trainees in a concise yet understandable fashion and include examples of its applications to the various divisions of laboratory medicine as an indicator of what the future of diagnostic medicine will be.

William B. Coleman
Gregory J. Tsongalis

Dedications

Over the years, many individuals have played crucial roles in our successes, but none greater than those members of our families who gave continuous support in an unselfish manner.

This book is dedicated to our parents, Alice and Byrns Coleman and Mary and Demetrios Tsongalis for believing in higher education and helping make dreams come true.

To our wives, Monty and Nancy, for their unprecedented support, understanding, and appreciation for what we do.

To our children, brothers, sisters, and extended families for the many years of love, friendship, and tolerance.

W. B. C.

G. J. T.

Contents

Preface .... *v*

List of Contributors .... *ix*

PART I   BASIC MOLECULAR BIOLOGY *1*

1 A Historical Perspective on the Clinical Diagnostic Laboratory
   Robert E. Moore *3*

2 An Overview of Nucleic Acid Chemistry, Structure, and Function:
   The Foundations of Molecular Biology
   William B. Coleman *15*

3 Basic Nucleic Acid Procedures
   R. Keith Esch *35*

PART II   MOLECULAR TECHNOLOGIES *61*

4 Nucleic Acid Blotting Techniques: *Theory and Practice*
   Sharon Collins Presnell *63*

5 DNA Amplification Techniques: *An Overview*
   David H. Sorscher *89*

6 RT-PCR: *Quantitative and Diagnostic PCR in the Analysis
   of Gene Expression*
   Robert B. Sisk *103*

7 PCR-Based Methods for Mutation Detection
   Elizabeth M. Rohlfs and W. Edward Highsmith, Jr. *123*

8 Nucleic Acid Hybridization and Amplification *In Situ:
   Principles and Applications in Molecular Pathology*
   Matthew S. Cowlen *163*

9 Gene Therapy
   Jeffrey S. Bartlett *193*

PART III   APPLICATIONS TO MOLECULAR PATHOLOGY *215*

10 An Overview of Molecular Genetics
    Gregory J. Tsongalis *217*

11 Genetic Basis of Neurologic and Neuromuscular Diseases
    *Myra J. Wick, Pamela A. Crifasi, Zhenyuan Wang,
       and Stephen N. Thibodeau* *229*

vii

12 Molecular Mechanisms of Endocrine Disorders
    Bruce F. Bower and Carl D. Malchoff 249

13 Molecular Pathogenesis of Cardiovascular Disease
    John H. Contois and Juch Chin Huang 271

14 Molecular Mutations in Human Neoplastic Disease:
    Application of Nucleic Acid Technology in the Assessment
    of Familial Risk, Diagnosis, and Prognosis of Human Cancers
    William B. Coleman and Gregory J. Tsongalis 293

15 Molecular Genetics and the Diagnosis
    of Hematological Malignancies
    William N. Rezuke and Evelyn C. Abernathy 317

16 Molecular Techniques in Laboratory Diagnosis
    of Infectious Diseases
    Jaber Aslanzadeh 341

PART IV   ISSUES FOR THE CLINICAL MOLECULAR PATHOLOGY LABORATORY 361
17 Quality Control Issues for the Clinical Molecular Pathologist
    Daniel H. Farkas 363

18 Prospects for the Future Role of the Clinical Laboratory
    Lawrence M. Silverman 373

    Index 379

Contributors

EVELYN C. ABERNATHY • *Department of Pathology and Laboratory Medicine, Hartford Hospital, Hartford, CT*

JABER ASLANZADEH • *Department of Laboratory Medicine, University of Connecticut School of Medicine, Farmington, CT*

JEFFREY S. BARTLETT • *Gene Therapy Center, University of North Carolina School of Medicine, Chapel Hill, NC*

BRUCE F. BOWER • *Department of Clinical Endocrinology, Hartford Hospital, Hartford, CT; University of Connecticut School of Medicine, Farmington, CT*

WILLIAM B. COLEMAN • *Department of Pathology and Laboratory Medicine, University of North Carolina School of Medicine, Chapel Hill, NC*

JOHN H. CONTOIS • *Department of Pathology and Laboratory Medicine, Hartford Hospital, Hartford, CT*

MATTHEW S. COWLEN • *Department of Pathology and Laboratory Medicine, McLendon Clinical Laboratories, University of North Carolina Hospitals, Chapel Hill, NC; Present Address: Pathology Associates International, Frederick, MD*

PAMELA A. CRIFASI • *Department of Laboratory Medicine, Molecular Genetics Laboratory, Mayo Clinic, Rochester, MN*

R. KEITH ESCH • *Department of Biochemistry and Biophysics, University of North Carolina, Chapel Hill, NC. Present Address: Department of Biology, Ursinus College, Collegeville, PA*

DANIEL H. FARKAS • *Department of Clinical Pathology, William Beaumont Hospital, Royal Oak, MI*

W. EDWARD HIGHSMITH, JR. • *Department of Pathology, University of Maryland, Baltimore, MD*

JUCH CHIN HUANG • *Department of Pathology and Laboratory Medicine, Hartford Hospital, Hartford, CT*

CARL D. MALCHOFF • *Department of Medicine and Surgery, Surgical Research Center, University of Connecticut Health Center, Farmington, CT*

ROBERT E. MOORE • *Department of Pathology and Laboratory Medicine, Hartford Hospital, Hartford, CT*

SHARON COLLINS PRESNELL • *Department of Pathology and Laboratory Medicine, University of North Carolina School of Medicine, Chapel Hill, NC*

WILLIAM N. REZUKE • *Department of Pathology and Laboratory Medicine, Hartford Hospital, Hartford, CT*

ELIZABETH M. ROHLFS • *Department of Pathology and Laboratory Medicine, McLendon Clinical Laboratories, University of North Carolina Hospitals, Chapel Hill, NC*

LAWRENCE M. SILVERMAN • *Department of Pathology and Laboratory Medicine, University of North Carolina, Chapel Hill, NC*

ROBERT B. SISK • *Department of Marine Science, University of North Carolina School of Medicine, Chapel Hill, NC*

DAVID H. SORSCHER • *Department of Biochemistry and Biophysics, University of North Carolina, Chapel Hill, NC*

STEPHEN N. THIBODEAU • *Department of Laboratory Medicine, Mayo Clinic, Rochester, MN*

GREGORY J. TSONGALIS • *Department of Pathology and Laboratory Medicine, Hartford Hospital, Hartford, CT*

ZHENYUAN WANG • *Department of Laboratory Medicine, Molecular Genetics Laboratory, Mayo Clinic, Rochester, MN*

MYRA J. WICK • *Department of Laboratory Medicine, Molecular Genetics Laboratory, Mayo Clinic, Rochester, MN*

Part I
Basic Molecular Biology

A Historical Perspective
on the Clinical Diagnostic Laboratory

Robert E. Moore

1. INTRODUCTION

As the clinical diagnostic laboratory prepares to enter the 21st century, it is interesting to reflect on past scientific and social events that have influenced the current status of the laboratory, and anticipate future problems and opportunities. It would be a mistake to suggest that all the significant medical and social events that had an impact on the present laboratory function can be discussed or evaluated in a short introductory chapter. It is also possible to mistakenly attribute more influence to some events than they deserve simply because they are being interpreted with a 20th century bias. However, some threads of commonality have influenced the evolution of diagnostic laboratories from earliest times. It is the objective of this chapter to highlight events that, in my opinion, have shaped how and/or why clinical laboratories have arrived at their present position in the practice of medicine.

A history of diagnostic testing can be started by reviewing the evolution of diagnostic tests from isolated procedures to organized diagnostic laboratory testing. Originally, laboratory tests were performed at the side of the patient with small, simple equipment, rapid evaluation of the result, and a diagnostic opinion rendered. Test choice, performance, and interpretation were all left to the individual practitioner. There was no professional support staff to assist at any point in the process. Little exchange took place between practitioners, because the individual's success was directly related to which procedures were done and the manner in which they were done. A premium was paid for showmanship as well as successful treatments.

The modern laboratory is a physical place, either standing alone or as a component of a health care institution, with numerous pieces of complicated capital equipment, where hundreds and sometimes thousands of specimens per day are processed for dozens of tests. Usually the laboratory accepts a teaching and a research responsibility to accompany this patient service obligation. Today's laboratories are staffed by professionals trained in several subspecialties, who are available for consultation in all aspects of diagnostic testing. This structure underlines the current complexity and sophistication of the modern laboratory operation. There are a myriad of professional organizations, meetings, and publications that have developed to make information

From: Molecular Diagnostics: For the Clinical Laboratorian
Edited by: W. B. Coleman and G. J. Tsongalis Humana Press Inc., Totowa, NJ

exchange convenient and efficient. This exchange is also necessary to ensure a single level of care. The system that supports showmanship and theatrics has been replaced by one that only tolerates accepted medical practice.

Today's laboratory is in a state of flux, faced with issues of near-patient testing, outreach programs, utilization, extensive regulation, and stringent fiscal controls. The first three of these issues are reminiscent of the early beginnings of diagnostic testing. The laboratory organization has replaced the individual practitioner, but testing is moving back toward the patient in the form of near patient testing or outreach programs. In the past, a few individuals spoke about appropriate use of diagnostic testing, whereas today committees and organizations are dedicated to the control of laboratory utilization—an ontogeny recapitulating phylogeny phenomenon. A review of history gives some insight into relationships and similarities of past activity with current practice. What are perceived as new problems and opportunities can be traced to antiquity.

The development of the modern laboratory required several conditions to be met at appropriate times in history. Obviously, technology was and is the primary force behind advances in medicine. This has been both a blessing and a curse. It is a blessing because the understanding and treatment of disease require sophisticated tools that only technological advances can produce. It can be a curse because there is a direct relationship between sophistication and health care cost. Other social issues dealing with availability and ethics assume a much greater importance than in the past. Angiography, CAT scans, organ transplantation, and DNA analysis are just a few of the expensive but valuable technologies available to the modern physician. Such questions as when are they used, to whom are they available, and what is done with the result, are dilemmas of the 20th-century laboratory.

Another result of this technology is that it removes a large number of tests and procedures from the primary physician. The expertise required to perform these and other procedures combined with the significant cost of the equipment precludes the primary physician from being the laboratorian.

A second condition that had to be met was logistics. Laboratory testing had to be convenient. All the concerns of collection, preservation, testing, and reporting had to be easy and fast for both patient and physician. A practical consequence of this was the proliferation of laboratories with increased resources to deliver the service. In the beginning, these resources were human and consisted of having specimens transported to the primary laboratory site. This later became multiple collection sites, courier services, mechanical processing, and electronic reporting.

These logistical issues lead directly to a third condition for laboratory development: economics. There are two components to economic considerations. First, the laboratory service has to be an economically viable option for the ordering physician. The service must be delivered in such a way that the physician does not experience any cost or significant loss of income from referring tests to a diagnostic laboratory. Second, there must be a mechanism to support the cost of laboratory testing. This latter problem was solved, for a short time, by the third-party reimbursement system. As one of the social reform programs of the 20th century, the widespread availability of insurance made the cost of health services invisible to the patient. Without proper controls, the effect of this reimbursement system was to encourage the proliferation of technology and make service accessible to large segments of the population. The incentive was for every testing center to have all the best technology and make it available to everyone.

This chapter will highlight some historical events and practices that demonstrate how this evolution took place. The events outlined here are not absolute in defining the practice of laboratory medicine, but suggest how concepts could evolve and develop into the practice of diagnostic laboratory testing as it exists today.

2. EARLIEST MEDICINE

Long before there were laboratories there were accepted practices for patient evaluation. Early health care providers (not all were physicians) attempted to determine the health status of the person under evaluation by any means possible. The diagnosis and the prescribed treatment were not always an accurate or scientifically based pronouncement. It was a process that was motivated by a combination of altruism, vanity, greed, scientific thought, and philosophical and religious edict. This is not meant to imply that all was quackery and incantation. The procedures that had medical value are the ones that laid the foundation for legitimizing diagnostic medicine along with its subsequent support functions, one of which is the clinical diagnostic laboratory.

One major obstacle that physicians faced in ancient times was that it was illegal to practice invasive procedures. The patient could be observed and touched, but the only specimens that could be taken were those that naturally passed from the body. As a result of these limitations, urine has been the sample with the longest history of evaluation. There is some evidence that the Sumerians and Babylonians used urine for diagnosis as early as 4000 BCE *(1)*. The diagnosis of pregnancy was probably made by ancient Egyptians using the urine of the woman to germinate seeds *(1)*. Hindu medicine describes the sweet taste of urine and that black ants are attracted to this urine if it is poured on the ground *(1)*. Hippocrates (460–355 BCE) described the characteristics and colors of urine from his patients, and mentioned bubbles being present in urine from patients with long-standing kidney disease *(1–3)*. Over the next 600 years, the study of urine was advanced very little. Galen (129–200 AD) wrote and taught that urine was a filtrate of blood, and as such, could indicate the type and location of illnesses *(1)*. The teachings of these two men were the information base for urinalysis, or uroscopy, as it was called, for the next 9–10 centuries.

During this time, approx 800 AD, the first treatise on urine was written by Theophilus Protospatharius; in it is mentioned the first chemical test done on urine. The urine from patients with kidney disease was heated over a candle flame and became cloudy *(1)*. Other physicians repeated the process, some substituting acid for heat, and although it took centuries before the precipitating substance was identified as protein, the association with disease had been recognized *(3)*.

Other observations were made concerning the quality of the urine sample. The differences between morning and afternoon urine samples and factors like age, food, and medicaments exerted effects on the composition of urine. These were noted as early as the 10th century by Avacinna *(1)*. It was realized as early as the 11th century that the first voided specimen in the morning was the best urine specimen for analysis, and that when 24-h urine collections were required, they should be protected from light and heat *(1)*.

Urinalysis continued to be such a focus of study that Gilles de Corbeil developed a glass vessel (called a matula), shaped like a urinary bladder, specifically for the examination of urine. The concept was that the urine sediments and discoloration would occur in the vessel at a place that corresponded to the site of pathology in the body. These early urine vessels were among the first pieces of laboratory equipment and were so common and identifiable that they were one of the predecessors to the caduceus as the symbol of medicine.

Other tests and procedures were added to urinalysis and various aides were developed to make the process easier. One device of this type was the urine wheel. This wheel was the original color chart similar in purpose to those that accompany most modern dipstick packages. Along with matching the urine color on the wheel, there was an interpretive text included to assist in making a diagnosis *(3)*.

Uroscopy soon took on a life of its own. Samples were sent to physicians without any explanation of the patient's complaint, and it was expected the physician would return a diagnosis and therapy *(3)*. Expectedly, uroscopy was ripe for abuse, and assuredly this happened. The prominence of the practitioner was enhanced if he was perceived as being able to do more than other uroscopists. Consequently, claims were made concerning the interpretive powers of the analyst that far exceeded the limits of observation. It was during this period, when there was an opportunity to make a handsome income from urine analysis, that Joannes Actuarius began to write about the limitations of urine examination. He was one of the first to caution that urine examination, independent of how well it was done, could not be used to the exclusion of all other clinical findings *(3)*.

It should not be inferred that uroscopy was always a questionable effort. Proteinuria, although protein as such had not been identified, nephritis, type I diabetes, hematuria, infection, concentration, and limited assessment of liver disease were all recognized through urinalysis. In most cases it took centuries to identify the specific component in urine and its association with a disease. Nevertheless, urine testing was a valuable diagnostic tool *(3)*.

These early attempts to diagnose disease through the study of the only practical body fluid available gives some insight into the development of laboratory medicine. First, the progression from pure observation to the use of some elementary aids and procedures suggests that the seed of intellectual curiosity was germinating. If simple observation was useful, then employing procedures to define components was better. Second, equipment was being generated for a specific medical application. The equipment was primarily small and portable, but with such procedures as distillation, precipitation, and evaporation, the need for a place to do this work was becoming an issue. A permanent site or address for the practitioner to do laboratory work enabled patients to "send" their urine for analysis (an early precursor to the outpatient laboratory). Third, since uroscopy was becoming a routine practice, some members of the legitimate medical community were discussing the appropriate use of these procedures. This may be the first suggestion of test utilization in history.

3. THE TRANSITION

Progress requires an advance in technology or the appearance of a gifted individual. Science and technology had advanced to a point where a breakthrough on some other front was required. Two historic events that meet this requirement are the invention of movable type by Johann Gutenberg in the 15th century and the Reformation. Moveable type and the printing press had the potential to make information available to large numbers of scholars. Experiments and data could be corroborated by other professionals, and foundless claims could become less common. Education, in all its forms, would be a benefactor. Education needs an appropriate environment. The Reformation provided that environment. The individual was acquiring more freedom in life, and the old way or restricted and regimented thought was passing. In this time of change, there were individuals of the proper education and personality to take advantage of the situation.

Andreas Vesalius, who is credited as the founder of modern anatomy, was such an individual. He was the first to do extensive dissections and accurately document the anatomical information in text and illustration *(4)*. The importance of this lies in the transition from animal to human dissections. Accurate anatomical data would become available and true progress in the other anatomical sciences, histology and zoology, could take place *(4)*. Another individual of this type was Giovanni Battista Morgagni, a successor to Vesalius, who combined anatomic dissection with clinical history to describe pathologic anatomy *(4)*. This is arguably the beginning of modern pathology.

It was during the 17th century that the science of laboratory medicine began to acquire the characteristics that are easily recognized today. Laboratories were being established in homes in which research and development were being conducted *(4)*. The results of this cottage industry were the development of equipment for laboratory and diagnostic use. Thermometers and hydrometers were two such pieces of equipment. *(4)*. Although the thermometer was described by Galileo in the late 1500s, it was not used for patient evaluation until the 17th century. The arguments waged concerning which fluid was the best indicator of change and the best way to calibrate the instrument *(4)*. Given these and other practical problems, some physicians were quick to realize that a quantitative measure of body temperature was an improvement over using one's hand. For other physicians, the problems with obtaining and using the thermometer were too great. After this brief flurry of activity, the thermometer returned to a quiescent state until the 1800s. By the 1800s, many of the original problems had been either resolved or minimized, so it became a more practical matter to measure temperature. Articles appeared regarding the value of temperature in diagnosis and prognosis in major medical journals *(5)*.

The hydrometer had relatively little difficulty in its acceptance. The instruments were made small and reliable, so they could be taken on home visits to the sick. Specific gravity was one of the well-entrenched measurements of uroscopy. A reliable and simple instrument catered to the needs of the common practitioner. Urinalysis was still king.

The home lab contributed to the refinement of equipment and methods. It should be remembered that alchemy was slowly giving way to organic chemistry, which was defined as the chemistry of living organisms *(6)*. It was not until the synthesis of urea in 1828 that organic chemistry became the chemistry of carbon compounds. Consequently, the efforts of the more inquisitive chemist-physicians turned to chemical procedures on body fluids *(6)*. Paracelsus and later Willis, suggested chemical analysis of urine *(6)*. To separate the fluid into its component parts was thought to yield better diagnostic or prognostic information *(6)*. True to history, a new hypothesis always has its detractors. Perseverance by the investigators and positive, predictable results from the applications generated broader acceptance.

It was an extension of this philosophy of active investigation instead of passive observation that led Robert Boyle to analyze blood. He had done chemical analysis on urine and continued this approach on human blood *(6,7)*. Boyle had the disadvantage of not being a physician and so did not have the opportunity to analyze the blood of sick patients *(7)*. He did have the insight to propose that knowing the results of his chemical analysis on healthy people, the evaluation of the sick would be made easier *(7)*. Robert Boyle was obviously an early proponent of normal reference intervals. This concept was carried further by the French physician Raymond Vieussens, who chemically analyzed the blood of large numbers of people of all descriptions *(7)*. Normals, abnormals, men, women, and those of different temperments were included in his study. These studies of defined populations were exceptional in their time.

Diagnostic testing had achieved a credibility that made it acceptable to perform chemical analysis on blood and urine and use the information in a diagnostic workup. Laboratories were beginning to grow in number and they were developing techniques that could be applied to medicine. Laboratory skills were gaining respectability along with laboratory testing and laboratory data.

4. EARLY MODERN MEDICINE

Chemistry as a science was developing rapidly in the 18th and early 19th centuries. Diabetes was the subject of intensive investigation by the medical chemists. Physicians like John Rollo and William Cruikshank demonstrated the presence or absence of sugar in the urine of diabetics, depending on the state of the patient's disease *(7)*. They were proponents of being able to monitor a patient's status by knowing if there was sugar in the patient's urine *(7)*. The conventional wisdom of the time was that most of the practicing physicians were not sophisticated enough to do this type of analysis routinely *(7)*. However, the concept of monitoring through repeated testing was being considered.

In 1827, Richard Bright published his *Reports of Medical Cases*, in which he described albumin in the urine of patients with dropsy, which is the collection of serous fluid in body cavities or cellular tissue. Bright was aware of the anatomical lesions that were associated with this condition, and made the link between chemical findings and anatomic findings *(7,8)*. This condition was later referred to as Bright's disease in honor of the association made by Bright *(8)*. This undoubtedly gave considerable credence to the analysis of specimens to diagnose disease. The test was simple. Just heat the urine and observe the white precipitate that formed. The presence of kidney disease could be predicted by the outcome of the test. The test was not perfect, and as more people performed the test conflicting results were obtained. Some "albuminous" material did not precipitate unless chemicals were added, and some normal people had precipitates in their urine *(7)*.

These and other arguments were responsible for the slow acceptance of Bright's albumin procedure and its use in diagnostic medicine. However, the principle of laboratory testing and the additional insight that it gave the physician was developing slowly. Progress was on the front side of a geometric curve, and by the end of the first half of the 19th century greater utilization and faster development of laboratory diagnostic medicine would be commonplace.

A major driving force for this increased activity was the work of Gabrial Andral. Recognizing the value of chemical analysis of body fluids, he argued effectively for increased research by the medical community *(6,7)*. He was a believer in chemical and microscopic examination of the liquid as well as the solid components of the body *(6,7)*. His work, *Pathological Hematology*, examined blood chemically, microscopically, and visually in both the healthy and diseased populations *(6)*. He measured or calculated the major components of blood and was able to demonstrate a decreased red cell mass in anemia and a decreased blood albumin in albuminuria *(6)*. The success of Andral's work coupled with his enthusiasm led other workers to pursue similar investigations. The studies of sugar in the blood of diabetics and uric acid in the blood of those who suffered from gout are prime examples of this effort *(7)*.

The hematology specialties were benefiting from Andral's work. The invention of counting chambers for red cell quantitation and their use in diagnosing anemia were discussed in medical publications *(7)*. All the work in chemical analysis of fluids and the microscopic analysis of blood was facilitated because bloodletting was still an acceptable form of therapy. This was a catch 22 situation. As more information was gained about diseases like anemia through these new methodologies, it became apparent that bloodletting was not appropriate therapy, and this inexhaustible source of study material would become less available.

The last half of the 19th century was a prolific time for the development of laboratory methods. So many methods began to appear that the practicing physician had difficulty in choosing which assays were reliable and which were not *(7)*. Time and equipment were also becoming impediments to the routine use of these new tests. Physicians complained that the time required to conduct these analyses and the expertise involved in their performance exceeded their capabilities *(7)*. The problem would get worse before it ever got better. Chemistry was becoming a tool to be used by all the medical disciplines. Paul Ehrlich used chemical dyes to test urine in the diagnosis of typhoid fever and aniline dyes to distinguish different types of leukocytes *(7,8)*. The study of gastric disturbances was accomplished by chemical analysis of stomach contents removed by gastric tubes *(7)*.

The medical literature was replete with discussions of new methods and of the failures and shortcomings of older ones. If technological advances were the only requirement for legitimacy, then laboratory medicine was an established discipline. However, true acceptance can only be established through academic credentials. Throughout the 19th century, there was a parallel development of the academic and political status of diagnostic laboratories. Initially, medical schools did not have the status of universities, and it was well into the 19th century before they became equivalent to colleges *(9)*. Around the same time, medical chemistry was being split from chemistry, which was now general or organic chemistry *(9)*. The latter subjects were considered to be more pure science and, therefore, more prestigious. The result was that physiological chemistry was the domain of physiology, with no academic standing of its own *(9)*. There were notable exceptions, one being the University of Tübingen, at which the first chair of physiological chemistry was established in 1845 *(9)*. The first chairman was Julius Schlossberger, who was responsible for all the chemistry teaching in the medical facility *(9)*. He was followed by Felix Hoppe-Seyler, under whom the chair was transferred to the philosophical faculty *(9)*. The chair survived until the 20th century primarily because of the stature of the chairmen, all of whom were both organic and physiologic chemists *(9)*. Similar academic structures were not as successful at other universities. It was not until the position was established in the medical schools of the United States that physiological chemistry became secure.

The first laboratory of physiological chemistry in the United States was established in 1874 at the Sheffield Scientific School of Yale University under the direction of Russell H. Chittenden *(10)*. This was rapidly followed by similar laboratories being established at other major universities. Faculty were expected to teach and conduct research, and professional positions were awarded on the academic credentials of the applicant *(10)*. These facilities were a permanent part of universities and, later, medical schools. The premedical and medical training of physicians included laboratory training in the biological and chemical sciences.

Another development in the late 1800s was the appearance of hospitals in the United States. By midcentury, these hospitals were designing laboratory space for purposes of urinalysis *(8)*. Resources were being made available for laboratory work, of which the overwhelming volume was urinalysis *(8)*. There is some indication that urinalysis was routine in at least one prestigious Eastern hospital *(8)*. At the end of the century, the hospital laboratory had been joined by the ward laboratory *(7)*, a smaller and less extensive version of the main laboratory. The rationale was that a small lab space near patients would reduce the length of time required to obtain results, and could be staffed by physicians and house staff. In practice, these two types of laboratories grew, each requiring more resources to keep them operational.

Two physicians added considerable credence to the concept of a professionally staffed, hospital based laboratory. Otto Folin, at a lecture in 1908, proposed that laboratories should be hospital based and staffed by professional physiological chemists *(11)*. William Osler judged the value of the laboratory to be indispensable to the clinical physician. When physicians as influential and respected as these were become proponents of laboratory testing, the position of the laboratory was permanently secured *(7)*.

With the continued acceptance of the laboratory, and hospitals considering them to be integral to their service, a subtle change began to take place. Once the lab became established, work was generated. A review of several hospital's records at the beginning of the 20th century indicates that urine testing was being done on most patients even if there were no indications for such a test *(8)*. These urine tests were being refined by investigators that now had positions in the laboratory. New tests were being added for blood and other body fluids. Many of the famous names associated with clinical laboratory medicine, such as Folin, Benedict, Garrod, Koch, Van Slyke, and Ehrlich, among others came from this era. This was a very productive time for research and development; many of these findings were being transferred to the diagnostic service laboratory.

Urine and diabetes have been studied for centuries in the hope of providing better care. There are records at the Pennsylvania Hospital that urine sugar measurements were used to monitor the therapy for a diabetic woman *(8)*. The end point was a negative urine sugar finding, so urine was analyzed every day. This was one of the first records of using lab tests to monitor treatment. After insulin was discovered, it became more important to monitor sugar owing to the difficulty in controlling insulin therapy. Insulin preparations were of different purities, and external factors, such as exercise and diet, made insulin dosing very difficult. Blood sugar analysis was possible, but difficult, and so it became routine to do regular urine sugar measurements *(8)*.

Methods continued to be developed and clinical applications were tested. Each test or procedure found its way into the service offerings of the clinical lab. It was apparent that at least two problems were continuing to plague the lab. First, the volume of work was increasing and projections indicated that the trend would continue. Second, laboratory tests were difficult and tedious to do, and as a result showed significant variability because of imprecision. A partial solution to these issues came from Leonard Skeggs. His design of a continuous-flow analyzer was the first practical unit for the laboratory *(12)*. These first designs were essentially mechanical duplicators of hand procedures, but enabled the lab to increase throughput and improve the precision of the analysis. Automation for laboratory testing has undergone several generations of change. These instruments are now found in all sections of the laboratory and encompass a wide spectrum of methodologies.

5. THE NEW ERA

As the end of the 20th century approaches, the clinical diagnostic laboratory is entering into a new phase. Biotechnology, in all its forms, is the fastest-growing discipline in the modern clinical laboratory. From the original experiments of Gregor Mendel in 1865 describing hybridization of plants to the Human Genome Project, molecular biology is presenting the laboratory professional with new challenges. As in the past, the volume of research work being done is translating to a growing list of diagnostic tests for the service laboratory.

Molecular biology has developed, more than any other science, by the cooperative effort of many diverse disciplines. Mendel described the hereditary units as algebraic units and presented more of a mathematical discussion of heredity than a biological one *(13)*. Subsequent contributions have come from all the sciences. The isolation of protein-free nucleic acid by Richard Altman and the experiments to convert nonvirulent to virulent bacteria by Fred Griffith in 1923 and Oswald Avery in 1940 are significant developmental landmarks *(14)*. The application of the principles of theoretical chemistry by Max Delbrück and Erwin Schrödinger allowed others to proceed using the principles of physical science *(13)*. James Watson and Francis Crick elucidated the mathematically satisfying structure of DNA *(15)*. There were many investigators who have contributed to the underlying science of the laboratory procedures for molecular biology.

For the first time in the history of the diagnostic laboratory, molecular biology is extending the range of information available. Until this time, the laboratory had been descriptive in nature. It could measure events that were currently going on by evaluating the chemistry or hematology or anatomical pathology. Molecular biology allows the laboratory to be predictive in nature. Now statements can be made about events that may occur in the future. This is different from an elevated value for blood glucose when the diagnosis of diabetes can be made. This new technology returns results that give an indication that the patient may be at risk for the disease. Ethical considerations and genetic counseling have become an inseparable part of the laboratory procedure. Preventive medicine will benefit from the new technology. In cases of a family history that suggests high risk for a particular disease, a lab test may indicate that there is no risk to a specific family member. If there is a significant risk, then medical care may be able to intervene at a much earlier stage. This has significant financial benefits for those that have to control the costs of health care.

6. OTHER FACTORS

As has been discussed, the laboratory has developed through a series of advances and setbacks. Until recently, the volume of testing has gone up dramatically every year in excess of what is predicted for diagnostic purposes. One contributing factor may be that in the mid-20th century, health insurance became available to a large portion of the working population. Under this type of program, medical care was delivered with little concern about the cost. These costs were passed along to the insurance company, who paid the charges. This put the laboratory in a revenue-generating position, and more tests translated to more income. There was no incentive to control costs; in fact, there was an incentive to do more tests, hire more staff, and buy more equipment. This led to a considerable growth in laboratory services, and although test costs were coming down, the increased volume made the total cost higher. As the new technology matures, there may be a paradoxical financial shift. That is, the individual laboratory tests may currently be more expensive to perform than more traditional assays, but the benefit from earlier intervention and genetic counseling may reduce the long-term aggregate cost of health care.

The subsequent chapters will outline a wide variety of diagnostic testing that is available along with the benefits and medical options that are available to the patient and the health care team. This is the technology that will carry laboratory diagnostic medicine into the 21st century.

REFERENCES

1. Haber, M. H. Pisse prophecy: a brief history of urinalysis. *Clin. Lab. Med.* **8:**415–430, 1988.
2. Rubin, L. P. A young woman taken to the doctor by her family. Mezzotint by Johann Andreas Pfeffel after an original painting by Jan Josef Horemans. *J. Hist. Med. Allied Sci.* **36:**488–489, 1981.
3. White, W. I. A new look at the role of urinalysis in the history of diagnostic medicine. *Clin. Chem.* **37:**119–125, 1991.
4. Camac, C.N.B. *Imhotep to Harvey: Backgrounds of Medical History.* Milford House, Boston, 1973.
5. Flint, A. Remarks on the use of the thermometer in diagnosis and prognosis, in *Technology and American Medical Practice 1880–1930*, Howell, J. D., ed., Garland Publishing, New York, pp. 1–14, 1988.
6. Caraway, W. The scientific development of clinical chemistry to 1948. *Clin. Chem.* **19:**373–383, 1973.
7. Reiser, S. J. *Medicine and the Reign of Technology.* Cambridge University Press, Cambridge, 1978.
8. Howell, J. D. *Technology in the Hospital.* The Johns Hopkins University Press, Baltimore, 1995.
9. Kohler, R. E. *From Medical Chemistry to Biochemistry.* Cambridge University Press, New York, 1982.
10. Chittenden, R. H. *The Development of Physiological Chemistry in the United States.* The Chemical Catalog Company, New York, 1930.

11. Meites, S. First call for clinical chemists in U. S. *Clin. Chem.* **29:**1852–1853, 1983.

12. Lewis, L. Leonard Skeggs—a multifaceted diamond. *Clin. Chem.* **27:**1465–1468, 1981.

13. Miclos, D. A. and Freyer, G. A. Themes in the development of DNA science, in *DNA Science—A First Course in Recombinant DNA Technology.* Cold Spring Harbor Laboratory, Cold Spring Harbor, NY, pp. 4–9, 1990.

14. Blackburn, M. G. and Gait, M. J., eds. Introduction and overview, in *Nucleic Acids in Chemistry and Biology.* IRL Press at Oxford University Press, pp. 3,4, 1990.

15. Kay, L. E. *The Molecular Vision of Life, Caltech, The Rockefeller Foundation, and the Rise of the New Biology.* Oxford University Press, New York, 1993.

2

An Overview of Nucleic Acid Chemistry, Structure, and Function

The Foundations of Molecular Biology

William B. Coleman

1. INTRODUCTION

Chemists and early biochemists determined the essential building blocks of living cells and characterized their chemical nature. Among these building blocks were nucleic acids, long-chain polymers composed of nucleotides. Nucleic acids were named based partly on their chemical properties and partly on the observation that they represented a major constituent of the cell nucleus. That nucleic acids form the chemical basis for the transmission of genetic traits was not realized until about 50 years ago *(1)*. Prior to that time, there was considerable disagreement among scientists concerning whether genetic information was contained in and transmitted by proteins or nucleic acids. It was recognized that chromosomes contained deoxyribonucleic acid (DNA) as a primary constituent, but it was not known if this DNA carried genetic information or merely served as a scaffold for some undiscovered class of proteins that carried genetic information. However, the demonstration that genetic traits could be transmitted through DNA formed the basis for numerous investigations focused on elucidation of the nature of the genetic code. During the last half-century, numerous investigators have participated in the scientific revolution leading to modern molecular biology. Of particular significance were the elucidation of the structure of DNA *(2,3)*, determination of structure/function relationships between DNA and RNA *(4)*, and acquisition of basic insights into the processes of DNA replication, RNA transcription, and protein synthesis *(5–7)*. Molecular pathology represents the application of the principles of basic molecular biology to the investigation of human disease processes. Our ever broadening insights into the molecular basis of disease processes continues to provide an opportunity for the clinical laboratory to develop and implement new and novel approaches for diagnostic and prognostic assessment of human disease.

2. THE CENTRAL DOGMA OF MOLECULAR BIOLOGY

Molecular biology has developed into a broad field of scientific pursuit and, at the same time, has come to represent a basic component of most other basic research

From: Molecular Diagnostics: For the Clinical Laboratorian
Edited by: W. B. Coleman and G. J. Tsongalis Humana Press Inc., Totowa, NJ

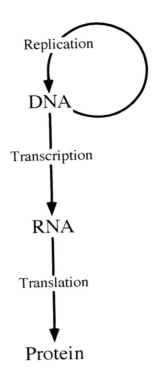

Fig. 1. The central dogma of molecular biology.

sciences. This has come about through the rapid expansion of our insights into numerous basic aspects of molecular biology and the development of an understanding of the fundamental interaction among the several major processes that comprise the larger field of investigation. A theory referred to as the "central dogma" describes the interrelationships among these major processes. The central dogma defines the paradigm of molecular biology that genetic information is perpetuated as sequences of nucleic acid, but that genes function by being expressed in the form of protein molecules *(8)*. The flow of genetic information among DNA, RNA, and protein that is described by the central dogma is illustrated in Fig. 1. Individual DNA molecules serve as templates for either complementary DNA strands during the process of replication or complementary RNA molecules during the process of transcription. In turn, RNA molecules serve as templates for the ordering of amino acids by ribosomes during protein synthesis or translation. This simple representation of the complex interactions and interrelationships among DNA, RNA, and protein was proposed and commonly accepted shortly after the discovery of the structure of DNA. Nonetheless, this paradigm still holds nearly 40 years later, and continues to represent a guiding principle for molecular biologists involved in all areas of basic biological, biomedical, and genetic research.

3. CHEMICAL NATURE OF DNA

DNA is a polymeric molecule that is composed of repeating nucleotide subunits. The order of nucleotide subunits contained in the linear sequence or primary structure of these polymers represents all of the genetic information carried by a cell. Each nucleotide is composed of:

1. A phosphate group;
2. A pentose (5 carbon) sugar; and
3. A cyclic nitrogen-containing compound called a base.

In DNA, the sugar moiety is 2-deoxyribose. Eukaryotic DNA is composed of four different bases: adenine, guanine, thymine and cytosine. These bases are classified based on their chemical structure into two groups: adenine and guanine are double-ring structures termed purines, thymine, and cytosine are single-ring structures termed pyrimidines (Fig. 2). Within the overall composition of DNA, the concentration of thymine is always equal to the concentration of adenine, and the concentration of cytosine is always equal to guanine *(9,10)*. Thus, the total concentration of pyrimidines always equals the total concentration of purines. These monomeric units are linked together into the polymeric structure by 3',5'-phosphodiester bonds (Fig. 3). Natural DNAs display widely varying sizes depending on the source. Relative molecular weights range from 1.6×10^6 Dalton for bacteriophage DNA to 1×10^{11} Dalton for a human chromosome.

4. STRUCTURE OF DNA

The structure of DNA is a double helix composed of two polynucleotide strands that are coiled about one another in a spiral *(2,3)*. Each polynucleotide strand is held together by phosphodiester bonds linking adjacent deoxyribose moieties. The two polynucleotide strands are held together by a variety of noncovalent interactions, including lipophilic interactions between adjacent bases and hydrogen bonding between the bases on opposite strands. The sugar-phosphate backbones of the two complementary strands are antiparallel, that is, they possess opposite chemical polarity. As one moves along the DNA double helix in one direction, the phosphodiester bonds in one strand will be oriented 5'-3', whereas in the complementary strand, the phosphodiester bonds will be oriented 3'-5'. This configuration results in base pairs being stacked between the two chains perpendicular to the axis of the molecule. The base-pairing is always specific: Adenine is always paired to thymidine, and guanine is always paired to cytosine. This specificity results from the hydrogen bonding capacities of the bases themselves. Adenine and thymine form two hydrogen bonds, and guanine and cytosine form three hydrogen bonds. The specificity of molecular interactions within the DNA molecule allows one to predict the sequence of nucleotides in one polynucleotide strand if the sequence of nucleotides in the complementary strand is known *(11)*. Although the hydrogen bonds themselves are relatively weak, the number of hydrogen bonds within a DNA molecule results in a very stable molecule that would never spontaneously separate under physiological conditions. There are many possibilities for hydrogen bonding between pairs of heterocyclic bases. Most important are the hydrogen-bonded base pairs A:T and G:C that were proposed by Watson and Crick in their double-helix structure of DNA *(2,11)*. However, other forms of base-pairing have been described. In addition, hydrophobic interactions between the stacked bases in the double helix lend additional stability to the DNA molecule.

Three helical forms of DNA are recognized to exist: A, B, and Z *(12)*. The B conformation is the dominate form under physiological conditions. In B DNA, the base pairs are stacked 0.34 nm apart, with 10 bp/turn of the right-handed double helix and a diameter of approx 2 nm. Like B DNA, the A conformer is also a right-handed helix. However, A DNA exhibits a larger diameter (2.6 nm), with 11 bases/turn of the helix, and

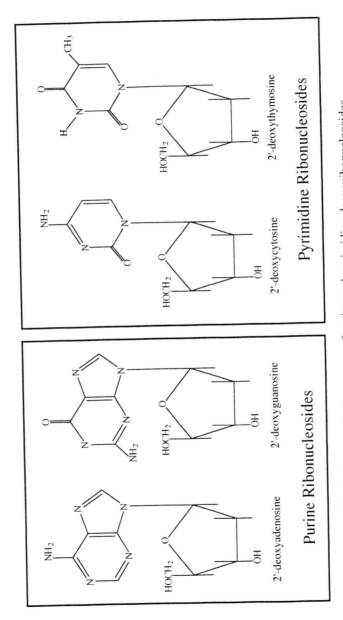

Fig. 2. The chemical structure of purine and pyrimidine deoxyribonucleosides.

18

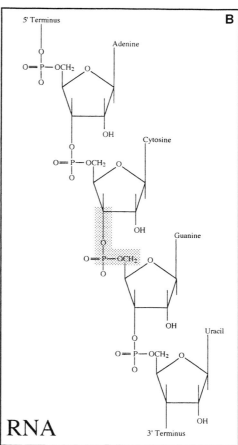

Fig. 3. The chemical structure of repeating nucleotide subunits in **(A)** DNA and **(B)** RNA. Each panel shows the sugar-phosphate backbone of a single polynucleotide strand of nucleic acid composed of four nucleotide subunits. The stippled area highlights a 3'-5' phosphodiester bond.

the bases are stacked closer together in the helix (0.25 nm apart). Careful examination of space-filling models of A and B DNA conformers reveals the presence of a major groove and a minor groove *(12)*. These grooves (particularly the minor groove) contain many water molecules that interact favorably with the amino and keto groups of the bases. In these grooves, DNA binding proteins can interact with specific DNA sequences without disrupting the base-pairing of the molecule. In contrast to the A and B conformers of DNA, Z DNA is a left-handed helix. This form of DNA has been observed primarily in synthetic double-stranded oligonucleotides, especially those with purine and pyrimidines alternating in the polynucleotide strands. In addition, high salt concentrations are required for the maintenance of the Z DNA conformer. Z DNA possesses a minor groove, but no major groove, and the minor groove is sufficiently deep that it reaches the axis of the DNA helix. The natural occurrence and potential physiological significance of Z DNA in living cells have been the subject of much speculation. However, these issues with respect to Z DNA have not yet been fully resolved.

5. ORGANIZATION OF GENOMIC DNA

The diploid genome of the typical human cell contains approx 7×10^9 base pairs of DNA that are subdivided into 23 chromosomes. A chromosome is defined as a single genetically specific DNA molecule to which are attached a large number of protein molecules that are involved in the maintenance of chromosome structure and regulation of gene expression. The actual number of genes contained in the human genome is not known. However, it has been estimated that the human genome contains 30–100,000 essential genes. Genomic DNA contains both "coding" and "noncoding" sequences. Noncoding sequences contain information that does not lead to the synthesis of an active RNA molecule or protein. This is not to suggest that noncoding DNA serves no function within the genome. On the contrary, noncoding DNA sequences have been suggested to function in DNA packaging, chromosome structure, chromatin organization within the nucleus, or in the regulation of gene expression *(13,14)*. A portion of the noncoding sequences represent intervening sequences that split the coding regions of structural genes. However, the majority of noncoding DNA falls into several families of repetitive DNA whose exact functions have not been entirely elucidated *(15)*.

Coding DNA sequences give rise to all of the transcribed RNAs of the cell, including mRNA. The organization of transcribed structural genes consists of coding regions that are interrupted by intervening noncoding regions of DNA (Fig. 4). Thus, the primary RNA transcripts contain both coding and noncoding sequences. The noncoding sequences must be removed from the primary RNA transcript during processing to produce a functional mRNA molecule appropriate for translation.

6. DNA FUNCTIONS

DNA serves two important functions with respect to cellular homeostasis: the storage of genetic information and the transmission of genetic information. In order to fulfill both of these functions, the DNA molecule must serve as a template. The cellular DNA provides the source of information for the synthesis of all the proteins in the cell. In this respect, DNA serves as a template for the synthesis of RNA. In cell division, DNA serves as the source of information inherited by progeny cells. In this case, DNA serves as a template for the faithful replication of the genetic information that is ultimately passed into daughter cells.

6.1. Transcription of RNA

Contained within the linear nucleotide sequence of the cellular DNA is the information necessary for the synthesis of all the protein constituents of a cell (Table 1). Transcription is the process in which mRNA is synthesized with a sequence complementary to the DNA of a gene to be expressed. The correct start- and end-points for transcription of a specific gene are identified in the DNA by a promoter sequence upstream of the gene and a termination signal downstream (Fig. 4). In the case of RNA transcription, only one strand of the DNA molecule serves as a template. This strand is referred to as the "sense" strand. Transcription of the sense strand ultimately yields an mRNA molecule that encodes the proper amino acid sequence for a specific protein.

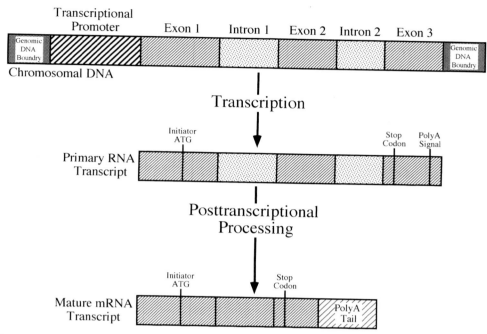

Fig. 4. Basic organization of a structural gene in DNA and biogenesis of mature mRNAs.

Table 1
The Universal Genetic Code

First position (5'-end)	Second position				Third position (3'-end)
	U	C	A	G	
U	Phe	Ser	Tyr	Cys	U
U	Phe	Ser	Tyr	Cys	C
U	Leu	Ser	Stop	Stop	A
U	Leu	Ser	Stop	Trp	G
C	Leu	Pro	His	Arg	U
C	Leu	Pro	His	Arg	C
C	Leu	Pro	Gln	Arg	A
C	Leu	Pro	Gln	Arg	G
A	Ile	Thr	Asn	Ser	U
A	Ile	Thr	Asn	Ser	C
A	Ile	Thr	Lys	Arg	A
A	Met	Thr	Lys	Arg	G
G	Val	Ala	Asp	Gly	U
G	Val	Ala	Asp	Gly	C
G	Val	Ala	Glu	Gly	A
G	Val	Ala	Glu	Gly	G

6.2. Replication of DNA

The double-stranded model of the structure of DNA strongly suggests that replication of the DNA can be achieved in a semiconservative manner *(16)*. In semiconservative replication, each strand of the DNA helix serves as a template for the synthesis of complementary DNA strands. The result is the formation of two complete copies of the DNA molecule, each consisting of one strand derived from the parent DNA molecule and one newly synthesized complementary strand. The utilization of the DNA strands as the template for the synthesis of new DNA ensures the faithful reproduction of the genetic material for transmission into daughter cells *(5)*.

6.3. Genetic Recombination

Genetic recombination represents one mechanism for the generation of genetic diversity through the exchange of genetic material between two homologous nucleotide sequences *(17)*. Such an exchange of genetic material often results in alterations of the primary structure (nucleotide sequence) of a gene and, subsequently, alteration of the primary structure of the encoded protein product. In organisms that reproduce sexually, recombination is initiated by formation of a junction between similar nucleotide sequences carried on the same chromosome from the two different parents. The junction is able to move along the DNA helix through branch migration, resulting in an exchange of the DNA strands.

6.4. DNA Repair

Maintenance of the integrity of the informational content of the cellular DNA is absolutely required for cellular and organismal homeostasis. The cellular DNA is continuously subjected to structural damage through the action of endogenous or environmental mutagens. In the absence of efficient repair mechanisms, stable mutations can be introduced into DNA during the process of replication at damaged sites within the DNA. Mammalian cells possess several distinct DNA repair mechanisms and pathways that serve to maintain DNA integrity, including enzymatic reversal repair, nucleotide excision repair, and postreplication repair *(18,19)*. Several steps in the process of DNA repair are shared by these multiple pathways, including:

1. Recognition of sites of damage;
2. Removal of damaged nucleotides; and
3. Restoration of the normal DNA sequence.

Each of these steps in DNA repair are accomplished by specific proteins and enzymes. Surveillance of the cellular DNA is a continual process involving specific aspects of the transcription and replication machinery. However, in each case where the restoration of the normal DNA sequence is accomplished through the replacement of damaged nucleotides, the undamaged DNA strand serves as a template in the repair process. This ensures the faithful reproduction of the primary structure of the DNA at the damaged site.

7. CHEMICAL NATURE OF RNA

Like DNA, RNA is composed of repeating purine and pyrimidine nucleotide subunits. However, several distinctions can be made with respect to the chemical nature of RNA and DNA. Unlike the 2'-deoxyribose sugar moiety of DNA, the sugar moiety in

RNA is ribose. Like DNA, RNA usually contains adenine, guanine, and cytosine, but does not contain thymidine. In place of thymidine, RNA contains uracil. The concentrations of purines and pyrimidine bases do not necessarily equal one another in RNA because of the single-stranded nature of the molecule. The monomeric units of RNA are linked together by 3',5'-phosphodiester bonds analogous to those in DNA (Fig. 3). RNAs have molecular weights between 1×10^4 Dalton for tRNA and 1×10^7 Dalton for rRNA.

8. STRUCTURE AND FUNCTION OF RNA

RNA exists as a long, regular, unbranched polynucleotide strand. The informational content of the RNA molecule is contained in its primary structure or nucleotide sequence. In spite of the fact that RNA exists primarily as a single-stranded molecule, significant higher-order structures are often formed in individual RNA molecules. In some cases, this higher-order structure is related to the actual function of the molecule. Three major classes of RNA are found in eukaryotic organisms: messenger RNA (or mRNA), transfer RNA (or tRNA), and ribosomal RNA (or rRNA). Each class differs from the others in the size, function, and general stability of the RNA molecules. Minor classes of RNA include heterogeneous nuclear RNA (or hnRNA), small nuclear RNA (or snRNA), and small cytoplasmic RNA (or scRNA).

8.1. Structure and Function of mRNA

The ability of DNA to serve directly as a template for the synthesis of protein is precluded by the observations that protein synthesis takes place in the cytoplasm, whereas almost all of the cellular DNA resides in the nucleus. Thus, genetic information contained in the DNA must be transferred to an intermediate molecule that is translocated into the cell cytoplasm, where it directs the ordering of amino acids in protein synthesis. RNA fulfills this role as the intermediate molecule for the transport and translation of genetic information. mRNA molecules represent transcripts of structural genes that encode all of the information necessary for the synthesis of a single-type polypeptide of protein. Thus, mRNAs serve two important functions with respect to protein synthesis: (1) mRNAs deliver genetic information to the cytoplasm where protein synthesis takes place, and (2) mRNAs serve as a template for translation by ribosomes during protein synthesis.

Mammalian cells (among others) express "interrupted" genes, that is, genes whose coding sequences are not intact in the DNA, and that require a posttranscriptional modification prior to translation of protein products (Fig. 4). The majority of structural genes in the higher eukaryotic organisms are interrupted. The average gene contains 7–10 exons, spread over 10–16 kb of DNA. The primary RNA transcript exhibits the same overall structure and organization as the structural gene, and is often referred to as the pre-mRNA. Removal of intronic sequences yields a mature mRNA that is considerably smaller with an average size of 1–3 kb. The process of removing the intronic sequences is called RNA splicing *(20)*.

The primary products of RNA transcription in the nucleus compose a special class of RNAs that are characterized by their large size and heterogeneity. These RNA molecules are referred to as hnRNA. hnRNAs contain both intronic and exonic sequences encoded in the template DNA of structural genes. These hnRNAs are processed in the nucleus *(21,22)* to give mature mRNAs that are transported into the cytoplasm where they participate in protein synthesis. Nuclear processing of RNA involves:

1. Chemical modification reactions (addition of the 5' CAP);
2. Splicing reactions (removal of intronic sequences); and
3. Polyadenylation (addition of the 3' polyA tail).

Additional processing of some specific mRNAs occurs in the cell cytoplasm, including RNA editing reactions *(23)*. It has been suggested that some snRNAs function in the processing of hnRNAs *(24)*. Mature mRNAs are transported into the cytoplasm of the cell, where they participate in the translational processes of protein synthesis.

In RNA splicing, intronic sequences are specifically removed from the primary RNA transcript and the remaining exonic sequences are rejoined into one molecule. There is no extensive homology or complementarity between the two ends of an intron precluding the general possibility that intronic sequences form extensive secondary structures (such as a hairpin loop) as a preliminary step in the splicing reaction. The splice junctions represent short well-conserved consensus sequences. The generic intron contains a GT sequence at the 5'-boundary and an AG sequence at the 3'-boundary (Fig. 5). The 5'- and 3'-splice junctions are often referred to as the splice donor and splice acceptor sites, respectively. Splice sites are generic in that they do not exhibit specificity for individual RNA precursors, and individual precursors do not convey specific information that is required for splicing. In principle, any splice donor site can react with any splice acceptor site. However, under normal conditions these reactions are restricted to the donor and acceptor sites of the same intron. Analysis of molecular intermediates formed during the splicing of large precursor RNAs suggests that the introns are removed in a definitive pattern or through a preferred pathway that dictates the general order of intron removal. This suggestion may imply a mechanism in which the conformation of precursor RNA molecules limits the accessibility of splice junctions, such that as specific introns are removed, the conformation of the molecule changes, and new splice sites become available. However, several other plausible mechanisms exists that could account for the observed patterns of splicing in RNAs that have been examined in detail *(20–22)*. The RNA sequences that are required for successful splicing include (1) the 5'-splice donor and 3'-splice acceptor consensus sequences, and (2) a consensus sequence known as the branch site. The branch site is located approx 20–40 bases upstream of the 3'-terminus of the intronic sequence, and conforms to the following consensus sequence: Py-N-Py-Py-Pu-A-Py. The role of the branch site is to identify the nearest splice acceptor site for connection to the splice donor site. The first step in splicing involves a cleavage of the RNA molecule at the 5'-end of the intron. The resulting intron-exon molecule forms a structure known as a lariat, through the formation of a 5'-2' bond between the G-residue located at the 5'-end of the intron and the adenine residue of the branch site. The second step involves cleavage of the RNA molecule at the 3'-splice site This cleavage releases the intron in lariat form, which is subsequently degraded.

The 5'-termini of all eukaryotic mRNAs are modified posttrascriptionally, through enzymatic reactions occurring in the nucleus and in the cytoplasm of the cell. Initially, a guanine residue is added to the 5'-terminus of primary mRNA transcripts through the action of an enzyme called guanylyl transferase. This reaction occurs in the nucleus

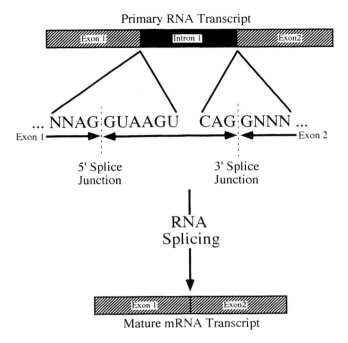

Fig. 5. Fundamental aspects of RNA splicing.

soon after the initiation of transcription. This guanine residue is linked to the first coded nucleoside triphosphate through a 5'-5' triphosphate linkage, rather than a 3'-5' phosphodiester bond. Thus, this guanine residue occurs in the structure of the mRNA in reverse orientation from all the other nucleotides. The modified 5'-terminus is referred to as a "CAP" and is the site of additional modification reactions involving the addition of methyl groups. These additional modifications are catalyzed by enzymes located in the cytoplasm of the cell. The first methylation occurs in all mRNAs and consists of the addition of a methyl group to the 7 position of the terminal guanine through the action of guanine-7-methyltransferase. Additional methylation reactions can occur involving the additional bases at the 5'-terminus of the mRNA transcript, and less frequently, internal methylation of bases within an mRNA molecule takes place.

The poly(A) tail possessed by most eukaryotic mRNAs is not encoded in the DNA. Rather, it is added to the RNA in the nucleus after transcription of the structural gene is complete. The addition of the poly(A) tail is catalyzed by the enzyme poly(A) polymerase, which adds approx 200 adenosine residues to the free 3'-OH terminus of the primary RNA transcript. The precise function of the poly(A) tail is unknown, but has been speculated to be involved in mRNA stability or in control of mRNA utilization. Although the removal of the poly(A) tail does precede degradation of certain mRNAs, a systematic correlation between mRNA stability or survival and the length or presence of the poly(A) tail has not been established. Removal of the poly(A) tail can inhibit the initiation of translation in vitro, suggesting a potential role for this structure in the control of mRNA translation. However, it is not clear whether this effect is related to a direct influence of poly(A) structures on the initiation reaction or the result of some indirect cause.

Some other forms of posttranscriptional RNA processing occur with respect to a small subset of eukaryotic mRNAs. The process of RNA editing involves a posttranscriptional alteration of the informational content of a specific mRNA *(23)*. The editing of RNA is revealed when the linear sequence of the mRNA molecule differs from the coding sequence carried in the DNA. In mammalian cells, there are examples in which substitution of a single base occurs in the mRNA, resulting in an alteration of an amino acid in the final protein product. Since no known template source mediates the RNA editing reaction, the most likely mechanism for mRNA editing would involve a specific enzyme that can recognize the sequence or secondary structure of the specific target mRNA and catalyze the specific base substitution. However, there are examples of RNA editing in some lower eukaryotes that utilize "guide RNA," which directs the RNA editing reaction *(25)*. The final result of RNA editing is the generation protein products representing more than one polypeptide sequence from a single coding gene. The different protein products may possess different biological activities, suggesting that RNA editing may represent a mechanism for controlling the functional expression of genes through a posttranscriptional process that does not impact the normal mechanisms for controlling levels of gene expression.

8.2. Structure and Function of Transfer RNA

tRNAs are small molecules consisting of approx 75–80 nucleotides. Like mRNAs, tRNA is generated through nuclear processing of precursor RNA transcripts. The structure of the tRNA molecule reflects its function as an adapter between the mRNA and amino acids during protein synthesis. Specific tRNAs correspond to each of the amino acids utilized in protein synthesis in any particular cell type. Although the specific tRNAs differ from each other with respect to their actual nucleotide sequence, tRNAs as a class of RNA molecules share several common structural features. Each tRNA contains information in the primary structure or nucleotide sequence that dictates the higher-order structure of the molecule. The secondary structure of the tRNA resembles a cloverleaf *(26)*. The folding of the cloverleaf structure is maintained through intrastrand sequence complementarity and base-pairing interactions between nucleotides. In addition, each tRNA contains an ACC sequence at the 3'-terminus and an anticodon loop *(26)*. Amino acids are attached to their specific tRNA through an ester bond to the 3'-hydroxyl group of the terminal adenine of the ACC sequence. The anticodon loop recognizes the triplet codon of the template mRNA during the process of translation. With the exception of the codons encoding methionine and tryptophan, there are at least two possible codons for each amino acid (Table 1). Nonetheless, each amino acid has only one corresponding tRNA. Thus, the hydrogen bonding between nucleotides of the codon and anticodon often involve "wobble" pairing. This form of base-pairing allows mismatches in the third base of a codon triplet. In the overall structure–function relationship in tRNA, the nucleotide sequence of the anticodon loop dictates which amino acid will be attached to the ACC sequence of the tRNA.

tRNAs serve as adapters between the mRNA template and the amino acids of growing polypeptide chains during the process of protein translation *(26)*, that is, the tRNA serves to ferry the appropriate amino acid into the active site of the ribosome, where it becomes incorporated into the growing polypeptide being synthesized. Amino acids are coupled to their specific tRNA through the action of enzymes called aminoacyl tRNA synthetases. The specificity of the "charging" reaction is critical to the integrity of the translation process, since the incorporation of amino acids at the level of the ribosome depends wholly on the sequence of the anticodon portion of the tRNA molecule. The charged tRNA interacts with the mRNA through the transient hybridization of the codon and anticodon RNA sequences in the ribosome complex as it moves along the mRNA. The entry of the charged tRNA into the active site of the ribosome brings its associated amino acid into juxtaposition with the nascent polypeptide, facilitating the formation of a peptide bond. In this manner the tRNA provides a link between the genetic information contained in the mRNA and the linear sequence of amino acids represented in the resulting polypeptide product.

8.3. Structure and Function of Ribosomal RNA

The ribosome is a nucleoprotein that serves as the primary component of a cell's protein synthesis machinery. The ribosome is a complex structure consisting of two subunit particle types (60S and 40S). The overall composition of the fully assembled ribosome includes at least four distinct rRNA molecules and nearly 100 specific protein subunits. The major rRNAs in mammalian cells were named for their molecular size as determined by their sedimentation rates. Three of these rRNAs (5S, 5.8S, and 28S) are components of 60S ribosomal particle. The smaller 40S ribosomal particle contains a single 18S rRNA. The 5.8S, 18S, and 28S rRNAs are the products of the processing of a single 45S precursor RNA molecule. The 5S rRNA is independently transcribed and processed. The rRNAs assemble with ribosomal protein subunits in the nucleus. The precise role of rRNA in the function of the ribosome is not completely understood *(27)*. However, it is recognized that interactions between the rRNAs of the ribosomal subunits may be important in the overall structure of the functioning ribosomal particle. In addition, rRNA sequences can interact with ribosome binding sequences of mRNA during the initiation of translation. Likewise, it is likely that rRNAs bind to invariant tRNA sequences when these molecules enter the active site of the ribosome *(27)*.

8.4. Special RNA Structures

Higher-order RNA structures exhibit hydrogen bonding between A:U and G:C base pairs. Several specific higher-order RNA structures have been recognized (Table 2) and characterized in detail *(28)*. Hairpin loops consist of a double-stranded stem and a single-stranded loop that bridges one end of the stem. These structures are essential components of more complex RNA structures and probably serve as nucleation sites for RNA folding. Loops may also function as recognition sites for protein–RNA interactions. Internal loops represent interruptions in double-stranded RNA caused by the presence of nucleotides on both strands that cannot participate in Watson-Crick base-pairing. Several important functions are associated with internal loops, including protein binding sites and ribozyme cleavage sites. In many cases, internal loops have been shown to represent highly ordered structures maintained by the formation of non-Watson-Crick base pairs. Bulges are structural motifs contained within double stranded RNA molecules with unpaired nucleotides on only one strand. RNA bulges contribute to the formation of more complex higher order RNA structures and can also serve as recognition sites for protein–RNA interaction. Nucleotide triples occur when single-

Table 2
Secondary and Tertiary Structural Motifs in RNA

Structure	Description	Functions
Hairpin loops	Single-stranded loop that bridges one end of a double-stranded stem	Component of more complex RNA structures; may serve as a nucleation site for RNA folding or recognition sites for protein–RNA interaction
Internal loops	Interruptions in double-stranded RNA caused by the presence of nucleotides on both strands that cannot participate in Watson-Crick base-pairing	Protein binding sites and ribozyme cleavage sites
Bulges	Double-stranded RNA molecules with unpaired nucleotides on only one strand	Contribute to the formation of more complex RNA structures; recognition sites for protein–RNA interactions
Nucleotide triples	Triple-helical structures that form through hydrogen bonding between nucleotides of a single-stranded RNA molecule and nucleotides within a double-stranded RNA molecule; hydrogen bonds can involve nucleotide bases, sugars, or phosphate groups	Orient regions of secondary structure in large RNA molecules and stabilize three-dimensional RNA structures
Pseudoknots	Results from base pairing between nucleotide sequences within an RNA loop structure and a complementary nucleotide sequence outside the RNA loop	RNA self-splicing, autoregulation of translational processes, and ribosome frameshifting

stranded RNA sequences form hydrogen bonds with nucleotides that are already base-paired. These interactions serve to stabilize three-dimensional RNA structures and to orient regions of RNA secondary structure in large RNA molecules. Pseudoknots are tertiary structural elements that result from base pairing between nucleotide sequences contained within a loop structure and sequences outside the loop structure. These are important in RNA self-splicing, translational autoregulation, and ribosomal frameshifting.

9. DNA DAMAGE, MOLECULAR MUTATIONS, AND THE CONSEQUENCES OF MUTATION

DNA damage can result from spontaneous alteration of the DNA molecule or from the interaction of numerous chemical and physical agents with the structural DNA molecule *(29)*. Spontaneous lesions can occur during normal cellular processes, such as DNA replication, DNA repair, or gene rearrangement *(18)*, or through chemical alteration of the DNA molecule itself as a result of hydrolysis, oxidation, or methylation *(30,31)*. In most cases, DNA lesions create nucleotide mismatches that lead to point mutations. Nucleotide mismatches can result from the formation of apurinic or apyrimidinic sites following depurination or depyrimidination reactions *(31)*, nucleotide conversions involving deamination reactions *(18)*, or in rare instances from the presence of a tautomeric form of an individual nucleotide in replicating DNA. Deamination reactions can result in the conversion of cytosine to uracil, adenine to hypoxanthine, and guanine to xanthine *(18)*. However, the most common nucleotide deamination reaction involves methylated cytosines, which can replace cytosine in the linear sequence of a DNA molecule in the form of 5-methylcytosine. The 5-methylcytosine residues are always located next to guanine residues on the same chain, a motif referred to as a CpG island. The deamination of 5-methylcytosine results in the formation of thymine. This particular deamination reaction accounts for a large percentage of spontaneous mutations in human disease *(32–34)*. Interaction of DNA with physical agents, such as ionizing radiation, can lead to single- or double-strand breaks resulting from scission of phosphodiester bonds on one or both polynucleotide strands of the DNA molecule *(18)*. UV light can produce different forms of photoproducts, including pyrimidine dimers between adjacent pyrimidine bases on the same DNA strand. Other minor forms of DNA damage caused by UV light include strand breaks and crosslinks *(18)*. Nucleotide base modifications can result from exposure of the DNA to various chemical agents, including N-nitroso compounds and polycyclic aromatic hydrocarbons *(18)*. DNA damage can also be caused by chemicals that intercalate the DNA molecule and/or crosslink the DNA strands *(18)*. Bifunctional alkylating agents can cause both intrastrand and interstrand crosslinks in the DNA molecule.

The various forms of spontaneous and induced DNA damage can give rise to a plethora of different types of molecular mutation *(35)*. These various types of mutations include both gross alteration of chromosomes and more subtle alterations to specific gene sequences in otherwise normal chromosomes. Gross chromosomal aberrations include:

1. Large deletions;
2. Additions (reflecting amplification of DNA sequences); and
3. Translocations (reciprocal and nonreciprocal).

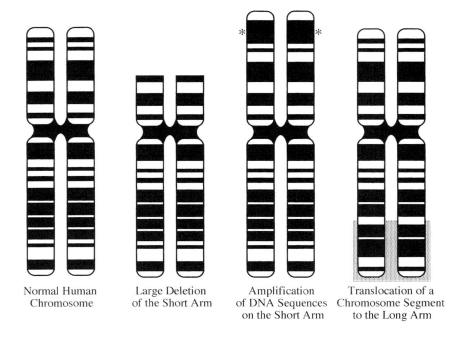

Normal Human	Large Deletion	Amplification	Translocation of a
Chromosome	of the Short Arm	of DNA Sequences	Chromosome Segment
		on the Short Arm	to the Long Arm

Fig. 6. Forms of gross chromosomal aberrations. Three examples of chromosomal aberrations are demonstrated using a standard G-band ideogram of human chromosome 11. The asterisks denote the chromosomal band that has expanded owing to DNA amplification. The stippled area highlights a region from another chromosome that has been translocated to the long arm of the starting chromosome, displacing the normal qter region without altering the overall size of the chromosome (note the differences in G-banding in this region).

All of these forms of chromosomal abnormality can be distinguished through standard karyotype analyses of G-banded chromosomes (Fig. 6). The major consequence of chromosomal deletion is the loss of specific genes that are located in the deleted chromosomal region, resulting in changes in the copy number of the affected genes. The deletion of certain classes of genes, such as tumor suppressor genes or genes encoding the proteins involved in DNA repair, can predispose cells to neoplastic transformation *(36)*. Likewise, amplification of chromosomal regions results in an increase in gene copy numbers, which can lead to the same type of circumstance if the affected region contains genes for dominant proto-oncogenes or other positive mediators of cell-cycle progression and proliferation *(36)*. The direct result of chromosomal translocation is the movement of some segment of DNA from its natural location into a new location within the genome, which can result in altered expression of the genes that are contained within the translocated region. If the chromosomal breakpoints utilized in a translocation are located within structural genes, then new hybrid genes can be generated.

The most common forms of mutation involve single nucleotide alterations, small deletions, or small insertions into specific gene sequences. These microscopic alterations very often can only be detected through DNA sequencing. Single nucleotide alterations that involve a change in the normal coding sequence of the gene are referred to as point mutations. The consequence of most point mutations is an alteration in the

Table 3
Forms and Consequences of Molecular Mutation

Normal coding sequence and amino acid translation										
. . . Phe	Phe	Glu	Pro	Gly	Ser	Asn	Val	Tyr	. . . . .	
. . . UUC	UUU	GAA	CCG	GGA	AGC	AAU	GUC	UAC	A . . .	
Missense point mutation resulting in amino acid change										
. . . Phe	Phe	Glu	Pro	**Val**	Ser	Asn	Val	Tyr	. . . . .	
. . . UUC	UUU	GAA	CCG	G<u>C</u>A	AGC	AAU	GUC	UAC	A . . .	
Missense point mutation without amino acid change (silent mutation)										
. . . Phe	Phe	Glu	Pro	Gly	Ser	Asn	Val	Tyr	. . . . .	
. . . UUC	UUU	GAA	CCG	GG<u>C</u>	AGC	AAU	GUC	UAC	A . . .	
Frameshift mutation resulting from a single base insertion										
. . . Phe	Phe	Glu	Pro	**Arg**	**Lys**	**Gln**	**Cys**	**Leu**	. . . . .	
. . . UUC	UUU	GAA	CCG	<u>A</u>GG	AAG	CAA	UGU	CUA	CA . .	
Frameshift mutation resulting from a single base deletion										
. . . Phe	Phe	Glu	Pro	**Glu**	**Asp**	**Met**	**Ser**	**Asn**	. . . . .	
. . . UUC	UUU	GAA	CCG	GAA	GCA	AUG	UCU	ACA	. . .	
Nonsense mutation resulting in a premature stop codon										
. . . Phe	Phe	Glu	Pro	**Stop**					. . . . .	
. . . UUC	UUU	GAA	CCG	<u>U</u>GA	AGC	AAU	GUC	UAC	. . .	

amino acid sequence of the encoded protein. However, some point mutations are "silent" and do not affect the structure of the gene product (Table 3). Silent mutations are possible, since most amino acids can be encoded by more than one triplet codon (Table 1). Point mutations fall into two classes, which are termed missense mutations and nonsense mutations. Missense mutations involve nucleotide base substitutions that alter the translation of the affected codon triplet. In contrast, nonsense mutations involve nucleotide base substitutions that modify a triplet codon that normally encodes for an amino acid into a translational stop codon. This results in the premature termination of translation and the production of a truncated protein product. Small deletions and insertions can usually be classified as frameshift mutations, because the deletion or insertion of a single nulceotide (for instance) alters the reading frame of the gene on the 3'-side of the affected site. This results in the synthesis of a polypeptide product that may bear no resemblance to the normal gene product (Table 3). In addition, small insertions or deletions can result in the premature termination of translation owing to the presence of a stop codon in the new reading frame of the mutated gene. Deletions or insertions that occur involving multiples of three nucleotides will not result in a frameshift mutation, but will alter the resulting polypeptide gene product, which will exhibit either loss of specific amino acids or the presence of additional amino acids within its primary structure. These types of alteration can also lead to a loss of protein function.

REFERENCES

1. Avery, O. T., MacLeod, C. M., and McCarty, M. Studies on the chemical nature of the substance inducing transformation of Pneumococcus types. *J. Exp. Med.* **79**:137–158, 1944.
2. Watson, J. D. and Crick, F. H. C. Molecular structure of nucleic acids: a structure for deoxyribose nucleic acid. *Nature* **171**:737–738, 1953.

3. Wilkins, M. H. F., Stokes, A. R., and Wilson, H. R. Molecular structure of deoxypentose nucleic acid. *Nature* **171**:738–740, 1953.

4. Watson, J. D. and Crick, F. H. C. Genetical implications of the structure of deoxyribonucleic acid. *Nature* **171**:738–740, 1953.

5. Coverly, D. and Laskey, R. A. Regulation of eukaryotic DNA replication. *Ann. Rev. Biochem.* **63**:745–776, 1994.

6. Kornberg, R. D. and Lorch, Y. Chromatin structure and transcription. *Ann. Rev. Cell Biol.* **8**:563–587, 1992.

7. Kozak, M. Regulation of translation in eukaryotic systems. *Ann. Rev. Cell Biol.* **8**:197–225, 1992.

8. Crick, F. H. C. On protein synthesis. *Symp. Soc. Exp. Biol.* **12**:548–555, 1958.

9. Chargaff, E., Vischer, E., Doniger, R., Green, C., and Misani, F. The composition of the desoxypentose nucleic acids of thymus and spleen. *J. Biol. Chem.* **177**:405–416, 1949.

10. Chargaff, E. Structure and function of nucleic acids as cell constituents. *Fed. Proc.* **10**:654–659, 1951.

11. Crick, F. H. C. and Watson, J. D. The complementary structure of deoxyribonucleic acid. *Proc. Royal Soc. A.* **223**:80–96, 1954.

12. Dickerson, R. E., Drew, H. R., Conner, B. N., Wing, R. M., Fratini, A. V., and Kopka, M. L. The anatomy of A-, B-, and Z-DNA. *Science* **216**:475–485, 1982.

13. Small, D., Nelkin, B., and Vogelstein, B. Nonrandom distribution of repeated DNA sequences with respect to supercoiled loops and the nuclear matrix. *Proc. Natl. Acad. Sci. USA* **79**:5911–5915, 1982.

14. Tsongalis, G. J., Coleman, W. B., Smith, G. J., and Kaufman, D. G. Partial characterization of nuclear matrix attachment regions from human fibroblast DNA using Alu-polymerase chain reaction. *Cancer Res.* **52**:3807–3810, 1992.

15. Jelinek, W. R. Repetitive sequences in eukaryotic DNA and their expression. *Ann. Rev. Biochem.* **51**:813–844, 1982.

16. Meselson, M. and Stahl, F. W. The replication of DNA in *Escherichia coli. Proc. Natl. Acad. Sci. USA* **44:** 671–682, 1958.

17. West, S. C. Enzymes and molecular mechanisms of genetic recombination. *Ann. Rev. Biochem.* **61**:603–640, 1992.

18. Friedberg, E. C. *DNA Repair.* Freeman, New York, 1985.

19. Sancar, A. and Sancar, G. B. DNA repair enzymes. *Ann. Rev. Biochem.* **57**:29–67, 1988.

20. Cech, T. R. Self-splicing of group I introns. *Ann. Rev. Biochem.* **59**:543–568, 1990.

21. Sharp, P. A. Splicing of messenger RNA precursors. *Science* **235**:766–771, 1987.

22. Padgett, R. A., Grabowski, P. J., Konarska, M. M., Seiler, S., and Sharp, P. A. Splicing of messenger RNA precursors. *Ann. Rev. Biochem.* **55**:1119–1150, 1986.

23. Powell, L. M., Wallis, S. C., Pease, R. J., Edwards, Y. H., Knott, T. J., and Scott, J. A novel form of tissue-specific RNA processing produces apolipoprotein-B48 in intestine. *Cell* **50**:831–840, 1987.

24. Mattaj, I. W., Tollervey, D., and Seraphin, B. Small nuclear RNAs in messenger RNA and ribosomal RNA processing. *FASEB J.* **7**:47–53, 1993.

25. Blum, B., Bakalara, N., and Simpson, L. A model for RNA editing in kinetoplastid mitochondria: "guide" RNA molecules transcribed from maxicircle DNA provide the edited information. *Cell* **60**:189–198, 1990.

26. Schimmel, P., and de Pouplana, L. R. Transfer RNA: from minihelix to genetic code. *Cell* **81**:983–986, 1995.

27. Noller, H. F. The structure of ribosomal RNA. *Ann. Rev. Biochem.* **53**:119–162, 1984.

28. Shen, L. X., Cai, Z., and Tinoco, I., Jr. RNA structure at high resolution. *FASEB J.* **9**:1023–1033, 1995.

29. Drake, J. W., and Balz, R. H. The biochemistry of mutagenesis. *Ann. Rev. Biochem.* **45**:11–37, 1976.

30. Lindahl, T. Instability and decay of the primary structure of DNA. *Nature* **362**:709–715, 1993

31. Ames, B. N., Shigenagan, M. K., and Gold, L. S. DNA lesions, inducible DNA repair, and cell division: three key factors in mutagenesis and carcinogenesis. *Environ. Health Perspect. Suppl.* **101**:35–44, 1993.

32. Cooper, D. N. and Youssoufian, H. The CpG dinucleotide and human genetic disease. *Hum. Genet.* **78**:151–155, 1988.

33. Rideout, W. M., Coetzee, G. A., Olumi, A. F. and Jones, P. A. 5-Methylcytosine as an endogenous mutagen in the human LDL receptor and p53 genes. *Science* **249**:1288–1290, 1990.

34. Jones, P. A., Buckley, J. D., Henderson, B. E., Ross, R. K. and Pike, M. C. From gene to carcinogen: a rapidly evolving field in molecular epidemiology. *Cancer Res.* **51**:3617–3620, 1991.

35. Bishop, M. Molecular themes in oncogenesis. *Cell* **64**:235–248, 1991.

36. Coleman, W. B., and Tsongalis, G. J. Multiple mechanisms account for genomic instability and molecular mutation in neoplastic transformation. *Clin. Chem.* **41**:644–657, 1995.

3

Basic Nucleic Acid Procedures

R. Keith Esch

1. INTRODUCTION

Nucleic acids are being increasingly employed in both analytical methods and in the creation of new tools for molecular biology and medicine. Our ability to use DNA and RNA in the laboratory effectively is directly tied to our understanding of the natural biochemical events involving these macromolecules. Knowledge of the in vivo processes continues to serve as a guide to the development and implementation of methods used in the laboratory manipulations of nucleic acids. In fact, many of the reagents used in nucleic acids techniques are identical to, or derived from, cellular components that perform the desired functions in nature.

Just as a firm grasp on the biology of nucleic acids facilitates their use in the laboratory, familiarity with the basic nucleic acids procedures allows the development of specialized techniques and clinical applications. The concepts and procedures presented in this chapter are often a prerequisite for the more advanced technologies presented in following chapters. These basic procedures are used in various combinations to synthesize complex procedures suitable for a vast array of molecular investigations.

2. ISOLATION OF DNA

2.1. Diversity of DNA as Genetic Material

Although the use of DNA as the source of genetic information is nearly universal, the molecular assemblies employed to comprise packages of genetic information are quite diverse. A genome is the package of genetic information contained within each cell of an organism. The genome structures of prokaryotic and eukaryotic cells are very different, and further variations are found among species within each group. Viruses, although their status as living organisms is debatable, contain units of genetic information that often are also referred to as genomes. Plasmids, although clearly not living organisms, define an additional class of DNA assemblies that are distinct packages of genetic information. The variations in assembly and structure of these genetic packages hold widespread implications for the isolation and use of DNA in laboratory procedures.

2.1.1. Prokaryotes

The use of nucleic acids and other cellular components from prokaryotes, particularly *Escherichia coli*, is common in many molecular laboratory investigations. The

From: Molecular Diagnostics: For the Clinical Laboratorian
Edited by: W. B. Coleman and G. J. Tsongalis Humana Press Inc., Totowa, NJ

relatively simple prokaryotic genome has been well characterized. Unlike eukaryotic cells, DNA that comprises the prokaryotic genome is not contained in a membrane-bound intracellular compartment. The entire prokaryotic genome is contained on one circular DNA molecule. Prokaryotes have only one copy of each gene and thus are haploid organisms. DNA in prokaryotic cells is often referred to as naked, because it is not associated with any complex system of repetitive protein structures, such as is found in eukaryotes. Although much smaller than higher eukaryotes, the DNA content of the prokaryotic genome is still extensive. For example, the *E. coli* chromosome contains approx 4.2 million bp, which represents approx 3500 individual genes.

A few major features stand out from the large body of knowledge amassed regarding the organization of prokaryotic genes themselves. Prokaryotic genes are expressed in either monocistronic or polycistronic transcriptional units. Monocistronic units encode a single gene product, whereas polycistronic units contain coding sequences for multiple proteins or RNA molecules. Polycistronic organization allows the coordinated expression of multiple gene products. Although prokaryotic protein-encoding genes include transcribed sequences that precede and follow the protein-coding sequence (5'-leader and 3'-trailer, respectively), with only rare exceptions, the protein-coding sequence itself is not interrupted (i.e., there are no introns).

2.1.2. Eukaryotes

The eukaryotic genome is much more complex than that of prokaryotes, and a basic knowledge of these complexities is central to the application of nucleic acids procedures. Perhaps the most recognized difference between eukaryotic and prokaryotic genomes is that the former is encased in a membrane-bound organelle within the cell. In eukaryotes, the genome is spread out among multiple chromosomes, each of which is a single linear DNA molecule. Eukaryotic DNA is tightly associated with proteins called histones that form a complex around which approx 200 bp of DNA are wound. Each molecule of DNA incorporates hundreds of these nucleosome structures in a continuous chain. This organization allows the DNA to be more compact and also plays a role in the regulation of transcription. Genome size varies in eukaryotes and generally correlates with the morphological complexity of the organism. However, mammalian genomes contain 4–8 billion bp, whereas the genomes of most amphibians and cartilaginous fish are much larger. In contrast to prokaryotes, a substantial portion of the eukaryotic DNA exists as long noncoding sequences between genes.

The typical structure of eukaryotic genes is also more complex than its prokaryotic counterpart. Multiple eukaryotic genes are rarely arranged in a single transcription unit. Proper expression of eukaryotic genes requires a much more extensive and diverse collection of DNA sequences functioning as regulatory elements. In addition to the noncoding sequences between genes, the coding sequences of most eukaryotic genes are themselves interrupted by lengths of noncoding DNA. These intervening sequences are called introns, and the coding sequences they interrupt are called exons.

2.1.3. Viruses

Both prokaryotes and eukaryotes serve as hosts for viruses, infectious agents that also contain genetic information in the form of DNA or RNA. Virus particles are generally comprised of the nucleic acid genome surrounded by a protein coat, and those that infect prokaryotes are usually termed phages. Viral genomes are small compared to those of their larger cellular hosts, and may be either linear or circular. The genomes of some DNA viruses are integrated into the host cell DNA, whereas others are replicated within the host independently from the host genome. Although viruses continue to act as sources for numerous pathologies, they also continue to be instrumental in the dissection of molecular mechanisms operating in living cells and in the development of molecular medical technologies.

2.1.4. Plasmids

Plasmids are naked circular DNA molecules that are smaller still than viral genomes. Like viruses, plasmids are dependent on their host cells for replication. Although a few eukaryotic plasmids have been identified, plasmids are much more commonly found, and used, in prokaryotes. Being particularly amenable to molecular cloning techniques, plasmids have become nearly indispensable for the laboratory manipulation of cellular DNA from any organism.

2.2. Isolation of Eukaryotic Genomic DNA

2.2.1. General Considerations and Procedures

The objective of DNA isolation is to obtain useful samples of DNA that are free from some or all contaminating molecules. In practical terms, this translates into separating the cells of interest from their environment and then separating the DNA from other cellular components. In addition, undesired additives used to facilitate these separations may also need to be removed. Cellular components that interact with DNA, such as some DNA binding proteins, are often difficult to separate because of their abilities to associate with DNA tightly. Other cellular components, particularly RNA, often require specialized separation steps, because their chemical nature is so similar to that of DNA.

The combination of several parameters determines what type of isolation procedure is most suitable for a given application. First is the degree of purity: Contaminants that would interfere with the intended use of the DNA must be reduced to an acceptable level. Second, although no less important, is the integrity of the DNA. Cellular enzymes that degrade DNA (nucleases) and mechanical shearing, caused by physical manipulation, reduce the size of DNA molecules during isolation. Limiting these sources of DNA damage is therefore crucial for applications that require high-mol-wt DNA. The third parameter, yield, is especially important in cases where the availability of DNA-containing material is low. Fourth, the use of hazardous reagents is a parameter of increasing concern and is to be restricted whenever feasible. Finally, monetary expense is also a variable to be considered. Depending on circumstances of individual investigators, such as access to expensive equipment, the most cost-effective isolation procedures may vary. Although many improvements and novel developments have occurred over recent decades, the tremendous variations produced by differential consideration of the above parameters ensures that there is no one universally favored isolation procedure and that many different techniques, new and old, are maintained.

The common starting point for most DNA isolation procedures is with harvested cells. More specialized preliminary manipulations that may be required for cell harvest will be covered in following sections. Isolation of DNA was changed dramatically when the use of proteinase K was introduced *(1)*. In this method, cells are lysed by

Table 1
Isolation of Genomic DNA[a]

1. Harvest cells with method appropriate to sample type.
2. If necessary, wash cells free from media by resuspension in cold phosphate-buffered saline and centrifugation at 1500g for 5 min at 4°C, repeat wash.
3. Resuspend with 10X cell volume of lysis buffer containing 10 mM Tris-HCl, pH 8.0, 10 mM EDTA, pH 8.0, 10 mM sodium chloride, 0.5% sodium dodecylsulfate, 100 mg/mL Proteinase K.
4. Incubate with mild agitation at 50°C for 3 h.
5. Transfer to a centrifuge tube and add an equal volume of phenol saturated with 0.5M Tris-HCl, pH 8.0, mix the two phases by slowly and repeatedly inverting the tube.
6. Centrifuge at 5000g for 10 min at room temperature.
7. Remove aqueous layer with a wide-bore pipet and transfer to a fresh tube. Repeat extraction twice.
8. Transfer the final aqueous solution into dialysis tubing and place into a beaker containing 100X sample volume of dialysis buffer containing 50 mM Tris-HCl, pH 8.0, 10 mM EDTA, pH 8.0, 10 mM sodium chloride.
9. Incubate at 4°C with gentle stirring and repeat with fresh dialysis buffer until the optical density at 270 nm of the dialysate is <0.05.
10. Transfer the DNA sample to a centrifuge tube, add DNase-free RNAase A to 50 mg/mL, mix gently and incubate for 3 h at 37°C.
11. Repeat the phenol extractions and dialysis steps excluding sodium chloride from the dialysis buffer.

[a]This is based on the methods of Gross-Bellard et al. *(1)* and Blin and Stafford *(2)*.

incubation at 37°C for 12 h in a buffer that contains a detergent, proteinase K, and EDTA.* The detergent serves to dissolve the cell membrane and denatures proteins. EDTA chelates divalent cations that are required for the activity of nucleases. The basis for this method is that proteinase K, an enzyme that degrades proteins, is highly active in this mixture, whereas DNA-degrading nucleases are greatly inhibited. This incubation is followed by a series of organic extractions generally employing mixtures of phenol, chloroform, and isoamyl alcohol. The organics are mixed with the DNA-containing sample, creating an emulsion, to dissolve hydrophobic contaminants and further denature and remove proteins. Since the organics are not cosoluble with the aqueous sample, they separate from each other into two phases (this is often facilitated by centrifugation). The aqueous phase is less dense and thus can be removed from atop the organic phase. It is then placed into a bag composed of dialysis membrane, which is selectively permeable based on size. During incubations in an appropriate buffer, small molecules will diffuse across the membrane to reduce contaminants, such as residual organics, simple sugars, and products of protein degradation, effectively. RNA is degraded by the enzyme RNase, which is subsequently removed by repeating the organic extractions and dialysis. Although this method produces relatively pure DNA of approx 100-kb fragments in reasonable yields, many improvements and modifications were welcome.

An early modification simply shortened the initial incubation time to 3 h and raised the temperature to 50°C (*2, see also* Table 1). This reduced the amount of time in which

*See p. 58 for list of abbreviations used in this chapter.

nucleases could act while still allowing the degradation of proteins by proteinase K. To avoid nuclease activity still further during cell lysis, another protocol eliminates proteinase K and adds the organics immediately to the cell lysate *(3)*. This procedure, however, tends to leave some cellular macromolecules in the aqueous phase. Further purification, which some applications necessitate, either involves lengthy and expensive procedures or results in low-mol-wt DNA.

Several DNA isolation procedures do not involve the use of organic extractions. A major limitation incurred with these extractions is that the physical agitation required for sufficient mixing of the organic and aqueous phases introduces significant DNA shearing. Another disadvantage is that organic solvents used in extractions, particularly phenol, present both potential health hazards and difficulty in handling and disposal. One procedure employs formamide, which denatures protein and dissociates it from DNA, followed by extensive dialysis *(4)*. Another protocol specifies dialysis of the lysate against a buffer containing polyethyleneglycol in order to remove small contaminants and greatly concentrate the DNA-containing solution *(5)*. Both of these procedures produce high yields of very high-mol-wt DNA (200–500 kb); however, the dialysis steps are quite lengthy and cumbersome.

Disruption of cells with chaotropic agents, such as guanidine hydrochloride, is featured in a rapid method (approx 3 h) that includes no centrifugation, organic extraction, or dialysis *(6)*. Although this method is quite convenient for processing multiple samples simultaneously, the resulting preparations yield DNA fragments that are relatively small (approx 80 kb) and include significant amounts of RNA. Multiple samples of comparably sized DNA can be rapidly obtained with very little RNA contamination by adding cesium chloride to the lysate and carrying out ultracentrifugation *(7)*. The convenience of this procedure relies on access to an expensive ultracentrifuge and use of the costly reagent, cesium chloride. A rapid method for multiple samples that is less expensive uses formamide following lysis and then precipitation with lithium chloride, which greatly reduces the levels of RNA *(8)*. Although DNA produced with this method is suitable for most Southern blotting applications and enzyme treatments, it is quite small (about 25 kb). Realizing that proteinase K is quite active and subsequently autoinactivates at 65°C, a method was developed that uses a 2-h proteinase K treatment following lysis *(9)*. Since this incubation is relatively short and there are no vigorous mixing steps, the resulting DNA has an average size of >300 kb. This method also produces high yields, is convenient for processing many samples, and results in DNA suitable for most enzymatic manipulations and amplification. Proteolytic digestion products are not removed, however, and may interfere with some subsequent techniques.

2.2.2. New Products and Procedures

Recently introduced products of pharmaceutical and biotechnology companies provide additional alternatives that generally increase the convenience of genomic DNA isolation. The expense of such products is often offset by the savings realized in time and labor. Two new isolation procedures are based on the ability of chaotropic reagents to disrupt cellular components and inhibit nucleases without causing excessive damage to the DNA. One procedure specifies a short (approx 30 min) incubation of cells with the chaotrope, guanidinium isothiocyanate. This is coupled with the use of a conveniently prepared small-scale anion-exchange column, which purifies DNA based on its negative charge. Kits employing this method are available in different sizes for isolation of various amounts of DNA (Pharmacia Biotech, Piscataway, NJ). A novel guanidine-detergent solution is the chaotropic reagent used in the lysis step of the second procedure. Following lysis, the DNA is simply precipitated away from cellular contaminants and resuspended. This procedure can be completed in <30 min and is suitable for processing many samples. The quantity of the reagent needed depends on the source of DNA and the amount to be isolated (Gibco-BRL, Gaithersburg, MD). Both of these methods produce good yields of DNA with molecular weight and purity sufficient for Southern blots, PCR amplification, and molecular cloning. Another new method is based on the incorporation of a membrane that selectively retains nuclei into a modified pipet tip. Following nuclear disruption and protein degradation, DNA is removed by centrifugation. Although this procedure produces very high-mol-wt DNA (>1000 kb), each tip yields only 10–20 μg (Amersham, Arlington Heights, IL).

Automation of DNA isolation has been made possible by incorporating the processes of cell lysis, organic extraction, ethanol precipitation, and filtration into a single apparatus *(10)*. These DNA extractors process multiple samples simultaneously, require relatively little attention from the operator, and produce DNA suitable for Southern blot analysis.

2.2.3. Isolation of DNA from Cultured Cells

Cells cultured in artificial vessels are readily accessible sources of genomic DNA. For the purposes of cell preparation prior to DNA isolation procedures, they may be divided into two categories. Cells attached to a substrate in a monolayer can be disassociated by either gently scraping them from the surface or by treatment with the protease, trypsin *(11)*. Cells grown in suspension simply require centrifugation for harvest. In either case, it is generally advisable to wash and recentrifuge the cells to remove components of the growth media and permit resuspension in an appropriate buffer at the desired density.

2.2.4. Isolation of DNA from Blood Samples

Genomic DNA is readily extractable from either fresh or frozen blood samples. Although DNA can also be isolated from clotted blood, homogenization of the clot is required, and yields are lower. It is therefore preferable to collect blood samples in the presence of an anticoagulant. Although EDTA and heparin are effective and commonly used for this purpose, it has been determined that the use of acid citrate dextrose produces higher yields of DNA from blood stored at room temperature. In addition, heparin is not recommended, because it tends to inhibit DNA binding enzymes used in subsequent DNA manipulations *(12)*. The nucleated leukocytes are only a small minority of total blood cells, but are easily separated from plasma and red blood cells by centrifugation. The resulting layer of white blood cells is removed and resuspended in an appropriate buffer for DNA isolation.

2.2.5. Isolation of DNA from Primary Tissue Samples

Samples of solid tissue need to be disrupted prior to initiating DNA isolation procedures. This is generally accomplished by subjecting such samples to mechanical forces that yield dissociated individual cells, but cause a minimum of lysis. This mechanical disruption is often achieved by use of a homogenizer. However, in cases where high-mol-wt DNA is sought, the inhibition of nucleases by maintaining tissue samples at extremely low temperatures has been shown to be beneficial *(2,3)*. Immediately following excision, the sample is frozen in liquid nitrogen. Disruption is then performed by pulverizing the tissue in the presence of dry ice by using either an electric blender or a mortar and pestle. Immediately after the dry ice sublimes from the resulting powder mixture, the cells can be resuspended for the initiation of the DNA isolation procedure.

2.2.6. Other Sources of DNA and Applications Requiring Special Consideration

2.2.6.1. PRESERVED TISSUE SAMPLES

The vast stores of diseased tissue that have been preserved represent an important resource for molecular genetic analysis. The DNA from such samples may provide information pertinent to the causes of their pathologies. Procedures using routinely treated tissue fixed with formalin or formaldehyde and embedded in paraffin have yielded DNA that is of sufficient quality for Southern blot analysis, amplification, and molecular cloning techniques. The preserved samples are sliced into fine sections and incubated with detergent and proteinase K. The DNA is collected by precipitation in ethanol following organic extractions *(13)*.

2.2.6.2. FORENSIC SAMPLES

Procedures have also been developed for the extraction of genomic DNA from a wide variety of samples used in forensic studies: whole blood; blood clots; blood stains; semen stains; oral, anal, and vaginal swabs; and hair. In many instances, a preliminary separation of the cells of interest from contaminating cells is necessary *(14)*. DNA isolation may be successful even when the source is in extremely limiting quantity (such as one hair) and in poor condition, as is often the case for forensic samples. Isolated DNA may be used in molecular procedures, including DNA fingerprinting and restriction fragment length polymorphism analysis. Such procedures are being increasingly applied to relationship determination, accident investigation, and identification of individuals committing violent and sexual crimes.

2.2.6.3. PULSED-FIELD GEL ELECTROPHORESIS

Pulsed-field gel electrophoresis is used to separate very large DNA molecules (on the order of 1000 kb). It is essential, therefore, that DNA be isolated in a manner that preserves its integrity. This is most widely achieved by incorporating cells into gelatinous agarose blocks prior to lysis with detergent and treatment with protease *(15)*. This technique virtually eliminates hydrodynamic shearing while still permitting access to enzymes and convenient introduction of samples into the gel apparatus.

2.2.6.4. VIRAL DNA

DNA from animal virus genomes is important in pathogen diagnosis as well as in the construction of mammalian plasmid vectors (*see below* for discussion of plasmid isolation). Many viruses infect only a subset of cell types. Therefore, appropriate sources of viral DNA are dictated by the types of cells infected by the particular virus being investigated. Isolation of DNA from tissue samples or cultured cells for identification of viral infection is performed using the relevant methods described above for genomic DNA. Subsequent diagnostic procedures, often based on viral DNA hybridization and amplification, generally do not require the methods producing high-mol-wt DNA.

2.3. Preparation of Plasmid DNA

2.3.1. Properties and Uses of Plasmid DNA

Plasmids are naturally occurring genetic elements that serve as convenient tools for the isolation and manipulation of cloned DNA fragments. Replication of plasmid DNA is carried out by host enzymes and requires the presence of an origin of replication *(ori)* in the plasmid. The number of plasmid molecules in a host cell (copy number) is determined by sequences adjacent to the *ori*. Although copy numbers of plasmids in bacteria vary from just 1 to over 500, most plasmids commonly used in current molecular biology have copy numbers of approx 100.

Plasmids generally encode genes that have functions beneficial to their hosts. Many such genes confer to the host the ability to grow in the presence of an antibiotic. When plasmid DNA is introduced into a population of bacterial cells in the laboratory (transformation), the cells that actually internalize plasmid molecules (transformants) can be distinguished based on the antibiotic resistance supplied by the plasmid-borne gene. Such genes are known as selectable markers.

The usefulness of plasmids has been greatly enhanced by the engineering of convenient cloning sites into their DNA sequences. These sites serve as locations for insertion of foreign DNA fragments. Several different sites are often clustered together to form a polylinker, which allows the same plasmid to harbor a wider variety of foreign DNA fragments depending on which site(s) is used.

In addition to simply carrying heterologous DNA in an accessible genetic unit, some plasmids are designed to facilitate further molecular manipulations. For example, promoter sequences adjacent to insertion sites direct transcription of the inserted DNA to make RNA, which may, in turn, be translated into protein. Plasmids with these capabilities are termed expression vectors. Other plasmids contain sequences that direct one strand to be synthesized and packaged into phage particles. The single-stranded DNA can be easily isolated and used for determining the base sequence of an inserted fragment. Some plasmids have two replication origins and two selectable markers. One set functions in bacteria and the other functions in the unicellular fungus, yeast. These plasmids, called shuttle vectors, can be manipulated in vitro, propagated in bacteria, and transformed into yeast cells where they are stably maintained and useful for genetic and biochemical investigations. Likewise, prokaryotic plasmids are combined with DNA elements of higher eukaryotes to create mammalian expression vectors. Some mammalian vectors are only transiently present in host cells, whereas more stable vectors employ viral sequences in the control of replication and incorporate genes encoding mammalian selectable markers.

2.3.2. Isolation Procedures for Plasmid DNA

Plasmid DNA is routinely isolated from liquid cultures of its bacterial hosts, usually *E. coli*. A plethora of plasmid isolation protocols are available. Many of these, including that presented in Table 2, are variations of the commonly used alkaline lysis method, which can be scaled up or down to suit the magnitude of the preparation needed *(16)*. After harvesting by centrifugation, the cells are treated with a detergent and sodium hydroxide in the presence of EDTA. This causes cell lysis and denaturation of the relatively large chromosomal DNA of the host. Base-pairing is disrupted, but because of its small, circular, supercoiled structure, the strands of plasmid DNA remain associ-

Table 2
Preparation of Plasmid DNA[a]

1. Grow plasmid-containing cells to saturation in 50 mL of selective media containing appropriate antibiotics.
2. Transfer cells to a tube and centrifuge at 3000g for 5 min to pellet bacterial cells.
3. Discard the supernatant and resuspend the cell pellet in 2.5 mL of solution I containing 50 mM glucose, 25 mM Tris-HCl, pH 8.0, and 10 mM EDTA, pH 8.0.
4. Add 5 mL of solution II containing 1.0 % sodium dodecyl sulfate and 0.2N NaOH.
5. Mix by repeatedly inverting the tube and then incubate on ice for 5–10 min.
6. Add 3.75 mL of solution III containing 3M potassium acetate and 2M acetic acid.
7. Mix by repeatedly inverting the tube and then incubate on ice 5–10 min.
8. Centrifuge at 3000g for 5 min and collect supernatant by filtering through several layers of cheesecloth into a fresh tube.
9. Add 12 mL of isopropanol, mix, and incubate on ice for 5–10 min or at –20°C until procedure is resumed.
10. Centrifuge at 3000g for 15 min and discard supernatant.
11. Resuspend the pellet in 300 μL of buffer containing 10 mM Tris-HCl, pH 7.5, and 1 mM EDTA.
12. Transfer sample to a microfuge tube and add 200 μL 6M lithium chloride, incubate on ice for 15 min.
13. Microcentrifuge for 10 min and transfer supernatant to a fresh tube.
14. Add 1.0 mL absolute ethanol, mix, and incubate on ice 5–10 min or at –20°C until procedure is resumed.
15. Microcentrifuge for 15 min, remove supernatant, and resuspend the pellet in 100 μL of buffer containing 10 mM Tris-HCl, pH 7.5, and 1 mM EDTA.

[a]This procedure is based on the methods of Birnboim and Doly *(16)*.

ated. In addition to inhibiting nucleases, EDTA aids in the destruction of the bacterial cell wall. The preparation is neutralized by the addition of acetic acid, at which time base-pairing in the plasmid is restored and the chromosomal DNA precipitates out of solution with other cellular components. The supernatant of the subsequently centrifuged mixture contains the plasmid DNA, which can be further purified by a variety of methods.

Choice of purification method, if any, depends on many of the same parameters discussed above for genomic DNA. Primary considerations are the scale of the isolation and the extent of purity required for the intended use of the plasmid DNA. Organic extraction is a quick and effective way to eliminate protein from crude plasmid samples, but includes all the disadvantages associated with using harmful solvents. A somewhat longer procedure uses polyethylene glycol to precipitate plasmid DNA selectively away from contaminants. For isolating substantial amounts of very pure plasmid DNA, cesium chloride equilibrium centrifugation may be undertaken *(17)*.

2.3.2.1. NEW PRODUCTS AND ALTERNATIVE METHODS IN PLASMID DNA PREPARATION

Many companies that supply products for molecular biological investigations produce reagents, apparatuses, and kits for the purification of plasmid DNA. Most of these are used following alkaline lysis and rely on either a silica-based resin or anion-exchange chromatography. The silica-based products selectively bind DNA in the presence of high concentrations of chaotropic salts. The resin–DNA complexes are then easily separated from unbound contaminants by centrifugation or filtration. Plasmid DNA is recovered by elution in buffer of low salt concentration (Pharmacia, Promega, Bio-Rad). Products for anion-exchange purification are generally used for plasmid preparations of larger scale and are available in formats suitable for column centrifugation or HPLC processing (Pharmacia, Bio-Rad). More recently, the attributes of alkaline lysis, silica-based resins, and anion-exchange chromatography have all been combined in the formation of automated plasmid extraction and purification devices (Pharmacia).

2.4. Extraction of DNA from Gels

It is often useful, particularly in molecular cloning and probe preparation, to purify DNA fragments that have been separated by gel electrophoresis. Several different methods are commonly used to extract DNA from agarose *(18,19)*. Agarose containing the band of interest may again be subjected to electrophoresis, such that the DNA travels through the agarose and into a containment medium. This process is called electroelution. Examples of containment media are:

1. A well of high-density buffer;
2. A membrane that binds DNA and can subsequently release it into a salt solution; and
3. A buffer-containing dialysis bag.

Agarose containing the band of interest may also be dissolved by virtue of it being a specially formulated low-melting-point agarose or by treatment with sodium iodide. Finally, DNA may be physically eluted from agarose by either allowing it to diffuse out of crushed pieces or by using the force of centrifugation to drive the DNA outward through the gel matrix.

Either simple diffusion or electroelution is generally used for extraction of DNA from polyacrylamide gels. In the case of the latter, the DNA binding membrane is placed in contact with the slice of polyacrylamide gel that contains the band of interest. This may be sandwiched between two agarose gel blocks to facilitate application of an electric field in a horizontal electrophoresis apparatus.

Reduction of contaminating gel material is frequently beneficial with any of the above extraction methods. This is generally accomplished by purifying the recovered DNA using a silica-based resin procedure.

2.5. Analysis of Prepared DNA

2.5.1. Nonselective Methods

Two methods are commonly used to determine the general quality and quantity of isolated DNA. These methods do not provide information about the identity of any specific DNA species, but instead provide information concerning the population of DNA molecules as a whole. The total DNA content of a sample can be determined by measuring its optical density at 260 and 280 nm with a spectrophotometer. The absorbance at 260 nm is used to calculate the concentration of DNA (50 μg/mL for OD = 1; note: contaminating RNA also absorbs at 260 nm). The 260/280 absorbance ratio is used to estimate the purity of the preparation (ratio <1.8 indicates impurities). The second nonselective method, gel electrophoresis, differs from spectrophotometry in that it fractionates the isolated DNA based on size. By staining DNA in the gel with ethidium bromide and comparing to standards, one can estimate the concentrations of individual bands and calculate the total concentration. Although this is obviously problematic for samples with a multitude of different sizes, such as genomic DNA, this method provides valuable information concerning the size distribution of DNA molecules within a preparation.

2.5.2. Selective Methods

In order to determine the presence or quantity of a particular subset of DNA molecules within a sample, methods based on sequence-specific hybridization to probes of known identity are employed. A nonfractionating method, known as dot or slot blotting, immobilizes the sample to be analyzed such that the quantity of the DNA sequence of interest can be readily assayed by its ability to hybridize with labeled probe molecules. Fractionation by gel electrophoresis followed by DNA transfer to a nylon membrane allows quantitation and size determination for DNA molecules that hybridize to a selected probe *(20)*. This method is clearly advantageous when the presence or quantities of different sized DNA species is to be determined individually.

3. RNA

3.1. Types of RNA

RNA molecules are divisible into three major classes: messenger RNA (mRNA), ribosomal RNA (rRNA), and transfer RNA (tRNA). mRNAs are the products of the transcribed genes and therefore carry the genetic information that specifies amino acid sequences of proteins. Long chains of adenosine (poly-A) are added to the 3'-ends of mRNA molecules and may provide protection from cellular nucleases. The presence of introns in mRNA transcribed from eukaryotic genes necessitates the process of splicing, removal of introns, and rejoining of exons, in order to produce a complete, continuous coding segment. rRNAs account for the bulk of cellular RNA and are essential structural components of ribosomes, the cellular complexes that perform translation. tRNAs are small RNAs that function in protein synthesis by matching mRNA sequences (codons) with appropriate amino acids. Neither rRNA nor tRNA has a 3' polyA tail structure as are found on mRNA.

3.2. RNA Isolation

3.2.1. RNA Instability

A significant problem often encountered in the isolation of RNA is its degradation by ribonucleases (RNases). RNases, many of which are extremely hardy enzymes, are required in cells to insure appropriate turnover of RNA. In addition to those endogenous to the organism from which RNA is to be extracted, RNases can also be introduced through laboratory materials and human hands. Numerous precautions may be instituted in order to minimize degradation by RNases. Of primary importance is to avoid contamination of RNA samples by contact with materials used in the course of, or following, RNase treatment of DNA preparations. Many investigators have found it beneficial to use disposable plasticware when feasible and to reserve a set of solutions, instruments, apparatuses, and so forth, strictly for use with RNase-sensitive samples. Several inhibitors of RNases may be used, but none of these is universally effective throughout RNA isolation procedures *(17)*. Laboratory equipment and materials may be baked or treated with DEPC as appropriate *(21)*. To minimize risk of contamination from the hands of investigators, disposable gloves should be worn throughout procedures involving RNA samples or materials that may potentially contact RNA samples. Frequent changing of gloves reduces introduction of RNase from contaminated objects and surfaces in the laboratory.

3.2.2. Procedures for Preparation of Cellular RNA

A commonly used approach to RNA isolation employs a detergent lysis step that includes RNase inhibitors. EDTA is also added to chelate divalent cation cofactors of nucleases. The presence of high-mol-wt DNA causes the lysate to be highly viscous, and therefore, reduces its amenability to manipulation and mixing. Since intact DNA is not needed and RNA is not damaged by hydrodynamic shearing, the lysate may be subjected to mechanical disruption, such as repeatedly being forced through a needle attached to a syringe. Proteins and cellular debris are removed by subsequent proteinase K treatment and organic extractions. Since RNase inhibitors are separated from RNA during organic extractions, they are again added prior to incubation with DNase. After a second series of organic extractions (to remove DNase), the RNA is recovered by ethanol precipitation *(22)*. A related method eliminates the proteinase K step, a potential opportunity for RNase-mediated degradation, and includes modified organic extractions. The pH of the lysate is lowered before extraction with phenol, so although the RNA remains in the aqueous solution, the DNA precipitates and gathers at the aqueous-organic interphase *(23)*. These types of RNA isolation methods are generally applicable to cells cultured on plates or in suspension.

Since the disruption of solid tissue inevitably causes some cell lysis, it is recommended that RNA isolation from tissue be initiated by homogenization in the presence of a strong chaotropic denaturant, such as guanidine cyanate. Tissue cut into small pieces should be used immediately or frozen with liquid nitrogen for storage. The inclusion of detergent in the homogenization buffer permits effective disruption of tissue, cell lysis, and DNA shearing in the same step *(24,25)*. The useful properties of chaotropic salts have led to their general employment in RNA isolation procedures (Table 3). In fact, chaotropic salts are key components of the numerous commercially available kits and reagents designed to simplify RNA isolation.

3.3. mRNA Purification

Although the above procedures for isolation of total RNA are sufficient for many RNA-based laboratory applications, effective performance of others, particularly cDNA synthesis, necessitates the purification of mRNA. Depending largely on tissue type, mRNA accounts for 1–5% of total cellular RNA. Fortunately, the presence of poly-A tails on nearly all eukaryotic mRNA molecules allows their biochemical distinction from other RNAs in the laboratory. Selective hybridization of the mRNA poly-A tails to single-stranded nucleotide sequences consisting of either multiple Ts or Us serves as the basis for separating this small fraction of RNA from rRNA and tRNA.

The aqueous product of the total RNA isolation is incubated with either oligo dT-cellulose *(26)* or poly U-sepharose *(27)* in a buffer of high sodium chloride concentration. The abundance of cations shields the negative charges of the phosphate groups in the nucleic acid backbones. This reduces interstrand repulsion and permits base-

Table 3
Isolation of Cellular RNA[a]

1. Harvest and wash 100 mg of cells with method appropriate to sample type.
2. Homogenize/resuspend with 1 mL of denaturation buffer containing $4M$ guanidinium thiocyanate, 25 mM sodium citrate, pH 7.0, 100 mM 2-mercaptoethanol, and 0.5% sarcosyl.
3. Transfer to a polypropylene centrifuge tube and add sequentially with mixing:
a. 0.1 mL $2M$ sodium acetate (4.0).
b. 1.0 mL water-saturated phenol.
c. 0.2 mL chloroform/isoamyl alcohol (49:1).
4. After vigorous agitation, incubate on ice for 10 min.
5. Centrifuge at 10,000g for 15 min at 4°C.
6. Remove aqueous layer and transfer to a fresh tube.
7. Add an equal volume of isopropanol and incubate at –20°C for at least 1 h.
8. Centrifuge at 10,000g for 15 min at 4°C and remove supernatant.
9. Resuspend pellet in 0.3 mL of denaturation buffer and transfer to a microfuge tube.
10. Add an equal volume of isopropanol, incubate at –20°C at least 1 h.
11. Microcentrifuge for 15 min at 4°C, remove supernatant.
12. Wash RNA pellet with 70% ethanol.
13. Microcentrifuge for 5 min at 4°C and remove supernatant.
14. Resuspend the pellet in 50 μL buffer containing 10 mM Tris-HCl, pH 7.5, and 1 mM EDTA.
15. Store at –70°C.

[a]This procedure is based on methods described by Chomczynski and Sacchi (25).

pairing with the poly-A stretches of RNA in solution. Nonhybridizing RNA molecules are removed by repeated washing of the mixture with the same buffer. When RNA is no longer detected in the washes, the mixture is treated with a buffer containing little or no salt. The lack of shielding cations causes mutual repulsion of the nucleic acid backbones and dissociation of the previously hybridized sequences. The eluted RNA should consist primarily of mRNA; however, this affinity purification process may be repeated to increase the mRNA proportion further.

The conventional format for using the poly-A binding materials is in a packed vertical cylinder that forms a column. The sample and various buffers are added to the top of the column and allowed to flow through the affinity matrix by the force of gravity. When processing multiple samples, it is often more convenient to use these materials in batches where they can be freely mixed with liquids and subsequently separated by centrifugation. Oligo-dT strands may also be attached to filters that can readily be moved as one piece from solution to solution. Commercially available kits and reagents based on these affinity purification principles feature additional formats. For example, "spin columns" require little preparation and allow the use of centrifugal force to separate solutions from the affinity matrix. Use of these products, some of which combine total RNA isolation with mRNA purification, generally simplifies and accelerates these processes.

3.4. Plasmid-Directed RNA Synthesis

In addition to being isolated from cells, RNA can be synthesized in vitro using engineered template molecules and the purified components required for transcrip-

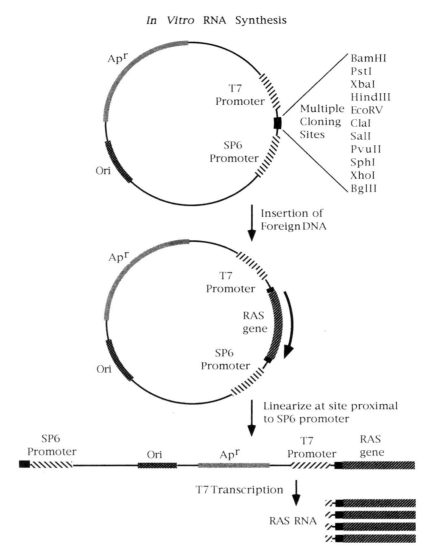

Fig. 1. In vitro synthesis of RNA using engineered template molecules and the purified components required for transcription.

tion (Fig. 1). In this way, RNA encoded by cloned DNA segments can be produced and easily isolated in large quantities. The DNA encoding the RNA of interest is inserted into a plasmid vector specialized for this purpose. These plasmids contain *ori* sequences for replication in bacteria as well as a selectable marker for antibiotic resistance (*see* Section 2.3.1.). In addition, multiple cloning sites (restriction enzyme cleavage sites) are grouped together in one location on the plasmid, such that the foreign DNA segment of interest can be efficiently inserted. Promoter elements positioned adjacent to the multiple cloning sites are capable of directing transcription by commercially available RNA polymerases. The resulting plasmid can be used as the template for transcription of the inserted DNA. For example, the *RAS* gene insert depicted in Fig. 1 is flanked by the T7 promoter upstream and the SP6 promoter downstream. Either strand of the *RAS* gene RNA can be produced by incubating the plasmid with ribonucleotides and either SP6 polymerase or T7 polymerase in the appropriate buffer. Termination of transcription is assured by cleavage of the plasmid, prior to incubation, at the end of the insert proximal to the promoter not selected. RNA synthesized in vitro may be used as a probe, as a target for RNA processing analysis, and as a template for in vitro protein synthesis.

3.5. RNA Analysis

3.5.1. Nonselective Methods

Just as with DNA, spectrophotometry and electrophoresis are two common approaches to determining general quality and quantity of RNA samples. The concentration of an RNA sample can be calculated from its optical density at 260 nm (40 μg/mL for OD = 1). Several gel systems have been developed for the electrophoresis of RNA *(17)*. RNA molecules of the same length migrate together as a band, and thus in cases, such as plasmid-directed RNA synthesis, in which samples contain a limited number of RNA species, the quantity and length of any particular RNA species can be calculated by comparison with standards after staining with ethidium bromide. For more complex RNA samples, electrophoresis also provides the size distribution of RNA within a sample. This is often used to detect degradation and rRNA contamination in mRNA preparations.

3.5.2. Selective Methods

Also analogous to DNA, the presence or quantity of specific RNA molecules can be detected by hybridization to probes of known identity. This principle can be applied with or without prior fractionation of RNA samples. Nonfractionating hybridizations often take the form of dot blots or slot blots *(see* Section 2.5.2.), but also can be formed in solution. In the case of the latter, the quantity of the target RNA can be determined, because it is proportional to the quantity of the probe protected from degradation by a single-strand-specific nuclease *(22)*. The combination of gel electrophoresis, blotting, and probe hybridization (northern blot) allows the determination of both length and quantity of specific RNAs *(28)*.

Selective methods have also been developed for mapping the structures of RNA molecules. These methods are widely used to determine sites of transcription initiation and termination as well as splice junctions. Nuclease mapping is similar to solution hybridization described above, but must employ a complementary probe of precisely known sequence that overlaps the RNA position to be mapped. For example, the location of the transcription initiation site is calculated based on the length of the probe following nuclease treatment (Fig. 2). An alternative method for mapping 5'-ends of RNA, known as primer extension, requires only a short segment of complementary DNA to hybridize to RNA molecules of interest. This short fragment is then used as a primer for DNA synthesis by reverse transcriptase. Since synthesis continues only as far as the RNA template, the length of the DNA produced indicates the distance from the primer annealing site to the RNA terminus.

Nuclease Mapping

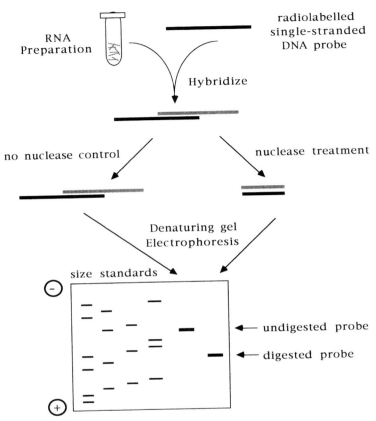

Fig. 2. Schematic illustrating the essential processes used in mapping RNA termini via nuclease digestion.

4. INTRODUCTION TO MOLECULAR CLONING

4.1. *Definition and Purpose*

Cloning, as applied to living organisms, is the process of producing a subpopulation that is derived from a single individual and is therefore genetically homogenous. In molecular cloning, segments of DNA from a source organism are inserted into vectors producing recombinant DNA molecules that are propagated in host cells. Individual host cells reproduce to give rise to subpopulations in which all cells contain identical segments of source DNA. It is molecular cloning that provides the opportunity to iso- late, analyze, and manipulate specific genes and their corresponding products. Taking advantage of this opportunity has revolutionized many aspects of medicine and bio- medical research. It is the foundation for molecular genetics that has produced innu- merable developments with respect to understanding biological mechanisms as well as the bases for many disease states. Here we will focus on the techniques used to create recombinant DNA molecules.

A

Cloning with Cohesive Ends

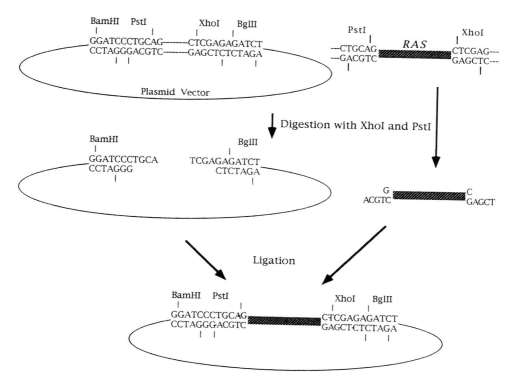

Fig. 3. (A) Cloning of DNA with cohesive (or sticky) ends. The plasmid DNA and insert DNA (RAS) are digested with restriction enzymes (*Pst*I and *Xho*I) that generate cohesive termini. Subsequent ligation of the hybridized plasmid and insert yields a stably cloned RAS gene and recreates the *Pst*I and *Xho*I restriction sites.

4.2. Basics of DNA Manipulation

4.2.1. Restriction Enzymes

Restriction enzymes are naturally occurring DNA endonucleases that comprise a fundamental set of tools for molecular cloning. By recognizing specific sequences of DNA and cleaving at precisely defined locations, restriction enzymes allow the consistent creation of DNA molecules with distinct identities *(29)*. There are now well over 100 commercially available restriction enzymes, most of which recognize specific six base-pair sites that are symmetrical (Fig. 3A,B). Some restriction enzymes cleave both strands of the DNA at the same exact location and thus produce DNA molecules with flush, or blunt, ends. Others cut the two strands at slightly different positions and produce staggered ends. Some of these leave 5'-protruding ends, whereas others leave 3'-protruding ends.

4.2.2. DNA Ligation Reactions

The power of molecular cloning is dependent not only on the ability to create distinct segments of DNA, but also on the ability to fuse the ends of different DNA molecules together. This biochemical fusion process is referred to as ligation, and the

B   Cloning with Blunt Ends

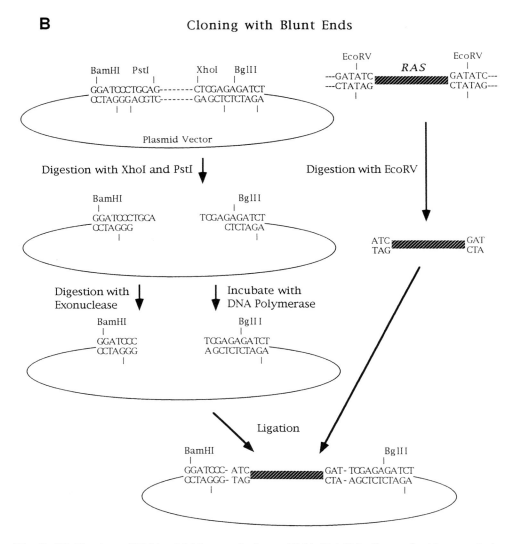

Fig. 3. (B) Cloning of DNA with blunt ends. Insert DNA (RAS) is digested with a restriction enzyme (EcoRV) that creates blunt termini, whereas the plasmid DNA is digested with *Pst*I and *Xho*I, which give cohesion ends. The cohesive ends are converted to blunt ends by either "filling in" (with DNA polymerase), or "chewing back" (with exonuclease). Subsequent ligation of the plasmid and insert DNAs produces a stably cloned RAS gene. However, none of the restriction sites used in this cloning reaction have been recreated. Nonetheless, the cloned RAS DNA can be liberated from the plasmid utilizing the *Bam*HI and *Bgl*II sites flanking the insert.

enzyme that accomplishes it is DNA ligase *(30)*. DNA ligase functions in both DNA replication and DNA repair systems in vivo by covalently joining 3'-terminal hydroxyl groups and 5'-terminal phosphates of separate DNA molecules with phosphodiester linkages. This biochemical activity is exploited in vitro to synthesize recombinant DNA molecules from selected DNA fragments. Although their ideal reaction conditions vary, both flush ends and complementary staggered ends can be ligated *(17; see* Section 4.3.).

4.2.3. Polymerases, Exonucleases, and Phosphatases

Molecular cloning is facilitated in many instances by the modification of restriction enzyme-generated fragments. It is often beneficial to convert staggered ends of restriction fragments to blunt ends. This task is made relatively straightforward by the availability of naturally produced DNA-modifying enzymes. DNA polymerases, which synthesize in the 5' to 3' direction, are used to add nucleotides to recessed 3'-ends using the protruding 5'-ends as templates *(17)*. Exonuclease activities are used to degrade protruding 3-ends *(17)*. Thus, blunt ends can be created by either "filling in" or "chewing back," depending on which type of protruding ends result from restriction enzyme cleavage. Fragments are sometimes more efficiently ligated into vectors from which the terminal 5'-phosphate residues have been removed. This modification is carried out by a phosphatase, another naturally occurring and commercially available enzyme *(17)*.

4.3. Molecular Cloning Examples

4.3.1. Cloning DNA with Cohesive Ends

The simplest form of molecular cloning is performed by creating a restriction fragment with staggered ends and ligating it into a vector with complementary staggered ends. This can more frequently be accomplished when available vectors contain many unique restriction sites from which to choose. Figure 3A illustrates an example of a cohesive end cloning process that shows details of an *RAS* gene insertion into a vector such as that seen in Fig. 1. The plasmid vector has a region of multiple cloning sites identical to that of Fig. 1. The sequences of the two restriction sites at each end of this region are displayed and labeled. The positions of cleavage are indicated by short vertical lines. For this example, the *RAS* gene is flanked by *Pst*I and *Xho*I sites. Digestion of the plasmid with *Pst*I and *Xho*I linearizes it, releasing the small DNA fragment between the sites that can readily be removed, and generating 3'- and 5'-protruding ends, respectively. Digestion of the foreign DNA containing the *RAS* gene with *Pst*I and *Xho*I disconnects the *RAS* sequence, leaving ends complementary to those of the plasmid. When the two prepared molecules are incubated together, the complementary bases anneal and the two molecules are joined by DNA ligase. Annealing of complementary ends is facilitated by incubation at approx 15°C. Note that additional DNA fragments with cohesive ends may be generated from digestion of the foreign DNA. If not separated from the *RAS* gene prior to ligation, these fragments would also be inserted into the vector. Also note that the vector cannot be self-ligated only because the two restriction enzymes used generate different staggered ends. The *RAS* gene can at this point be removed and manipulated using either of the upstream flanking restriction sites in conjunction with either of the downstream flanking restriction sites.

4.3.2. Cloning DNA with Noncohesive or Blunt Ends

Unfortunately, restriction sites compatible with those found in available vectors are not always located at positions useful for a desired cloning operation. In some such instances, restriction sites can be attached to blunt-ended fragments, but in other cases, this proves impractical. Blunt ends are created by some restriction enzymes, by shearing, and by enzymatic conversion of staggered ends. Figure 3B illustrates an example of a blunt-end cloning process related to that described above for cohesive ends. In this example, the same plasmid restriction sites are used, but the *RAS* gene is flanked by sites for the *Eco*RV restriction enzyme which leaves blunt ends. In order to accept the *RAS* gene insert, the ends of the digested vector must be made flush. The *Xho*I cleavage leaves a 5'-protruding end and thus the other strand can be synthesized by a DNA polymerase. The *Pst*I cleavage, however, leaves a protruding 3'-end that must be removed by an enzyme with exonuclease activity specific for single-standed substrates. Ligation of these prepared vector and fragment molecules is generally less efficient than for those with compatible staggered ends and does not benefit from incubation at lower than room temperature. Although *Pst*I, *Xho*I, or EcoRV sites were not re-created, the *RAS* gene can be removed and manipulated as a *Bam*HI-*Bgl*II fragment, since these sites flanked the site of insertion.

4.4. Clone Libraries

A collection of genetic elements containing representative DNA fragments derived from a particular organism is referred to as a clone library. Plasmids and viral genomes, as well as other genetic elements, serve as receptacles for the cloned DNA fragments. Clone libraries, therefore, can be propagated in populations of bacteria from which clonal subpopulations (colonies) may be isolated. Each such isolate will uniformly contain a single member of the clone library. To identify particular genes or sequences within a clone library, a screen of the library is performed. Such screens are based on:

1. Hybridization of the cloned segment to a probe of known identity;
2. Recognition of the encoded protein by antibodies of known specificity; or
3. Any assay that can detect the function of the encoded protein.

Creation and analysis of clone libraries allows the selection of particular sequences and novel genes in a cloned form that facilitates further manipulation and analysis.

4.4.1. Genomic DNA Libraries

For investigations that would benefit from a clone library in which all sequences of a given genome are represented, a genomic library is indicated. By fragmenting purified DNA using methods that approach the production of random segments, a collection that includes all sequences can be obtained. These methods include mechanical shearing and restriction enzyme digestion under conditions that permit cleavage at only a small fraction of the recognition sites. The collection of genomic fragments is often fractionated by size to exclude those that are too small, and thus would lower the efficiency of subsequent screening, as well as those that are too large to be propagated with the appropriate vector. Finally, the genomic fragments are ligated into a suitable vector and introduced into bacteria for replication. Much of a genomic library is made up of fragments partially or totally consisting of intergenic regions. Although this necessitates the screening of more clones to identify a particular gene, it also affords the opportunity to clone noncoding sequences important for genome structure as well as transcriptional and translational regulation.

4.4.2. cDNA Libraries

In cases where cloning the coding sequence of a particular gene is the immediate objective, use of cDNA libraries is usually advantageous. Construction of a cDNA library begins with isolation of RNA followed by mRNA purification *(see above)*. Oligonucleotides containing deoxythymidines are then hybridized to the poly-A tails of the mRNA molecules and used as primers for the syntheses of single strands of complementary DNA by reverse transcriptase. This "first strand" of DNA then serves as the template for synthesis of the complementary, mRNA-displacing "second strand" by DNA polymerase. Convenient restriction sites can be positioned on the ends of the cDNAs by ligation of oligonucleotide linkers containing the restriction enzyme recognition sequence. cDNAs are the ligated into appropriate vectors and propagated in bacteria.

The foundation of cDNA libraries being in purified mRNA produces several important implications for cloning. Whereas an ideal genomic library equally represents every sequence of a genome, an ideal cDNA library represents protein-coding sequences unequally, depending on the abundance of their mRNAs. Because genes are differentially expressed, some cDNAs may be common and others may be rare or nonexistent. For this reason, the source of mRNA for cDNA synthesis is of paramount importance. Some parameters that affect relative mRNA levels, and thus cDNA representation in a library, include tissue type, developmental stage, cell-cycle phase, nutritional state, and response to environmental stimuli. These parameters are taken into consideration, and often manipulated, to produce an mRNA source likely to yield high levels of desired cDNAs while restricting levels of undesired cDNAs.

Clone libraries are valued tools that are applied in a wide variety of investigations. For example, the gene corresponding to a purified protein can be isolated by using specific antibodies generated from the purified protein to screen a clone library expressed in bacteria. Genes encoding particular functions of interest are often identified by selecting library clones on the basis of their ability to reverse a specific mutant phenotype in yeast cells. Finally, novel genes encoding proteins that contain conserved structural motifs can be cloned by virtue of the hybridization of the corresponding conserved DNA sequences with appropriately designed probes.

5. INTRODUCTION TO DNA SEQUENCING

The ability to determine nucleotide sequences of DNA molecules has been, and continues to be, fundamental to the success of molecular approaches to biological research and medicine. In addition to its role as a complementary tool to cloning techniques, DNA sequencing is indispensable in the identification of mutations as well as the construction of data bases that catalog DNA segments based on their structure. These data bases permit enlightening comparisons useful in the characterization of novel genes, the study of evolution, and the delineation of DNA and protein structure–function relationships. Currently used DNA sequencing protocols are derived from two methods, depicted in Fig. 4, that rely on some common techniques, but are based on different principles.

5.1. The Chemical Cleavage Method

The method of DNA sequencing developed by Maxam and Gilbert is founded in the specific cleavage of DNA molecules at positions directly adjacent to chemically modified nucleotides *(31)*. A homogeneous sample of DNA radiolabeled at one end is treated in four (or sometimes five) separate chemical reactions, each of which modifies a particular type or types of bases. Conditions of the subsequent cleavage reactions are set such that cleavage occurs an average of only once for each DNA molecule. Each reaction, therefore, contains a mixture of DNA molecules of different lengths, each ending with the same subset of bases. The products of each reaction are subjected to denaturing polyacrylamide gel electrophoresis, which fractionates the populations of fragments

DNA Sequencing

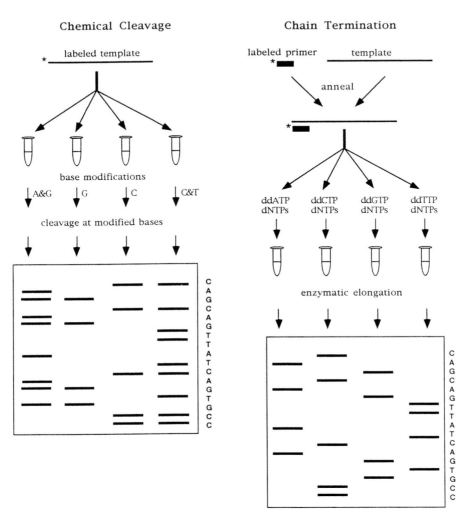

Fig. 4. Manual DNA sequencing methods: **(left)** the chemical cleavage method of Maxam and Gilbert *(31)*; **(right)** the chain termination method of Sanger and colleagues *(32)*.

by length with resolution sufficient to detect single nucleotide differences. The separate reaction products are electrophoresed in adjacent lanes such that following the detection of radiolabeled fragments with X-ray film, one can "read" the sequence of nucleotides. This is accomplished by recording the identity of the terminal nucleotide starting with the shortest fragment and proceeding with successively larger fragments.

5.2. The Chain Termination Method

The sequencing method developed by Sanger relies on enzymatic DNA synthesis from a specific oligonucleotide primer *(32)*. The primer is annealed to the complementary sequence adjacent to the DNA of interest on a genetic element. DNA polymerase is used to extend the primer through the target segment, synthesizing a single strand of DNA while using the opposite strand as a template. In addition to the customary dNTP used to synthesize DNA, each of four separate reactions contains a different ddNTP. These analogs can be incorporated into growing DNA strands, but owing to their lack of a 3'-hydroxyl cannot form a phosphodiester bond with an incoming dNTP. Therefore, the incorporation of a ddNTP causes the single-strand synthesis to terminate. The ratio of the specific ddNTP to dNTPs in each reaction is manipulated such that ddNTPs are incorporated only periodically and thus produce a mixture of synthesis products varying in length, but always ending with the same ddNTP. These single-stranded fragments are specifically labeled by using either labeled primers or, more generally, a labeled dNTP during synthesis. The products of the four reactions are fractionated, visualized, and analyzed using the same techniques described for the chemical cleavage method.

Prior to the availability of myriad cloning vectors, the chain termination method was significantly disadvantaged by the requirement for flanking sequence of known identity for primer annealing. However, the availability of appropriate vectors and the increasing ease with which high quality oligonucleotide primers are synthesized have contributed to the growing popularity of this method. Sequencing with this method is most simply accomplished with a template that is single-stranded. DNA to be sequenced, therefore, is often isolated from genetic elements that are packaged into phage particles as single-stranded DNA. Double-stranded templates can be used, but require denaturation to permit access of the primer to its complementary sequence. In addition, impurities in small, rapidly prepared samples of double-stranded plasmids interfere with enzymatic sequencing. Small DNA and RNA molecules function as competitors of primers during reannealing and direct DNA synthesis from unintended starting positions. Other contaminants inhibit polymerase activity. Many of these problems have been somewhat alleviated by new plasmid purification methods. The flexibility of effectively using either single-stranded or double-stranded templates is now widely enjoyed.

Developments in DNA polymerase usage have also increased the power of chain termination sequencing. The Klenow fragment of *E. coli* DNA polymerase I was used to develop the method and is still used in many instances despite significant drawbacks. Klenow fragment is not a highly processive enzyme and therefore occasionally creates "false termination" fragments by dissociating with the template at random positions. The length of sequence produced by Klenow fragment is limited by its inability to travel long distances on the template. Finally, Klenow fragment is often ineffective at synthesizing DNA in stretches containing a single dNTP which often form extensive secondary structure. A phage T7 polymerase lacking its 3' to 5' exonuclease activity (also known as Sequenase) is a much more processive enzyme and is capable of sequencing longer segments of DNA *(33)*. A *Taq* polymerase is active at temperatures high enough to eliminate most secondary structure and is therefore successful at sequencing through homopolymeric stretches *(34)*. Thermal-tolerant DNA polymerases have also permitted the development of protocols that produce multiple ddNTP-terminated fragments from each template molecule. This cyclic sequencing reaction is achieved by repetitive cycles consisting of primer annealing at a relatively low temperature, DNA synthesis at an intermediate temperature, and denaturation at a high temperature.

5.2.1. Automated DNA Sequencing

Combining technological advancements in chain termination sequencing has led to substantially automated procedures. Perhaps the crucial advancement was the ability to accurately detect DNA in gels during electrophoresis. This was made possible through the use of flourescently labeled nucleotides that emit light of a characteristic color when stimulated by a laser. The DNA synthesis products of each termination reaction may be uniformly labeled and electrophoresed in separate lanes or may be distinctly labeled and electrophoresed together in a single lane *(35,36)*. As electrophoresis proceeds, bands reaching a designated position are illuminated by a laser and identified by a fluorescence detector. The DNA sequence is determined by the temporal order of nucleotides passing the detection system and is recorded automatically by a computer. Although still incomplete, sequencing automation has thus far eliminated the need for the time-consuming processes of X-ray film exposure, manual gel reading, and manual recording of sequence data. Automated sequencers are often located in centralized facilities within institutions or departments such that access is available to many investigators.

ABBREVIATIONS

ddNTP, 2'3'-dideoxynucleoside triphosphate; DEPC, diethyl pyrocarbonate; dNTP, 2'-deoxynucleoside triphosphates; EDTA, ethylenediaminetetraacetic-acid; *Taq*, *Thermus aquaticus* DNA polymerase.

REFERENCES

1. Gross-Bellard, M., Oudet, P., and Chambon, P. Isolation of high-molecular-weight DNA from mammalian cells. *Eur. J. Biochem.* **36**:32–38, 1973.
2. Blin, N. and Stafford, D. W. A general method for isolation of high molecular weight DNA from eukaryotes. *Nucleic Acids Res.* **3**:2303–2308, 1976.
3. Graham, D. E. The isolation of high molecular weight DNA from whole organisms or large tissue masses. *Anal. Biochem.* **85**:609–613, 1978.
4. Kupiec, J. J., Giron, M. L., Vilette, D., Jeltsch, J. M., and Emanoil-Ravier, R. Isolation of high-molecular-weight DNA from eukaryotic cells by formamide treatment and dialysis. *Anal. Biochem.* **164**:53–59, 1987.
5. Longmire, J. L., Albright, K. L., Lewis, A. K., Meincke, L. J., and Hildebrand, C. E. A rapid and simple method for the isolation of high molecular weight cellular and chromosome-specific DNA in solution without the use of organic solvents. *Nucleic Acids Res.* **15**:859, 1987.
6. Bowtell, DD. Rapid isolation of eukaryotic DNA. *Anal. Biochem.* **162**:463–465, 1987.
7. Weeks, D. P., Beerman, N., and Griffith, O. M. A small-scale five-hour procedure for isolating multiple samples of CsCl-purified DNA: application to isolations from mammalian, insect, higher plant, algal, yeast, and bacterial sources. *Anal. Biochem.* **152**:376–385, 1986.
8. Reymond, C. D. A rapid method for the preparation of multiple samples of eucaryotic DNA. *Nucleic Acids Res.* **15**:8118, 1987.
9. Grimberg, J., Maguire, S., and Belluscio L. A simple method for the preparation of plasmid and chromosomal *E. coli* DNA. *Nucleic Acids Res.* **17**:8893, 1989.
10. Landegren, U., Kaiser, R., Caskey, C. T., and Hood, L. DNA diagnostics—molecular techniques and automation. *Science* **242**:229–237, 1988.
11. Freshney, R. I. *Culture of Animal Cells: A Manual of Basic Technique.* Liss, New York, 1987.

12. Gustafson, S., Proper, J. A., Bowie, E. J., and Sommer, S. S. Parameters affecting the yield of DNA from human blood. *Anal. Biochem.* **165**:294–299, 1987.
13. Cooper, C. S. and Stratton, M. R. Extraction and enzymatic amplification of DNA from paraffin-embedded specimens, in *Methods in Molecular Biology, vol. 9, Protocols in Human Molecular Genetics.* Mathew, C. G., ed. Humana, Clifton, NJ, pp. 133–140, 1991.
14. Sullivan, K. M. DNA fingerprinting and forensic medicine, in *Methods in Molecular Biology, vol. 9, Protocols in Human Molecular Genetics.* Mathew, C. G., ed. Humana, Clifton, NJ, pp. 273–285, 1991.
15. Schwartz, D. C. and Cantor, C. R. Separation of yeast chromosome-sized DNAs by pulsed field gradient gel electrophoresis. *Cell* **37**:67–75, 1984.
16. Birnboim, H. C. and Doly, J. A rapid alkaline extraction procedure for screening recombinant plasmid DNA. *Nucleic Acids Res.* **7**:1513, 1979.
17. Sambrook, J., Fritsch, E. F., and Maniatis, T., eds. *Molecular Cloning: A Laboratory Manual*, Cold Spring Harbor Laboratory Press, Cold Spring Harbor, New York, 1989.
18. Smith, H. O. Recovery of DNA from gels. *Methods Enzymol.* **65**:371–380, 1980.
19. Lucotte, G. and Baneyx, F. *Introduction to Molecular Cloning Techniques.* VCH, New York, 1993.
20. Southern, E. M. Detection of specific sequences among DNA fragments separated by gel electrophoresis. *J. Mol. Biol.* **98**:503, 1993.
21. Kumar, A. and Lindberg, U. Characterization of ribonucleoprotein and messenger RNA from KB cells. *Proc. Natl. Acad. Sci. USA* **69**:681–685, 1977.
22. Favaloro, J., Treisman, R., and Kamen, R. Transcription maps of Polyoma virus-specific RNA: Analysis by two-dimensional nuclease S1 gel mapping. *Methods Enzymol.* **65**:718–749, 1980.
23. Stallcup, M. R. and Washington, C. D. Region specific initiation of mouse mammary tumor virus RNA synthesis by endogenous RNA polymerase II in preparations of cell nuclei. *J. Biol. Chem.* **258**:2802–2807, 1983.
24. Chirgwin, J. M., Przybyla, A. E., McDonald, R. J., and Rutter, W. J. Isolation of biologically active ribonucleic acid from sources enriched in ribonuclease. *Biochemistry* **18**:5294–5299, 1979.
25. Chomczynski, P. and Sacchi N. Single-step method of RNA isolation by acid guanidinium thiocyanate-phenol-chloroform extraction. *Anal. Biochem.* **162**:156–159, 1987.
26. Aviv, H. and Leder, P. Purification of biologically active globin messenger RNA by chromatography on oligi-thymidylic acid-cellulose. *Proc. Natl. Acad. Sci. USA* **69**:1408–1412, 1972.
27. Lindberg, U. and Persson T. Isolation of mRNA from KB-cells by affinity chromatography on polyuridylic acid covalently linked to Sepharose. *Eur. J. Biochem.* **31**:246–54, 1972.
28. Alwine, J. C., Kemp, D. J., and Stark, G. R. Method for detection of specific RNAs in agarose gels by transfer to diazobenzyloxymethyl-paper and hybridization with DNA probes. *Proc. Natl. Acad. Sci. USA* **74**:5350–5354, 1977.
29. Roberts, R. J. Restriction and modification enzymes and their recognition sequences. *Nucleic Acids Res.* **11**:135–167, 1983.
30. Engler, M. J. and Richardson, C. C. in *The Enzymes*, vol. 5, Boyer, P. D., ed., Academic, San Diego, 1982.
31. Maxam, AM. and Gilbert, W. Sequencing end-labeled DNA with base-specific chemical cleavages. *Methods Enzymol.* **65**:499–560, 1980.
32. Sanger, F., Nicklen, S. and Coulson, A. R. DNA sequencing with chain-terminating inhibitors. *Proc. Natl. Acad. Sci. USA* **74**:5463–5467, 1977.
33. Tabor, S. and Richardson, C. C. DNA sequence analysis with a modified bacteriophage T7 DNA polymerase. *Proc. Natl. Acad. Sci. USA* **84**:4767–4771, 1987.

34. Barnes, W. M. The fidelity of Taq polymerase catalyzing PCR is improved by an N-terminal deletion. *Gene* **112:**29–35, 1992.

35. Smith, L. M., Sanders, J. Z., Kaiser, R. J., Hughes, P., Dodd, C., Connell, C. R., Heiner, C., Kent, S. B. H., and Hood, L. E. Flourescence detection in automated DNA sequence analysis. *Nature* **321:**674–679, 1986.

36. Ansorge, W., Sproat, B. S., Stegemann, J., and Schwager, C. A non-radioactive automated method for DNA sequence determination. *J. Biochem. Biophys. Methods* **13:**315–23, 1986.

Part II
Molecular Technologies

4

Nucleic Acid Blotting Techniques

Theory and Practice

Sharon Collins Presnell

1. INTRODUCTION

This chapter deals with basic concepts and techniques in nucleic acid blotting. In principle, the techniques of Southern blotting (DNA) and northern blotting (RNA) are very similar. Negatively charged, purified nucleic acid from prokaryotic or eukaryotic cells is separated according to size by electrophoresis through an agarose gel matrix. The RNA or denatured DNA is subsequently transferred and immobilized onto a membrane composed of nitrocellulose or nylon. The nucleic acids on the membrane are then hybridized to a specific labeled "probe," which consists of homologous single-stranded nucleic acids that carry molecules allowing detection and visualization of the hybridized probe. Hybridization between the immobilized nucleic acids and labeled probe allows detection of specific DNA or RNA sequences within a complex mixture of DNA or RNA. The specific method of detection and visualization is dependent on the nature of the labeled probe; radioactive probes enable autoradiographic detection, and probes labeled with enzymes facilitate chemiluminescent or colorimetric detection. Nucleic acid blotting yields valuable information pertaining to gene integrity and copy number (Southern blot) and provides a means of analyzing gene expression (northern blot). These methods are widely used to characterize tissues and cultured cells in the laboratory, and often provide valuable information for clinical evaluation of patient samples.

2. THE SOUTHERN BLOT

The DNA blot was developed by Southern in 1975 *(1)*, and it remains the method of choice among many researchers for reliable, quantitative detection of specific DNA sequences. The Southern blot can detect the presence of homologous genes across species. For example, if a biologically relevant gene has been located in the rat, it is possible to construct a labeled probe from the rat gene and use it to search for a homologous gene in humans by Southern blot analysis. The DNA blot can also be used to assess the relative copy number of a specific gene. This particular application of the Southern blot is useful in detecting gene amplification, which is a common response to environmental pressure and often accounts for drug resistance in mammalian cells *(2,3)*. South-

From: Molecular Diagnostics: For the Clinical Laboratorian
Edited by: W. B. Coleman and G. J. Tsongalis Humana Press Inc., Totowa, NJ

ern analysis can identify mutations, deletions, or rearrangements that alter the integrity of a specific gene, which can be useful in the prognosis of certain types of cancer and in the prenatal diagnosis of genetic diseases. In addition, the DNA blot is a valuable tool for molecular cloning, providing a mechanism for localization of specific sequences to defined fragments within larger bacteriophage and cosmid genomic DNA clones.

3. METHODOLOGY OF SOUTHERN BLOT ANALYSIS

3.1. Preparation of DNA for Southern Blotting

Most basic techniques for purification of DNA produce material appropriate for Southern analysis. Standard Southern blot protocols recommend the use of 10 µg of DNA when analyzing single-copy genes *(4)*. However, when the amount of DNA is limiting, smaller quantities may be used without compromising the signal by altering the geometry of the sample well during electrophoresis (decreasing the width of the well will increase the intensity of the final signal) *(5)*. In situations where multiple copies of the gene are present or if the gene constitutes a high percentage of the DNA (plasmid DNA containing the gene of interest is being analyzed), the quantity of DNA can be dramatically reduced to as little as 200 ng. Under optimal conditions, rare sequences (single copy genes) can be detected when just 10 µg of genomic DNA are analyzed *(4)*.

DNA that is to be analyzed by Southern blot must first be fragmented into small pieces that can migrate through an agarose gel matrix. Restriction enzymes are bacterial enzymes that recognize specific DNA sequences (four to six nucleotides long) in DNA and cleave the DNA at these restriction sites. Digestion of genomic DNA with a given restriction enzyme produces a reproducible set of fragments that are easily separated by agarose gel electrophoresis. In order to determine which restriction enzyme(s) to use, it is helpful to know which restriction sites are present within and around the gene of interest. Generally, when evaluating the presence or copy number of a particular gene, one should avoid using restriction enzyme(s) that cut the gene of interest into a large number of small fragments. Ideally, the gene of interest should be cleaved into a few fragments (one to three) that range in size from 1.0–10.0 kb. A different approach may be desirable when evaluating the integrity of a specific gene. A normal gene contains many restriction sites, and cleavage of the gene with a particular restriction enzyme produces a distinct number of fragments of a defined size. Mutations, deletions, or rearrangements occurring within a gene may result in a disruption of the normal nucleotide sequence, possibly altering the number of restriction sites within the gene or altering the size of the restriction fragments produced. Such a change in the size pattern of DNA fragments produced by enzymatic cleavage is referred to as a restriction fragment length polymorphism (or RFLP). A detailed restriction map of a gene is generated by cleaving the DNA with several restriction enzymes (separately) and then performing a Southern analysis of the fragmented DNA with a probe for the gene of interest. Restriction maps are useful for identifying subtle differences between homologous genes. Hundreds of restriction enzymes are commercially available (Gibco-BRL [Grand Island, NY], Sigma [St. Louis, MO], New England Biolabs [Beverly, MA]), and manufacturers typically provide the proper buffer necessary for digestion as well as instructions for the quantity of enzyme, temperature, and duration

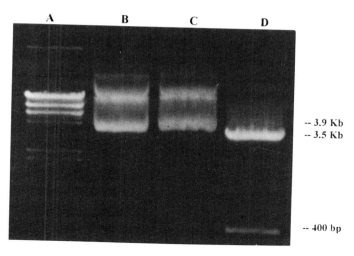

Fig. 1. Agarose gel electrophoresis of plasmid restriction digests. Five micrograms of a 3.9 kb plasmid containing a 400-bp insert of the c-*met* gene were digested with the restriction enzyme *Bst*XI for 1 h at 37°C. Lane **A** contains DNA mol-wt standards (*Hind*III-digested γ DNA). Lane **B** contains plasmid that was not incubated with a restriction enzyme. Lane **C** contains plasmid that was incubated at a temperature of 4°C instead of 37°C, demonstrating the importance of incubation temperature. Lane **D** contains fully digested plasmid DNA. Notice the disappearance of the 3.9-kb DNA band corresponding to the intact plasmid, and the appearance of a 400-bp DNA band representing the insert and a 3.5-kb DNA band representing the plasmid remnant. The very high-mol-wt band present in lanes B and C is likely to consist of aggregates of circular plasmid DNA, and disappears with enzymatic digestion (lane D).

of reaction required for thorough digestion. One unit of an enzyme is defined as the amount required to cleave 1.0 µg of DNA in 1 h. Complete cleavage of the DNA is essential for Southern blotting, especially when single-copy genes are being analyzed. A small aliquot (0.5–1.0 µg) of the digested DNA sample can be subjected to agarose gel electrophoresis and stained with ethidium bromide to determine whether enzymatic digestion of the DNA is complete (*see* Figs. 1 and 2). Thorough digestion of plasmid DNA is evidenced by total disappearance of the uncut plasmid and the appearance of specific bands. Digestion of genomic DNA is confirmed by the appearance of distinct bands, usually in the lower portion of the gel. These bands are produced from enzymatic fragmentation of repetitive elements within the DNA and are characteristic of the restriction enzyme utilized. After fragmentation, the DNA is typically concentrated by ethanol precipitation and resuspended in a small volume of electrophoresis buffer in preparation for electrophoretic separation (*see* Table 1).

3.2. Electrophoresis of Restriction Digested DNA

Nucleic acids are negatively charged at a neutral pH, which allows their migration through an electric field *(6)*. Agarose is a highly porous polysaccharide that acts as a sieve, allowing the fragments of DNA to be separated according to length. Under low-voltage conditions, the electrical resistance of all components remains constant, and the linear DNA fragments move through the agarose gel at a velocity proportional to

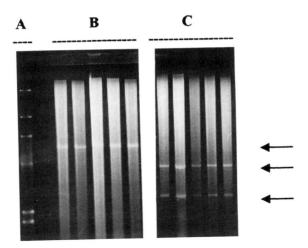

Fig. 2. Agarose gel electrophoresis of genomic DNA restriction digests. Genomic DNA samples were isolated from cultures of rat liver epithelial cells. Lane **A** contains DNA mol-wt standards (*Hin*dIII-digested γ DNA). Lanes **B** and **C** show 10-µg DNA samples that were digested with either *Hin*dIII (B) or *Bam*HI (C) for 18 h at 37°C. Agarose gel electrophoresis was carried out for 18 h at 22 V. The gel was stained with ethidium bromide and photographed under a UV lamp. The distinct bands (indicated with an arrow) within the digested DNA represent repetitive sequences or elements in the DNA. Note that this banding pattern differs depending on the restriction enzyme employed. Thorough digestion of the DNA produces a "smear" of DNA fragments that range in size from very large (>23 kb) to very small (<0.5 kb).

the voltage applied. The driving force for nucleic acid migration in the gel is the voltage gradient, which is dependent on the geometry of the electrophoresis chamber, geometry and composition of the gel, and the volume and ionic strength of the buffer used. The velocity of DNA migration can be increased by decreasing the distance between electrodes, decreasing gel thickness, or decreasing buffer volume. A practical approach is to keep the gel geometry, buffer composition, and volume constant and determine the optimal running voltage empirically. The gel should be covered by 3–4 mm of buffer and high voltage settings should be avoided, since they will lead to melting of the agarose and the appearance of artifacts on the final blot. The gel can be run overnight (12–16 h) at a low voltage (20–30 V) without compromising the quality of electrophoretic separation. Because the electrophoresed DNA should be transferred to a solid support (nylon or nitrocellulose) as soon as possible, overnight electrophoresis is often a desirable option for workers with time limitations.

Agarose electrophoresis of DNA allows separation of fragments ranging from 200 to 1×10^7 bp, although it is not possible to separate such a wide range of lengths on a single gel. A classical Southern analysis (as presented in Table 1) allows separation of fragments ranging from 200 bp to 20 kbp. Fragments smaller than 200 bp are typically analyzed by utilizing polyacrylamide gels (7–9), and DNA larger than 20 kbp may be analyzed by pulsed-field gel electrophoresis (10).

The percentage and composition of agarose used to prepare the gel are determined based on the size of the fragment(s) of interest. Good electrophoretic separation of small DNA fragments (0.2–1.0 kbp) can be accomplished using 2–4% agarose gels

Table 1
Southern Blot Analysis

1. Restriction enzyme digestion:
   a. Digest 10–20 µg genomic DNA with an appropriate enzyme (use 3–5 U enzyme/µg DNA).
   b. Check the efficiency of the digest by analyzing a 1-µg aliquot of DNA on an agarose gel.
   c. Precipitate the remaining digested DNA overnight with 1/10 vol 2.5M sodium acetate and 2 vol cold ethanol (100%).
   d. Resuspend precipitated DNA in 30 (l TPE and add 6 µL of DNA sample buffer (Table 2).
2. Electrophoresis of the DNA:
   a. Prepare a 0.9% agarose gel with TPE buffer (add ethidium bromide to 0.5 µg/mL).
   b. Place the gel in the electrophoresis tank and fill with TPE to 3–4 mm above gel surface.
   c. Load the samples into the sample wells. Include appropriate DNA size standards.
   d. Run the gel overnight at 22–30 V (or until the bromophenol blue migrates 8 cm).
   e. Photograph the gel and carefully measure migration distances of mol-wt standards.
3. Denaturation and neutralization of the DNA:
   a. Denature the DNA by soaking the gel 2 × 15 min in 0.5M sodium hydroxide.
   b. Neutralize the DNA by soaking the gel 3 × 10 min in 1.0M Tris, pH 7.5.
4. Capillary transfer of the DNA to a nylon membrane:
   a. Cut a piece of nylon membrane to the exact size of the gel; prewet in dH_2O.
   b. Equilibrate the gel and nylon membrane in 20X SSPE transfer buffer for 15 min.
   c. Assemble the capillary transfer apparatus as shown in Fig. 3. Take care to remove any air bubbles between the gel and the nylon membrane.
   d. Fill the buffer chamber with 20X SSPE and transfer overnight.
   e. Check the efficiency of transfer by staining the gel with ethidium bromide.
   f. Let the membrane air-dry briefly and then fix the DNA to the filter by UV crosslinking.
5. Hybridization with labeled nucleic acid probe
   a. Prepare the probe utilizing manufacturer's instructions.
   b. Prehybridize the membrane for 1 h in prehybridization solution option 1 (Table 2), at 42°C.
   c. Hybridize the membrane overnight in hybridization solution option 1 (Table 2), at 42°C.
   d. Wash the membrane 2 × 15 min in 2X SSPE, 0.1% SDS, at 42°C. If additional washing is needed, wash for 30 min in 1X SSPE, 0.1% SDS, at 42°C. If necessary, subsequent washes can be performed (3 × 10 min) with 0.5X SSPE, 0.1% SDS, at 42°C.
   e. Visualization (radiolabeled probes): Rinse the membrane briefly in 1X SSPE, blot excess fluid from the membrane, wrap securely in plastic wrap, and expose to X-ray film for 24 h at −70°C. Develop the film and adjust exposure time as necessary.

prepared with a 3:1 mixture of low-melting-point agarose and standard agarose (FMC BioProducts, Rockland, ME). Low-melting-point agarose consists of hydroxyethylated agarose, which has better sieving properties than standard agarose and results in greater clarity of DNA bands. These high-percentage gels are useful when analyzing PCR products or cloned DNA. For Southern analysis of genomic DNA, 0.7–1.2% standard agarose gels are recommended *(4)*. The efficiency of DNA transfer to a solid support is increased with decreasing agarose concentration, but low-percentage agarose gels are delicate and difficult to manipulate. The ideal sample well size should be determined empirically. Although a weak signal can be amplified by decreasing the width of the sample well, the use of wider sample wells results in better resolution of bands.

The inclusion of a DNA size standard on analytical DNA gels containing DNA fragments of known length is recommended because such standards provide a means of extrapolating the size of a positive signal from target DNA. A popular choice for a DNA size standard in a classical Southern blot is Lambda (λ) phage DNA, which has been digested with the restriction enzyme *Hin*dIII, which provides a pattern of fragments ranging from 125 bp to 23.1 kb. Various DNA size standards are commercially available (Amersham [Arlington Heights, IL], Gibco-BRL), and can be obtained prelabeled with molecules, such as biotin, that aid in their visualization. When choosing DNA standards, it is important to be sure that the target DNA sequences are within the range of kilobase lengths represented in the DNA standards. Most protocols recommend staining the electrophoresed agarose gels with ethidium bromide to visualize the DNA standards and the digested DNA. Gels can be stained after electrophoresis by soaking in a 2 μg/mL solution of ethidium bromide. Alternatively, ethidium bromide (0.5 μg/mL) can be added to the melted agarose (after cooling to 55°C) and to the electrophoresis buffer. Staining with ethidium bromide permits photography of the gel, so the exact migration of DNA standards can be recorded along with the quality of the restriction enzyme digestion of the test DNA.

After electrophoresis, the double-stranded DNA fragments must be denatured into single strands. Denaturation of the DNA can be accomplished by soaking the gel in an alkaline solution containing sodium hydroxide (*see* Table 2). This step should be carried out on a rotary platform, which allows thorough, constant submersion of the gel. After denaturation, it is important to neutralize the gel, which is typically done by soaking the gel in a neutral (pH 7.4) solution of Tris buffer. The single strands of DNA are then ready to be transferred to a solid support, such as nitrocellulose or nylon membrane, where they can be hybridized to a complementary, labeled nucleic acid probe.

3.3. Transfer of DNA to a Solid Support

3.3.1. Choice of Hybridization Membrane

Immobilization and hybridization of nucleic acid was first carried out with nitrocellulose *(1)*. However, nitrocellulose is not ideal for nucleic acid hybridization. Because the nucleic acids are attached by hydrophobic rather than covalent interactions, they are slowly leached out of the nitrocellulose matrix during hybridization and washing at high temperatures. In addition, the fragile filters cannot survive more than one or two cycles of hybridization and washing. The shortcomings of nitrocellulose have led to the development of several alternative matrices, the most versatile of which is positively-charged nylon *(11)*. Nylon membranes bind nucleic acids irreversibly and are much more durable, allowing sequential hybridizations with several different probes without a loss of membrane integrity. Nylon membranes also allow highly efficient electrophoretic transfer of small amounts of nucleic acid when capillary or vacuum transfer is insufficient. The single disadvantage to nylon membranes is the propensity for higher background hybridization, but this problem can be eliminated by increasing the amount of blocking agents during prehybridization and hybridization.

3.3.2. Methods of DNA Transfer

Single-stranded (denatured) DNA can be transferred to a solid support, such as a nitrocellulose or nylon membrane. If nitrocellulose membranes are used, the recommended method of transfer is capillary transfer. With the more versatile nylon membrane, several methods of transfer are available, including capillary transfer,

Table 2
Solutions used in Nucleic Acid Blotting

Solution	Composition	Use
TAE (Tris-acetate buffer)	0.04M Tris-acetate, 0.1 mM EDTA, pH 8.0	Agarose gel electrophoresis; Electrophoretic transfer of nucleic acids to a nylon membrane
TPE (Tris-phosphate buffer)	0.09M Tris-phosphate, 0.2M EDTA, pH 8.0,	Agarose gel electrophoresis (Southern blot)
TBE (Tris-borate buffer)	0.045M Tris-borate, 0.1M EDTA, pH 8.0,	Agarose gel electrophoresis
MOPS buffer (3-[N-morpholino] propanesulfonic acid)	(5X stock) 0.1M MOPS, pH 7.0, 40 mM sodium acetate 5 mM EDTA, pH 8.0	Electrophoresis of RNA through formaldehyde gels in Northern blotting
SSC (salt-sodium citrate buffer)	(20X stock) 3.0M NaCl, 0.3M sodium citrate, pH 7.0	Capillary transfer of nucleic acids to nylon or nitrocellulose membrane; washing hybridized filters
SSPE (salt-sodium phosphate-EDTA buffer)	(20X stock) 3.6M NaCl, 0.2M NaH$_2$PO$_4 \cdot$ H$_2$O 20 mM EDTA, pH 7.7	Capillary transfer of nucleic acids to nylon or nitrocellulose membrane; washing hybridized filters
DNA gel denaturation solution	0.5M sodium hydroxide	Denaturation of electrophoresed DNA prior to Southern blot transfer
Neutralization buffer	1.0M Tris-HCl, pH 7.5	Neutralization of DNA gels after sodium hydroxide denaturation
Alkaline transfer buffer	3M sodium chloride 8 mM sodium hydroxide, pH 11.4–11.45	Rapid alkaline capillary transfer of nucleic acids to nylon membranes
Denhardt's reagent	(50X stock) 1% Ficoll, 1% polyvinylpyrrolidine, 1% bovine serum albumin	A blocking agent added to hybridization solutions in Southern and Northern blots to reduce background
Prehybridization solution (option 1)	5X SSPE, 5X Denhardt's reagent, 200 µg/mL denatured salmon sperm DNA, 0.1% SDS, 50% formamide	Prehybridization of Northern and Southern blots prior to hybridization with labeled probe
Hybridization solution (option 1)	5X SSPE, 2.5X Denhardt's reagent, 200 µg/mL denatured salmon sperm DNA, 0.1% SDS, 50% formamide	Hybridization of Northern and Southern blots to labeled probe
Hybridization and prehybridization solution (option 2)	6X SSC, 2X Denhardt's reagent, 0.1% SDS	Prehybridization and hybridization of Northern and Southern blots
Hybridization and pre-hybridization solution (option 3)	5X Denhardt's reagent, 0.5% SDS, 100 µg/mL denatured salmon sperm DNA	Useful for reducing high background hybridization in northern and Southern blots
DNA and RNA sample buffer	50% Glycerol, 1 mM EDTA, 0.25% bromophenol blue, 0.25% xylene cyanol FF	Electrophoresis of RNA through formaldehyde gel

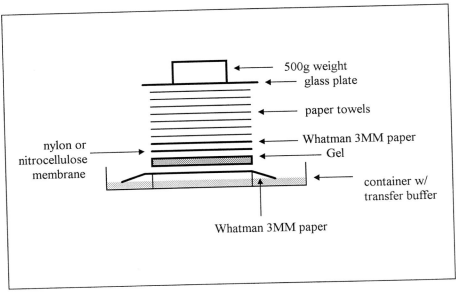

Fig. 3. Capillary transfer of nucleic acids to hybridization membranes.

electrotransfer, and vacuum transfer. Although nitrocellulose can be used for vacuum transfer or electrotransfer, these methods are optimal with nylon membranes. Regardless of the method of transfer, it is recommended that the gel and the membrane be equilibrated in transfer buffer prior to transfer. The composition of buffer is dependent on the method of transfer employed (*see* Table 2).

In capillary transfer *(1)*, nucleic acid fragments are eluted from the gel and deposited onto the membrane by transfer buffer that is drawn through the gel by capillary action (*see* Fig. 3). Rate of transfer is dependent on the size of the fragments, with larger fragments transferring less efficiently. The disadvantage of traditional capillary transfer is the length of time required for efficient transfer of large nucleic acid fragments (usually overnight). When large (>5 kb) fragments of DNA are to be analyzed, many protocols recommend depurinating the electrophoresed DNA prior to denaturation by soaking the gel in $0.2M$ hydrochloric acid for 5–15 min *(12)*. Depurination, along with denaturation, leads to the breakdown of long DNA fragments into shorter pieces, which transfer more efficiently. However, this nicking of the DNA has been reported to reduce the final hybridization signal significantly and decrease the clarity of bands on the autoradiograph *(5)*. Downward alkaline capillary transfer *(13,14)*, which can be completed in 1–3 h, offers a fast and efficient alternative to traditional capillary transfer and does not require special equipment (*see* Fig. 4).

Electrophoretic transfer *(15)* was developed as a faster alternative to capillary transfer. Size-separated nucleic acid fragments are transferred onto a membrane (preferably nylon) by placing the gel between porous pads that are inserted between parallel electrodes in a large buffer tank. These apparatuses are available from several manufacturers (Bio-Rad [Hercules, CA], Schleicher & Schuell [Keene, NH]). Electroblotting can be quite efficient, with complete transfer of high-mol-wt nucleic acids in 2–3 h. However, the electrophoresis apparatus must be equipped with a cooling mechanism for maintaining an acceptable buffer temperature, and large buffer volumes are required.

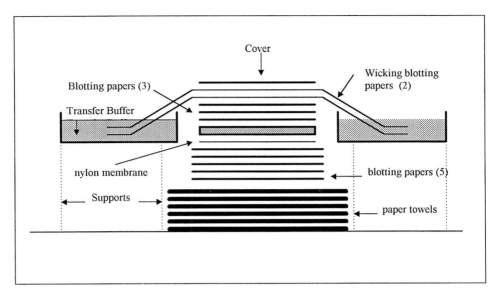

Fig. 4. Downward capillary transfer of nucleic acids to hybridization membranes.

The need for special equipment has largely limited the use of the electroblot to situations in which capillary transfer or vacuum transfer is not sufficient.

Vacuum blotting was recently introduced as another alternative to capillary transfer *(16,17)*, and involves the application of negative pressure to the gel. Nucleic acids are eluted by buffer that is drawn through the gel by application of negative pressure (a vacuum). Transfer of nucleic acids by vacuum blotting is more efficient than capillary transfer and has been reported to result in a two- to threefold increase in final hybridization signal obtained *(18)*. Vacuum blotting devices are commercially available (Bio-Rad) and work well when the vacuum is applied evenly over the gel surface. However, efficiency of transfer may be reduced if the vacuum exceeds 60 cm of water *(4)* owing to compression of the gel. When carried out properly, the vacuum blot provides a means for fast (approx 4 h), efficient, highly reproducible transfer of nucleic acids.

3.3.3. Fixing DNA onto Nitrocellulose or Nylon Membranes

After transfer, the DNA must be stably adhered to the membrane to ensure that it remains in place during hybridization and washing. If a nitrocellulose membrane was used, the DNA can be affixed by baking the damp membrane at 80°C for 2 h in a vacuum oven. Alternatively, nylon membranes may be exposed (DNA side up) to low-level UV irradiation (at 254 nm). Irradiation of the membrane results in crosslinks between the nucleic acid residues and positively charged amine groups on the membrane surface *(19)*. Overirradiation of the membrane may cause covalent attachment of a high percentage of the nucleic acid residues, resulting in a decreased hybridization signal. Special ovens for the irradiation of membranes are commercially available, and most manufacturers recommend 1.5 J/cm^2 for damp membranes and 0.15 J/cm^2 for dry membranes. Optimally, the ideal amount of irradiation should be determined empirically. Baked or irradiated Southern blots can be stored at room temperature until they are ready to be hybridized to a labeled nucleic acid probe.

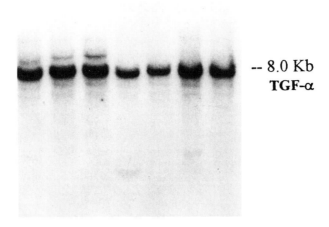

-- 8.0 Kb
TGF-α

Fig. 5. Southern blot analysis of transforming growth factor (TGFα). DNA was isolated from cultures of rat liver epithelial cells. Ten-microgram DNA samples were digested with the restriction enzyme *Bam*HI for 18 h at 37°C. The digested DNA was subjected to Southern blot analysis as described in Table 1. The ^{32}P-labeled probe was generated by random primer extension, utilizing a 1.8-kb fragment of the rat TGFα gene. The membrane was hybridized, washed, and exposed to X-ray film for 48 h. When rat liver epithelial cell DNA is digested with *Bam*HI, the TGFα gene is cut into an 8.0-kb fragment, which hybridizes to the radiolabeled probe and appears as a dark band in the 8.0-kb range on the autoradiograph.

4. INTERPRETATION OF THE SOUTHERN BLOT

Once the membrane that contains the target DNA sequences has been "probed" with a specific labeled probe, the results of the Southern analysis can be interpreted. Positive signals on the membrane are created when the labeled probe binds to complementary target DNA sequences, producing a band that can be visualized. If nonradioactive, colorimetric probing techniques were used, the bands will be visible to the naked eye. Chemiluminescent and radioactive probes must be visualized by exposing the hybridized membrane to X-ray film, producing an autoradiograph. Fig. 5 shows an autoradiograph generated by hybridization with a ^{32}P-labeled radioactive probe.

The autoradiographs that are produced are easily analyzed by a scanning densitometer—an instrument that provides a measure of the relative density of the bands that are present on the X-ray film. The end result is a numerical value which can be used to determine the relative number of target sequences present in one sample compared to another. For example, the relative density of a band produced by hybridization with a gene whose copy number has been amplified will be much higher than the relative density of the band corresponding to the normal gene copy number. Membranes that have been hybridized with radioactive probes may also be analyzed directly in a phosphorimager. This instrument provides a very accurate evaluation of the blot by measuring the amount of radioactive emission corresponding to each band on the membrane, generating a value expressed in counts per minute. The scanning densitometer and phosphorimager enable the user to evaluate the positive signals on a blot with concrete numerical data instead of guesswork.

Proper interpretation of Southern blots necessitates the use of controls throughout the procedure. In order to compare gene copy number between one sample and another, it is imperative that the same quantity of DNA be loaded onto the gel. This can be assured by carefully measuring the DNA concentration prior to loading and by evaluating the relative concentrations of DNA on the electrophoresed gel by staining with ethidium bromide. When analyzing patient samples that are suspected to be abnormal (i.e., gene deletion, rearrangement, or amplification), one should include DNA that is known to be normal for comparison.

5. TROUBLESHOOTING SOUTHERN BLOTS

There are several problems which may occur that will result in the failure of a signal to appear on the final blot. To help eliminate possibilities, consult this checklist:

Was enough DNA loaded onto the gel (10 µg)?
Was the DNA digested thoroughly prior to electrophoresis?
Was the electrophoresed DNA denatured and neutralized before transfer?
Was transfer complete? (Stain the gel after transfer to check for remaining DNA.)
Was the DNA properly immobilized onto the nitrocellulose or nylon membrane?
Was the DNA intact? (Has the membrane been probed and stripped multiple times?)
Was the probe prepared properly?
Was the hybridization time sufficient (overnight)?
Was the blot exposed to film for a sufficient amount of time?
Was the probe labeled sufficiently?

If the answer to all of the above questions is "yes," then the failure of a positive signal to appear could be related to the strength with which the probe hybridized to the target sequences on the membrane. If the probe is from a species other than the test DNA, weak hybridization may be the result of a lack of homology between the probe and the target gene sequence. A very weak signal can often be strengthened by decreasing the stringency of the posthybridization washes and/or increasing the length of exposure time while generating the autoradiograph. Alternatively, it may be necessary to try a different probe or a different probe-labeling technique.

High background on the final blot is usually indicative of insufficient blocking during the prehybridization and hybridization steps, or poor washing of the blot after hybridization. To eliminate the background, simply increase the amount of denatured salmon sperm DNA added to the prehybridization and hybridization solutions, and/or increase the stringency of the posthybridization washes by decreasing salt concentration or increasing temperature. When RNA probes (riboprobes) are utilized, the temperature of hybridization washes may need to be as high as 65°C to eliminate background hybridization.

6. THE NORTHERN BLOT

The northern blot allows identification of specific messenger RNA sequences within a mixture of RNA molecules. The final signal achieved on the blot is proportional to the number of specific sequences present, allowing for a quantitative analysis of gene expression. The RNA transcripts produced from a particular gene can vary in size owing to such phenomena as:

1. Utilization of a secondary transcription start site by RNA polymerase;
2. Premature termination of transcription resulting from nonsense mutation;

3. Posttranscriptional modifications, such as splicing; and
4. Deletions within the gene coding sequence.

These alternative transcripts can be detected by northern blot analysis. This information is routinely used to determine if the expression of a specific gene is altered in any way. Aberrations in gene expression are frequently studied in the laboratory to evaluate the cellular response to a particular stimulus or treatment at the molecular biology level. Because abnormal expression of specific genes is often reliably associated with certain disease states, the northern blot can also be a valuable tool for diagnosis/prognosis in the clinical setting.

7. GENERAL CONSIDERATIONS IN THE ANALYSIS OF RNA

7.1. The Importance of an RNase-Free Environment

Successful northern blot analysis requires a preparation of RNA that is intact and relatively free from contaminants, such as protein and DNA. When working with RNA, it is also imperative to maintain an environment that is free of RNases (ubiquitous enzymes that degrade RNA). This can be accomplished by treating deionized water and solutions that contact the RNA with 0.1% diethylpyrocarbonate for 24 h at 37°C prior to autoclaving *(4,11)*. Solutions containing Tris (tris[hydroxymethyl]aminomethane) cannot be treated with diethylpyrocarbonate. Therefore it is recommended to reserve a bottle of Tris that is used only for RNA work and is handled appropriately. Sterile, RNase-free tubes and pipet tips should be used at all times, and glassware should be baked or rinsed with chloroform to eliminate RNases *(4)*. Wash solutions are commercially available that destroy RNases and may be useful in cleaning glassware and work stations (*RNaseAWAY,* Gibco-BRL; *RNaseZAP,* Invitrogen [San Diego, CA]). The abundance of RNases in skin necessitates the use of gloves by personnel handling RNA samples, solutions, and labware.

7.2. Total Cellular RNA vs Messenger RNA

There are many variables to take into consideration when determining whether to analyze total cellular RNA or purified messenger RNA. The specificity and efficiency of the specific probe and the level of expression of the target gene contribute to the strength of the final signal observed on a northern blot. In a preparation of total cellular RNA, only about 2.5% is actually mRNA—the majority is composed of rRNA. The quantity of RNA that can be subjected to Northern analysis is limited to approx 30 µg by technical limitations related to the capacity of hybridization membranes for RNA binding. Therefore, detection of rare mRNAs frequently requires utilization of purified mRNA. There are many commercially available kits for purification of mRNA (Pharmacia Biotech [Uppsala, Sweden], Gibco-BRL, Promega [Madison, WI]), all of which take advantage of the polyadenylation signal on the 3'-end of mRNAs. The basic principle involves selection of the mRNA by binding the sequential adenosine residues to a synthesized stretch of deoxythymidine residues that have been affixed to a solid support (such as cellulose or magnetic beads). The unbound ribosomal RNA and other contaminants are washed away, and the mRNA is then eluted from the support matrix. Even rare mRNAs can be detected when as little as 1 µg of purified mRNA is subjected to northern analysis.

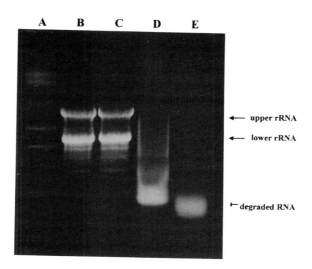

Fig. 6. RNA integrity gel. RNA was isolated from cultured rat liver epithelial cells by the acidic phenol extraction method *(21)*. Two micrograms of RNA per sample were run on an integrity gel for 2 h at 90 V. Lane **A** contains an RNA molecular size standard. Lanes **B** and **C** contain intact RNA (rRNA bands are clearly visible), whereas the samples in lanes **D** and **E** are degraded. The RNA in lane D was prepared in a small volume of tap water (instead of RNase-treated water) and the RNA in lane E came in contact with human skin during sample preparation.

8. METHODOLOGY OF NORTHERN BLOT ANALYSIS

8.1. Preparation of the RNA for Electrophoresis

The method of choice for RNA isolation in many labs is centrifugation through a cesium chloride cushion, followed by ethanol precipitation *(20)*. This method efficiently generates RNA of exceptional quality for northern blotting. However, alternative methods are available that address limitations of some investigators with respect to instrumentation. The acidic phenol extraction method described by Chomczynski *(21)* yields total cellular RNA of acceptable quality for northern blot analysis, can be performed in less time than a cesium chloride gradient, and does not require an ultracentrifuge. Commercial kits are available for the isolation of RNA (Gibco-BRL, Promega), most of which are based on variations of the acidic phenol extraction.

Regardless of the method utilized to generate total cellular RNA, it is advisable to check the quantity and quality of the samples by taking spectrophotometer readings at 260 and 280 nm and running a small aliquot (1 μg) through a 1.0% agarose integrity gel containing 0.5 μg/mL ethidium bromide. The ratio of the absorbance at 260 nm/280 nm is 1.8–2.0 in a clean RNA sample. Ratios <1.8 indicate contamination with protein or phenol. Visualization of the integrity gel with a UV light source is the best measure of RNA quality (*see* Fig. 6). DNA contaminants are revealed as very high-mol-wt bands that sometimes fail to migrate into the gel. Degraded RNA is identified as a smear in the very low-mol-wt range. When total cellular RNA is analyzed, 18S and 28S rRNA bands should be clearly visible, and a faint smear representing the heterogeneous mRNA population should be present as well. The eukaryotic 28S and 18S rRNAs are 5.0 and 1.87 kb in size, respectively *(5)*, and can serve as a convenient internal RNA size standard.

8.2. Electrophoretic Separation of RNA

A protocol for northern blot analysis is provided in Table 3. When analyzing total cellular RNA, the quantity of RNA loaded onto the gel can range from 5–30 μg. The ideal concentration should be determined empirically, and depends on the quantity and quality of target mRNA as well as specificity of the probe. Analysis of purified mRNA can be performed with as little as 1.0 μg, although a greater quantity (5–10 μg) is typically used to permit multiple uses of a single membrane. Just prior to electrophoresis, the single-stranded native RNA molecules must be denatured to abolish secondary structure (*see* Table 2). This is accomplished by heating the samples to 65°C in the presence of formaldehyde and formamide. The denatured state is maintained during electrophoresis by the addition of formaldehyde to the agarose gel *(22)*. Denaturation of RNA with glyoxal was introduced in 1977 as an alternative to formaldehyde denaturation *(23)*; Although glyoxal denaturation works well, additional steps are required to remove the glyoxal products after blotting. The standard RNA gel (1.2% agarose, 1.1% formaldehyde) allows separation of RNA from 0.5–6.0 kbp. It is advisable to run RNA mol-wt standards on every gel to aid in determining the mol-wt of bands present. Since RNA and DNA do not migrate at the same rate, DNA standards are not acceptable for RNA gels. RNA standards are commercially available in several size ranges (Amersham, Gibco-BRL). The addition of ethidium bromide to RNA gels is controversial. Although visualization of the RNA provides information on integrity and quantity, experimental evidence suggests that the subsequent transfer of RNA to nitrocellulose or nylon is impeded when ethidium bromide is present, resulting in a 12–18% decrease in final hybridization signal *(11,24)*. For this reason, many researchers remove and stain only the lane containing the RNA standards. However, the valuable information obtained from visualization of the RNA often outweighs the inconvenience of a reduced signal. Acridine orange *(23)* and Stains All (a cationic carbocyanine dye) *(25)* are alternative dye choices for staining and visualizing the RNA.

The recommended buffer for electrophoresis of RNA contains 3-(*N*-morpholino) propanesulfonic acid (or MOPS) *(4)*. A 5 or 10X stock of MOPS buffer (*see* Table 2) should be prepared in diethylpyrocarbonate treated water, brought to pH 7.0, filter-sterilized, and stored at room temperature in a dark bottle. Autoclaving or exposure to light can cause yellowing of the buffer. Although pale yellow buffer may still be used, buffer exhibiting a darker shade of yellow should not be used. Constant circulation of buffer during electrophoresis in the same direction as electrical flow prevents accumulation of buffer components and formaldehyde in the positive buffer chamber. The general rule for running RNA gels is 3–4 V/cm. The bromophenol blue (in the RNA sample buffer) should migrate at least 8 cm before electrophoresis is terminated. Because there is no reliable storage method for electrophoresed RNA gels, it is optimal to transfer the nucleic acids to a solid support immediately after electrophoresis. For this reason, many workers choose to run gels overnight at a low voltage (20–30 V).

If ethidium bromide is not included in the gel, the lane containing RNA standards must be excised and stained. The distance from the loading well to each band should be measured to generate a standard curve. A plot of the $\log_{10}$ of the RNA fragment sizes against distance migrated provides a curve by which sizes of RNA species detected by hybridization can be calculated. Prior to transfer of the RNA to a nitrocellulose or

Table 3
Northern Blot Analysis

1. Preparation of RNA samples:
   a. Combine an appropriate quantity of purified total RNA or mRNA with 2.0 μL 5X MOPS buffer, 3.5 mL 37% formaldehyde, pH > 4.0, 10.0 μL formamide, and RNase-free water to give a total vol of 20 ml.
   b. Add 4.0 μL of RNA loading dye (Table 2) and heat samples to 65°C for 10 min. Open the caps for 5–10 min prior to loading the samples to allow traces of ethanol to evaporate.
2. Preparation of the formaldehyde gel:
   a. Melt agarose (final concentration should be 1.2%) in RNase-free water by boiling in a microwave. Cool to 60°C, add 5X MOPS gel buffer (one-fifth final volume) and 37% formaldehyde (1/5.6 final volume). If desired, ethidium bromide may be added to the gel (0.5 μg/mL).
   b. Pour gel immediately into clean, level gel tray and insert the appropriate sample comb(s).
   c. When the gel has solidified (~20 min), place it in the electrophoresis tank, remove the sample comb, and fill the tank with 1X MOPS buffer until the liquid covers the gel by 3–4 mm. Prerun the gel for 5 min at 5 V/cm length.
3. Running the gel:
   a. Load the RNA samples carefully into the sample wells. Reserve one well for loading appropriate RNA size standards (1–3 μg are usually sufficient). If the samples "float" out of the well as they are loaded, they may still contain traces of ethanol. Reheating the samples briefly (uncapped) will eliminate this problem.
   b. The gel may be run overnight at 20–30 V, or at 3–4 V/cm length. Electrophoresis should continue until the bromophenol blue tracking dye has migrated a minimum of 8.0 cm.
   c. Once the samples have entered the gel (~20 min), begin circulating the buffer with a peristaltic pump in the same direction as the electrical flow.
   d. When electrophoresis is complete, record the migration distances of the RNA ladder (if ethidium bromide was not added to the gel, this lane should be cut away and stained in a 2 μg/mL solution of ethidium bromide). If ethidium bromide was added to the gel, the entire gel should be visualized with a UV light source and photographed. Remove the lane containing the RNA standards prior to transfer.
4. Capillary transfer of the RNA to a nylon membrane:
   a. Cut a piece of nylon membrane to the size of the gel and prewet it in RNase-free water. Equilibrate the membrane in 20X SSPE transfer buffer for at least 15 min.
   b. Remove formaldehyde from the gel by soaking 3 × 10 min in RNase-free water.
   c. Assemble the transfer setup as shown in Fig. 3 and allow the RNA to transfer for 12–18 h.
   d. Air-dry the nylon membrane briefly and then crosslink with UV irradiation.
5. Hybridization with nucleic acid probe:
   a. Prehybridize the filter for at least 1 h at 42°C in 10–20 mL of prehybridization solution.
   b. Prepare labeled probe as per manufacturer's instructions.
   c. Replace prehybridization solution with hybridization solution containing the labeled probe and incubate 12–14 h at 42°C.
6. Washing the hybridized filter:
   a. Wash the filter 2 × 15 min in 2X SSPE, 0.1% SDS at 42°C, and then 2 × 15 min in 1X SSPE, 0.1% SDS at 42°C.
   b. If a radioactive probe was used, check the filter with a Geiger counter. If additional washing is needed, wash 2 × 15 min in 0.5X SSPE, 0.1% SDS at 42°C.
7. Visualization of hybridized probe (radiolabeled probes): Wick excess buffer from the washed filter and then wrap the filter in plastic wrap; expose the membrane to film in a light-tight cassette at −70°C. Develop the autoradiograph after 24 h, adjusting the exposure time as needed.

nylon membrane, the formaldehyde should be removed from the gel. This is typically accomplished by soaking the gel in several changes of diethylpyrocarbonate-treated water or transfer buffer.

8.3. Transfer of RNA to a Solid Support

For optimal results, the electrophoresed RNA should be transferred to a nylon membrane. The methods of transfer (capillary, vacuum, and electrophoretic) are the same as for DNA transfer and are discussed in previous sections. Since the RNA molecules are already single-stranded, there is no need to denature the gel prior to transfer. However, both the gel and the nylon membrane should be equilibrated in the appropriate transfer buffer (*see* Table 2) prior to transfer. Traditional capillary transfer works well for most northern blots, although complete transfer takes 12–18 h (*see* Fig. 3). When time is limited, the downward alkaline transfer or vacuum transfer method may be used. Electrophoretic transfer is ideal when time is limited and when the target mRNA is present in a very low quantity. When fixing a northern blot, experimental evidence indicates that fixation by UV irradiation is superior to baking at 80°C *(19)*. As with DNA, overirradiation can cause extensive crosslinking of the RNA and diminish the final signal, so optimal UV exposure should be determined empirically. Irradiated, air-dried membranes may be stored at room temperature until they are ready to be hybridized to a nucleic acid probe.

8.4. Interpretation of the Northern Blot

When analyzing any experimental sample by northern blot, it is recommended to include a control on the gel consisting of RNA isolated from appropriate normal cells or tissue. Interpretation of a northern blot is most accurate when actual numerical values are assigned to the bands present on the final blot, which represent a positive signal. Colorimetric detection methods are the least sensitive, and should be avoided if comparisons are to be made between two test samples, in which differences in expression may be subtle. Both chemiluminescent and radioactive probes can be exposed to X-ray film to produce an autoradiograph. Figure 7 shows an autoradiograph generated from a northern blot that was probed with a ^{32}P-labeled cDNA probe. The autoradiograph can be analyzed by a scanning densitometer, which measures the density of each band and assigns a numerical value to the band. This analysis allows the detection of very small variations in expression. However, for interpretation to be accurate, a control must be included for the amount of mRNA that is present in the samples being compared. Some researchers rely on ethidium bromide staining of the gel prior to transfer and hybridization. However, visualization of the mRNA in formaldehyde-containing gels is difficult and not quantitative. A more reliable method is to perform a second hybridization reaction with the membrane, utilizing a probe (labeled in the same way as the probe used to detect the gene of interest) for a "housekeeping gene," such as actin (a structural protein) or cyclophilin (cyclosporin binding protein). Numerical values are then generated for the positive signal from the housekeeping gene via scanning densitometry. The expression of the gene of interest is then expressed as a function of the expression of the housekeeping gene, thereby "normalizing" each signal relative to the actual quantity of mRNA present in that particular lane of the gel. If radiolabeled probes are used, the blots may be analyzed directly in a phosphorimager, which detects positive signals on the blot and expresses the value as actual counts per minute of

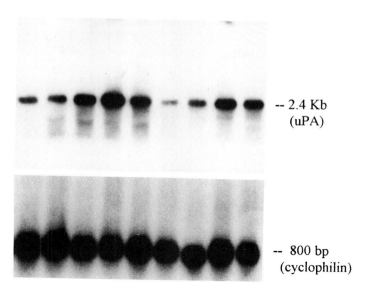

-- 2.4 Kb
(uPA)

-- 800 bp
(cyclophilin)

Fig. 7. Northern blot analysis of the urokinase plasminogen activator mRNA. RNA was isolated from nine different rat liver epithelial cell lines by acidic phenol extraction *(21)* and mRNA was subsequently purified by binding to oligo-dT. Two-microgram samples of mRNA from each cell line were subjected to northern blot analysis as described in Table 3. The radio-labeled probes were generated by random primer extension utilizing a 1.5-kb fragment of the urokinase plasminogen activator (uPA) gene and a 1.2-kb fragment of the cyclophilin gene. The blot was first probed with the probe for uPA and an autoradiograph was generated. Then the membrane was stripped in a solution containing 50% formamide and 2X SSPE and reprobed for the cyclophilin mRNA. Although the expression of the "housekeeping" gene (cyclophilin) remains relatively constant among the samples, the expression of the 2.4-kb uPA mRNA varies greatly among this group of cell lines.

radioactivity. This instrument is particularly useful in detecting very weak positive signals and can often shorten the time required to detect positive bands compared to generating traditional autoradiographs.

9. TROUBLESHOOTING NORTHERN BLOTS

Some genes are simply not expressed at any level in certain situations. However, if a known positive control was included on the gel and no positive signal was produced, there could be a technical problem. Consult the following checklist to eliminate some possibilities:

Was the RNA of good quality (integrity gel, ethidium bromide staining)?
Was electrophoresis of the RNA sufficient (migration of RNA bp ladder)?
Was the RNA transferred to the nylon membrane (stain the gel after transfer)?
Was the probe labeled properly?
Was hybridization time sufficient (overnight)?
Was the blot washed too stringently?

If no technical problems can be identified, the best solution is to reprobe the blot with a probe for a housekeeping gene that is known to be expressed. If no signal is present, the RNA may have been degraded or of too small a quantity to be effective.

High background signal may be reduced by increasing the amount of blocking agent (denatured salmon sperm DNA) in the prehybridization and hybridization reactions. However, background hybridization is frequently owing to insufficient washing of the blot after hybridization. Washing should be carried out in generous volumes (at least threefold volume of hybridization solution), and increasing the stringency of the wash (increasing temperature and/or decreasing salt concentration) will reduce background signal. A washing routine that works well for one probe may be insufficient for another, so optimal washing conditions must be determined separately for each probe used.

Sometimes a positive band on a northern blot creates a great deal of excitement until it is found to be the wrong size. Such occurrences lend a lot of support to the use of mol-wt standards, such as the RNA base-pair ladders, to prevent misinterpretation of data. If pure mRNA has been used and an unexpected band appears, it is possible that an alternative transcript has been identified. When mRNA is not pure (as when total cellular RNA is analyzed), nonspecific binding of probe to the rRNAs can be observed. For this reason, one should take great care in interpreting northern blots when rRNA is present. Any bands that appear at 5.0 or 1.87 kb may be attributed to binding of the probe to rRNA rather than hybridization with true target sequences. In situations in which these problems arise, it is advisable to repeat the blot utilizing highly purified mRNA.

10. PREPARATION OF LABELED NUCLEIC ACID PROBES

Once nucleic acids have been affixed to a membrane, specific sequences can be detected by hybridization with a labeled, denatured, single-stranded probe that binds to homologous RNA or DNA. These probes may be composed of either RNA or DNA, and labeling methods may be radioactive or nonradioactive.

10.1. Nick Translation

The method of nick translation relies on *Escherichia coli* DNA Polymerase I—a polymerizing enzyme that also possesses a 5' → 3' exonuclease activity that degrades double-stranded DNA and RNA:DNA hybrids *(26)*. First, discontinuities ("nicks") are generated in the phosphodiester backbone of the double-stranded DNA by brief treatment with pancreatic DNase I, producing free 3'-hydroxyl termini along the strand of DNA. DNA polymerase I then extends the 3'-OH termini in the presence of the four dNTPs, utilizing its exonuclease activity to hydrolyze nucleotides in the 5' → 3' direction *(see* Fig. 8). The use of radioactive nucleoside triphosphates in the reaction with DNA polymerase I produces uniformly labeled DNA. Disadvantages of nick translation include the strict requirements in the protocol to time and temperature limitations, and the large amount of template DNA (0.5 µg) required per reaction. It is also important to note that small DNA fragments (<200 bp) are not suitable for nick translation. Nick translation kits are commercially available and provide a reliable source for the buffers and enzymes to carry out the reaction (Promega, Amersham, Gibco-BRL). Most protocols recommend separating radiolabeled DNA from unincorporated dNTPs by centrifugation through a small column of Sephadex G-50 *(4,27)*.

10.2. Random Primer Extension

An alternative method for generating labeled DNA involves the utilization of oligonucleotide primers of random sequence *(26)*. The double-stranded DNA is denatured

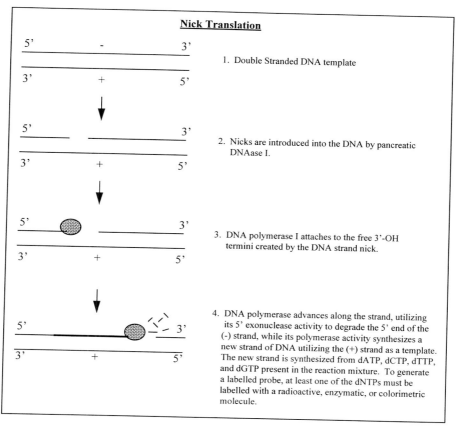

Fig. 8. Preparation of DNA probes by nick translation.

and random nanomers or hexamers are annealed to the template DNA strands (*see* Fig. 9). The primers are extended by the large fragment of DNA polymerase (Klenow fragment) or T7 DNA polymerase in the presence of radiolabeled dNTPs. Random-primed probes can be labeled to a higher specific activity than nick-translated probes, although they are typically shorter (~500 nucleotides). The reaction can also be carried out at room temperature with small quantities of template DNA (25–50 ng), and is not significantly affected by longer incubation times (overnight). This method may also be used to label small fragments (200 bp). Random primer extension kits are available commercially and provide the user with enzyme, cold dNTPs, and reaction buffers (Gibco-BRL, Amersham, Boehringer-Mannheim, [Indianapolis, IN]). Because the majority of radioactive dNTP is incorporated into DNA, purification of the probe is not usually necessary. However, if purification is needed, centrifugation through Sephadex G-50 is sufficient.

10.3. Generation of Strand-Specific Probes

The generation of radiolabeled probes from double-stranded DNA works well when the target sequences are present in sufficient quantity and the hybridization between the labeled DNA probe and target sequences is strong. When hybridization between probe and target is weak, hybrids form between the complementary DNA sequences of

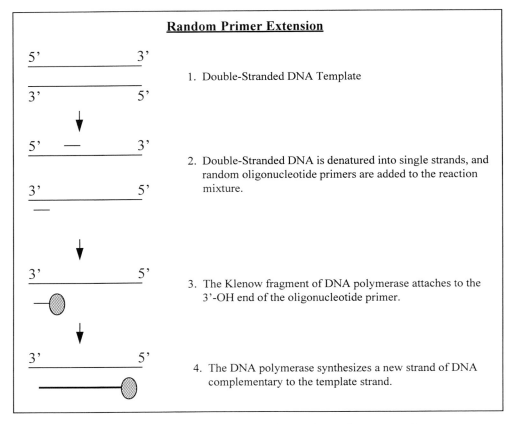

Fig. 9. Preparation of DNA probes by random primer extension.

the probe, resulting in segregation of the probe and decreased detection of target sequences. Single-stranded probes are composed of only one of two strands of a nucleic acid sequence, thus allowing detection of target sequences without unwanted reannealing of probe. These probes are particularly useful when analyzing target sequences that are only partially homologous to the probe (such as the detection of homologous genes in multiple species).

Radiolabeled cDNA probes are generated by primer extension of single-stranded DNA derived from a recombinant bacteriophage M13, and can yield probes of extremely high specific activity (1×10^9 cpm/µg) *(26)*. Primers are commonly chosen that anneal to the single-stranded viral DNA in a region upstream from the site of insertion. Extension of the annealed primers is typically accomplished with the Klenow fragment of DNA polymerase I in the presence of three nonradioactive dNTPs and one α-^{32}P-labeled dNTP. The major drawback of this method is the required separation of labeled probe from the template and smaller DNA fragments. Labeled probes can be separated by polyacrylamide gel electrophoresis, or by alkaline chromatography through Sepharose CL-4B (Pharmacia Biotech) *(27)*.

The ability to generate single-stranded RNA probes ("riboprobes") has been made possible by the development of plasmid vectors, which contain multiple cloning sites

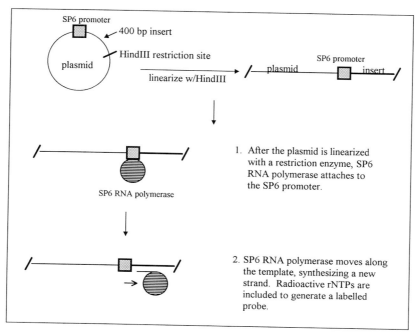

Fig. 10. Generation of riboprobes.

downstream from strong bacteriophage promoters (SP6, T7, and T3) *(28–30)*. These promoters are recognized by bacteriophage-specific, DNA-dependent RNA polymerases, which fail to recognize bacterial, plasmid or eukaryotic promoters that are present within the construct *(29)*. As a result, labeled RNA can be synthesized directly from these linearized plasmids at an extremely high efficiency and specific activity when radioactive NTPs are included in the reaction (*see* Fig. 10). The greater stability of RNA hybrids makes RNA probes superior to double-stranded and single-stranded DNA probes in Southern and northern analysis. In addition, the production of radiolabeled RNA is more efficient than generation of single-stranded cDNA probes, since unwanted template DNA can be eliminated by a simply treating the samples with RNase-free DNase I. When these RNA probes are to be applied to northern blots, it is important to generate the probe in the "antisense" direction, so that the probe is complementary and not identical to the mRNA of interest.

10.4. Generation of Nonradioactive Probes

Environmental concerns, cost, and safety are a few reasons that nonradioactive alternatives to ^{32}P-labeled probes are becoming more popular. Another advantage to nonradioactive probes is their long half-life, which permits them to be stored for extended periods of time. Several vendors provide kits for nonradioactive labeling and detection of probes, all of which employ the same basic concepts. Probes can be labeled by the traditional enzymatic methods (described above for radioactive probes), with the incorporation of alternatively labeled dNTPs or NTPs. Nonradioactive probes are typically labeled with haptens (such as digoxigenin), biotin, or fluorescein *(31–34)*. Detection of the hybridization signal depends on the type of label used, but is either colorimetric or chemiluminescent.

Biotin-labeled probes are usually detected by enzyme-conjugated streptavidin, and hapten-labeled probes are detected by enzyme-conjugated antihapten antibodies. The conjugated enzymatic activity (horseradish peroxidase or alkaline phosphatase) results in the production of a colored precipitate in the presence of a specific chemical substrate *(34)*, which allows direct visualization of hybridized bands on the membrane. However, colorimetric detection has several disadvantages that must be considered. Detection of rare sequences is limited and often requires long development times (>15 h). Furthermore, the colored precipitate cannot be efficiently removed from the membrane, thus preventing multiple uses of a single blot.

Chemiluminescent detection relies on the association of an enzyme-conjugated antibody with the digoxigenin, biotin, or fluorescein moieties of labeled probes. The reporter enzyme (horseradish peroxidase or alkaline phosphatase) dephosphorylates a chemiluminescent substrate, thus generating an unstable anion that emits light as it decomposes *(35)*. Positive signals are visualized by exposing the blot to X-ray film for short lengths of time. Chemiluminescence does not produce a precipitate, which allows blots to be stripped and reprobed by standard methods. Chemiluminescent detection is sufficiently sensitive for most applications and is currently the most accepted alternative to radioactive probes. The major drawback to chemiluminescent detection is the frequent observation of high background activity. However, strict adherence to the blocking steps provided in most protocols can significantly reduce background signal.

11. HYBRIDIZATION WITH LABELED PROBES

11.1. Factors Influencing Hybridization

The kinetics of nucleic acid hybridization rely heavily on such parameters as temperature, salt concentration, solvent concentration, and the relative strength of nucleic acid hybrids (RNA:RNA > RNA:DNA > DNA:DNA) *(4)*. Blots are typically prehybridized (at the hybridization temperature) in a solution that reduces nonspecific binding of labeled DNA during hybridization. The prehybridization solution is then replaced with hybridization solution, which contains the labeled probe. Composition of prehybridization and hybridization solutions can vary depending on the protocol and subsequent detection method. Two commonly used formulations are presented in Table 2. The temperature of hybridization largely determines the specificity of the signal obtained in northern and Southern analysis (high temperatures increase stringency). Many protocols recommend the use of formamide-based prehybridization and hybridization solutions to lower the required hybridization temperature without compromising stringency. Hybridization can be carried out in sealed plastic bags, although commercially available hybridization ovens are recommended as a safe and reliable alternative. Some protocols recommend the use of high-molecular-mass polyethylene glycol or dextran sulfate in the hybridization solution to concentrate the probe and enhance the final signal *(4,5)*.

11.2. Washing and Visualization of Nucleic Acid Blots

After hybridization, nonspecifically bound probe is removed by sequential washes with buffer (*see* Tables 1 and 3). The temperature and composition of the wash buffer have an effect on the specificity of the signal obtained. Higher temperatures and/or lower salt concentrations increase the stringency of the wash and remove probe that is not strongly hybridized to complementary sequences. When radioactive probes are utilized, the washing process can be easily monitored with a Geiger counter. Visualization of hybridized radiolabeled probes is accomplished by exposing the membrane to X-ray film. The use of tungstate-based intensifying screens can intensify a positive signal tenfold when applied at −70°C.

11.3. Removal of Bound Probes from Nucleic Acid Blots

If nitrocellulose or nylon membranes do not dry out during the blotting process, they may be stripped and reprobed. Probes can be removed from nitrocellulose by immersing the membrane in hot elution buffer *(4)* (*see* Table 2). Stripping of nylon membranes (DNA or RNA) can be accomplished using one of the following:

1. Immersion of the filter in 1 m*M* Tris-HCl, 1 m*M* EDTA, and 0.1X Denhardt's reagent for 2 h at 75°C;
2. Immersion of the membrane in a formamide-based stripping solution containing 2X SSPE and 50% formamide for one h at 65°C; or
3. By pouring boiling water over the membrane and letting it stand for 5–10 min.

Probes can also be removed from DNA blots by alkaline treatment with sodium hydroxide at 42°C, followed by neutralization in Tris buffer at 42°C *(5)*. Once the probe is removed, the hybridization membrane should air-dried briefly and sealed in a plastic bag. Sealed blots can be stored at 4°C for extended periods of time without deterioration.

12. SUMMARY

Nucleic acid blotting yields valuable information in both the research and clinical settings. More than 500 human genetic diseases are attributed to single-gene defects. For example, sickle-cell anemia is causes by a simple point mutation in the gene that codes for the β chain of hemoglobin *(36)*. By employing short oligonucleotide probes for mutant and normal gene sequences, it is possible to distinguish between the two forms of the gene by Southern blot analysis *(37)*. Pathological gene alterations can also be detected in diseases, such as Burkitt's lymphoma, Fragile X syndrome, familial hypercholesterolemia, the hemophilias, and inborn errors of metabolism *(38,39)*. The Southern blot provides a means of identifying a specific altered gene, thus allowing prenatal detection of many genetic diseases, many of which can be corrected by simply administering the functional protein that should be encoded by the defective gene. The northern blot provides information on gene expression that may be useful in establishing prognosis in diseases, such as colon cancer *(40)*. During embryonic development, large numbers of genes are switched "on" and "off" in elaborate, defined patterns. This is often true for the process of carcinogenesis as well, in which the expression patterns of specific genes become altered, contributing to the formation of a tumor. Northern blotting allows the expression of a specific gene to be examined so that one can determine if the gene of interest is underexpressed or overexpressed compared to normal. Experimental evidence supports the idea that carcinogenesis is the result of the loss of a cell or group of cells to control their growth. Such a phenomenon may be the result of overproduction of a growth-stimulatory factor, underproduction of a growth inhibitor, or altered production of cell-cycle regulatory molecules.

Nucleic acid blotting permits detailed characterization of a specific gene. Southern blots identify structural abnormalities, whereas northern blots show gene expression levels and allow detection of alternatively spliced transcripts. With modern improvements (such as nonradioactive probing techniques), nucleic acid blotting will remain a valuable tool in many molecular biology laboratories.

REFERENCES

1. Southern, E. M. Detection of specific sequences among DNA fragments separated by gel electrophoresis. *J. Mol. Biol.* **98**:503–517, 1975.
2. Stark, G. R. and Wahl, G. M. Gene amplification. *Ann. Rev. Biochem.* **53**:447–491, 1984.
3. Ruiz, J. C., Choi, K., Vontloff, D. D., Runinson, I. B., and Wahl, G. M. Autonomously replicating episomes contain mdr1 genes in a multidrug-resistant cell line. *Mol. Cell. Biol.* **9**:109–115, 1989.
4. Sambrook, J., Fritsch, E. F., and Maniatis, T., eds. *Molecular Cloning: A Laboratory Manual.* Cold Spring Harbor Laboratory, Cold Spring Harbor, NY, 1992.
5. Kroczek, R. A. Southern and northern analysis. *J. Chromator.* **618**:133–145, 1993.
6. Bostian, K. A., Lee, R. C., and Halvorson, H. O. Preparative fractionation of nucleic acids by agarose gel electrophoresis. *Anal. Biochem.* **95**:174–182, 1979.
7. Knowland, J. S. Polyacrylamide gel electrophoresis of nucleic acids synthesized during early development of *Xenopus laevis* daudin. *Biochem. Biophys. Acta* **204**:416–429, 1970.
8. Preat, T. High resolution southern analysis of genomic DNA using heat denatured acrylamide gels. *Nucleic Acids Res.* **18**:1073–1076, 1990.
9. Vesterburg, O. A short history of electrophoretic methods. *Electrophoresis* **14**:1243–1249, 1993.
10. Burmeister, M. and Ulanovsky, L. *Pulsed-Field Gel Electrophoresis.* Humana, Totowa, NJ, 1992.
11. Van Oss, C. J., Good, R. J., and Chaudhury, M. K. Mechanism of DNA (Southern) and protein (Western) blotting on cellulose nitrate and other membranes. *J. Chromator.* **391**:53–65, 1987.
12. Wahl, G. M., Stern, M., and Stark, G. R. Efficient transfer of large DNA fragments from agarose gels to diazobenzyloxymethyl paper and rapid hybridization by using dextran sulphate. *Proc. Natl. Acad. Sci. USA* **76**:3683–3687, 1987.
13. Chomczynski, P. One hour downward alkaline capillary transfer for blotting of DNA and RNA. *Anal. Biochem.* **201**:134–139, 1992.
14. Zhou, M. Y., Di, X., Gomez-Sanchez, P., and Gomez-Sanchez, E. Improved downward capillary transfer for blotting of DNA and RNA. *Biotechniques* **16**:58,59, 1994.
15. Smith, M. R., Devine, C. S., Cohn, S. M., and Liebermar, M. W. Quantitative electrophoretic transfer of DNA from polyacrylamide or agarose gels to nitrocellulose. *Anal. Biochem.* **137**:120–124, 1984.
16. Kroczek, R. A. and Siebert, E. Optimization of Northern analysis by vacuum blotting, RNA-transfer visualization, and ultraviolet fixation. *Anal. Biochem.* **184**:90–95, 1990.
17. Stacey, J. and Isaac, P. G. Restriction enzyme digestion, gel electrophoresis, and vacuum blotting of DNA to nylon membranes. *Methods Mol. Biol.* **28**:25–36, 1994.
18. Olszewska, E. and Jones, K. Vacuum blotting enhances nucleic acid transfer. *Trends Genet.* **4**:92–94, 1988.
19. Khandjian, E. W. UV crosslinking of RNA to nylon membrane enhances hybridization signals. *Mol. Biol. Rep.* **11**:107–115, 1986.
20. Kornguth, S. E., Anderson J. W., Scott, G., and Kubinski, H. Fractionation of subcellular elements from rat central nervous tissue in a cesium chloride gradient. *Exp. Cell Res.* **45**:656–670, 1967.

21. Chomczynski, P. and Sacchi, N. Single-step method of RNA isolation by acid guanidinium thiocyanate-phenol-chloroform extraction. *Anal. Biochem.* **162:**156–159, 1987
22. Lehrach H., Diamond, D., Wozney, J. M., Boedtker, H. RNA molecular weight determinations by gel electrophoresis under denaturing conditions, a critical reexamination. *Biochemistry* **16:**4743–4749, 1977.
23. McMaster, G. K. and Carmichael, G. G. Analysis of single and double-strand nucleic acids on polyacrylamide and agarose gels by using glyoxal and acridine orange. *Proc. Natl. Acad. Sci. USA* **74:**4835–4838, 1977.
24. Kroczek, R. A. Immediate visualization of blotted RNA in northern analysis. *Nucleic Acids Res.* **17:**9497–9499, 1989.
25. Wade, M. F. and O'Conner, J. L. Using a cationic carbocyanine dye to assess RNA loading in northern gel analysis. *Biotechniques* **12:**794–796, 1992.
26. Kaguni, J. and Kaguni, L. S. Enzyme-labelled probes for nucleic acid hybridization. *Bioanal. Appl. Enzymes* **36:**115–127, 1992.
27. Hagel, L. Properties, in theory and practice, of novel gel filtration media for standard liquid chromatography. *J. Chromatog.* **476:**329–344, 1989.
28. Krieg, P. A. and Melton, D. A. In vitro RNA synthesis with SP6 RNA polymerase. *Methods Enzymol.* **155:**397–415, 1987.
29. Butler, E. T. and Chamberlin, M. J. Bacteriophage SP6-specific RNA polymerase: isolation and characterization. *J. Biol. Chem.* **257:**5772–5778, 1982.
30. Studier, F. W., Rosenberg, A. H., Dunn, J. J., and Dubendorff, J. W. Use of T7 RNA polymerase to direct expression of cloned genes. *Methods Enzymol.* **185:**60–89, 1990.
31. Yamaguchi, K., Zhang, D., and Byrn, R. A. A modified nonradioactive method for northern blot analysis. *Anal. Biochem.* **218:**343–346, 1994.
32. Dubitsky, A., Brown, J., and Brandwein, H. Chemiluminescent detection of DNA on nylon membranes. *BioFeedback* **13:**392–399, 1992.
33. Murakami, A., Tada, J., Yamaguchi, K., and Takano, J. Highly sensitive detection of DNA using enzyme-linked DNA probes. *Nucleic Acids Res.* **17:**5587–5595, 1989.
34. Nakagami, S., Matsunaga, H., Oka, N., and Yamane, A. Preparation of enzyme-conjugated DNA probe and application to the universal probe system. *Anal. Biochem.* **198:**75–79, 1991.
35. Schaap, A. P., Akhaven, H., and Romano, L. J. Chemiluminescent substrates for alkaline phosphatase: applications to ultrasenstive enzyme-linked immunoassays and DNA probes. *Clin. Chem.* **35:**1863, 1864, 1989.
36. Ingram, V. M. A specific chemical difference between the globins of normal human and sickle-cell anemia hemoglobin. *Nature* **178:**792–794, 1956.
37. Chang, J. G. and Kan Y. W. A sensitive new prenatal test for sickle cell anemia. *New Engl. J. Med.* **307:**30–32, 1982.
38. Burkitt, D. and O'Connor, G. T. Malignant lymphoma in African children. A clinical syndrome. *Cancer* **14:**258–269, 1961.
39. Scriver, C. R., Beaudet, A. L., Sly, W. S., and Valle, D., eds. *The Metabolic Basis of Inherited Disease,* 6th ed., McGraw-Hill, New York, 1989.
40. Fearon, E. R. and Vogelstein, B. A genetic model for colorectal tumorigenesis. *Cell* **6:**759–767, 1990.

5

DNA Amplification Techniques

An Overview

David H. Sorscher

1. INTRODUCTION

The polymerase chain reaction (PCR) has revolutionized modern science. With the introduction of the PCR to the clinical laboratory, genetically based diseases are now diagnosed with an incredible level of sensitivity and accuracy. This chapter will review the original discovery of the PCR in which the synthetic cycles were driven by the Klenow fragment of DNA polymerase I, and the rapid development of this exciting technology after the introduction of the heat-resistant *Thermus aquaticus (Taq)* polymerase.

Various elegant nucleic acid amplification techniques derived from the PCR have been discovered and successfully applied to molecular medicine. For example, the ligase chain reaction has been applied to the characterization of gene mutations and the detection of infectious diseases. Nucleic acid sequence-based amplification and the related transcription-mediated amplification are especially useful techniques for the diagnosis of infection by RNA-based organisms, such as HIV, mycobacteria, or hepatitis virus. A divergent technique, branched DNA analysis, does not rely on amplification of the target molecule. Branched DNA-based detection has also been applied to HIV diagnostics. The PCR and each of these new diagnostic techniques will be discussed and illustrated.

2. THE PCR

During the last 10 years since the description of the PCR *(1,2)*, this powerful technique has attracted widespread attention. PCR technology has become essential to the clinical diagnostic and forensic laboratories as well as to basic research in molecular biology and evolution. In a typical PCR, 25–35 successive synthetic cycles are performed in which DNA polymerase copies the target DNA (or RNA) molecule in vitro. The products of each cycle provide new templates for the next round of polymerase activity. After 25 cycles, the concentration of starting material has increased exponentially.

The PCR is an incredibly sensitive and highly specific method of detection. It is possible to amplify a single copy of target sequence in the presence of surrounding

From: Molecular Diagnostics: For the Clinical Laboratorian
Edited by: W. B. Coleman and G. J. Tsongalis Humana Press Inc., Totowa, NJ

DNA from 1.5×10^6 cells that does not contain the gene of interest *(3)*. This specificity is integral to the analysis of mutations that predispose individuals to the development of cystic fibrosis or cancer *(4–7)*. A good example of the sensitivity and specificity of the PCR is a report describing the detection of one mutated *K-ras* allele in a background of 10^5 normal copies during diagnosis of pancreatic adenocaricinoma *(8)*.

Figure 1 illustrates the various components and mechanics of a PCR. The PCR mixture contains a thermostable DNA polymerase, gene-specific forward and reverse primers, each of the four deoxynucleotide triphosphates (dNTPs), reaction buffer, and genomic DNA or a cell lysate. The chain reaction proceeds by incubation at three different temperatures: 1 min at 94°C to unwind the DNA containing the gene of interest (unwinding), 1 min at 60°C for hybridization of primers to the single-stranded template (annealing), and 2 min at 72°C for polymerization (extension). These incubations are then repeated for 25–30 cycles. Since the copy number doubles after each successive cycle, an exponential increase of 2^n (*n* is the total number of cycles) is accomplished during the complete chain reaction.

3. EVOLUTION OF THE PCR

3.1. The PCR with Klenow Fragment of DNA Polymerase I

In the first experiments describing the PCR *(1,2)*, the Klenow fragment of *Escherichia coli* DNA polymerase I was used for DNA synthesis during each cycle. After the unwinding step, samples were quickly cooled before the addition of enzyme to avoid heat denaturation of the Klenow polymerase. It was necessary to add a fresh aliquot of Klenow enzyme after each denaturation cycle. Also, the primer hybridization and DNA synthesis steps were carried out at 30°C to preserve enzyme activity. Performing the annealing and extension cycles at 30°C resulted in hybridization of primer to nontarget sequences and considerable nonspecific reaction products *(2)*. Even with these drawbacks, the original PCR methodology was successfully applied to gene cloning and molecular diagnostic experiments *(1,2)*.

3.2. The Introduction of Thermostable Taq Polymerase

The major technological breakthrough in development of PCR came with the application of a thermostable polymerase (*Taq*) to the PCR *(3)*. The practicality of running the PCR reactions was greatly improved since *Taq* polymerase survived extended incubation at 95°C, thereby obviating the need to add new enzyme after each cycle. In addition, by using a heat block that automatically changes temperatures (a thermocycler), the PCR cycles became automated. The product yield was found to increase after using *Taq* when compared with Klenow polymerase, and during a 30 cycle PCR,

---

Fig. 1. *(opposite page)* The PCR *(3)*. A typical PCR cycle is shown beginning with the unwinding of double-stranded DNA to a single-stranded template (unwinding, 94°C). Gene-specific primers hybridize to the complementary sequence in the target during the annealing reaction (annealing, 60°C). The primer/template hybrid is a substrate for *Taq* polymerase, which extends each primer by incorporation of dNTPs (extension, 72°C). After one cycle, the copy number of target sequence is doubled. In cycle 2, both products from cycle 1 are substrates for the unwinding, annealing, and extension incubations. The yield is four copies after cycle 2. The concentration of target molecules is amplified by carrying out the chain reactions for 25–30 cycles.

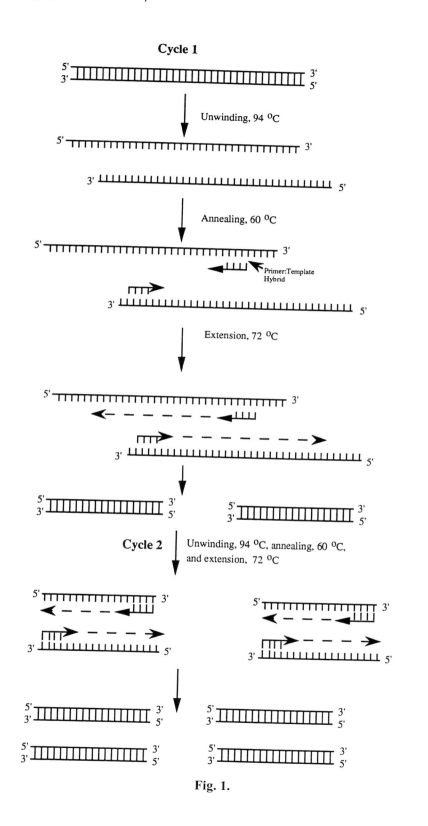

Fig. 1.

amplification of target sequence by 4×10^6 was observed *(3)*. The increase in copy number was limited only by diminishing polymerase activity after 25–30 cycles. Dilution of the PCR product after cycle 30 and reamplification for 30 additional cycles resulted in a $10^9–10^{10}$ increase in target sequence *(3)*.

The sensitivity of PCR employing *Taq* polymerase is limited only by the ability to obtain a single cell. An HIV-1 gene fragment was reliably detected and characterized after PCR-generated amplification using a single CD4$^+$ T-cell *(9)*. Also, the PCR was successfully performed with single blastomeres in an analysis of Duchenne muscular dystrophy gene mutations *(10)*.

Importantly, the specificity of the chain reaction was greatly improved by the introduction of *Taq* polymerase. Its high optimal reaction temperature of 72°C *(11)* ensured that only complete hybrids between the primer and target sequence persisted during extension cycles. Saiki et al. (3), demonstrated that the nonspecific hybridization and DNA synthesis previously observed at 30°C with Klenow polymerase was eliminated after using *Taq* polymerase. In these experiments the annealing and extension temperatures were 40°C and 70°C, respectively *(3)*. Often, the annealing step can be carried out at even higher temperatures. For example, primer hybridization can be carried out at 60°C when using a 30 base primer with 50% G/C content.

The reliability of PCR was dramatically optimized by the introduction of *Taq* polymerase. Since the PCR became an essential method for many different basic research disciplines and it was successfully applied to the diagnosis of genetic diseases, *Taq* polymerase was awarded Molecule of the Year status by *Science* in 1989 *(12)*.

3.3. The Long-Range PCR

Recent developments in PCR methods have extended the upper size limit for an efficient PCR product from 5–35 kb *(13,14)*. This finding has relevance to medical diagnostics because individuals carrying large deletions or insertions in clinically relevant chromosomal regions (e.g., Duchenne Muscular Dystrophy) can now be identified by using a single PCR.

The major obstacle to synthesis of long products during the PCR was found to be misincorporation by *Taq* polymerase at a frequency of 1×10^4 to 5×10^4 nucleotides *(15)*. Barnes *(13)* hypothesized that inhibition of extension by *Taq* polymerase at sites of mispairing would cause inefficient synthesis of full-length product. Reliable polymerization of long, accurate products was accomplished by adding a small amount of 3'–5'-exonuclease to a PCR mixture already containing *Taq* polymerase *(13,14)*. The 3'–5'-exonuclease activity recognized and removed misincorporated bases at the end of the growing DNA strand *(13,14)*. Optimal conditions for long PCR were obtained by using a modified *Taq* polymerase (termed Klentaq1) for DNA synthesis and a 3'–5'-exonuclease activity from either *Pfu*, Vent, or Deep Vent polymerase for excision of mispaired bases *(13)*. It was also necessary to increase the extension cycle in order to accommodate synthesis of molecules up to 35 kb in length *(13,14)*.

4. PCR COMPONENTS AND SAMPLE REACTION CONDITIONS

It is important to use sterile solutions and aerosol resistant pipette tips to provide an uncontaminated environment for execution of the PCR. Often, it is necessary to devote a laboratory bench or a small room to the PCR techniques. Because of the high sensitivity of the PCR assays, carryover contamination is commonly a problem. When distributing components between sample tubes, a nucleic acid molecule can be transferred, even after changing pipet tips.

4.1. Design of Oligonucleotide Primers

The oligonucleotide primers are usually 25–40 bases in length and are designed to flank the region of interest. They should be nonhomologous to each other and should not hybridize elsewhere in the gene being amplified. By convention, the forward primer anneals to the minus strand and directs synthesis downstream in a 5' to 3' direction. The reverse primer is located anywhere from 125 bp to 2.5 kb 3' of the forward primer, and will initiate polymerization upstream toward the forward primer. Often, the 5'-end contains additional GC sequences (a 3-bp "GC clamp") to exploit the increased melting temperature of G-C vs A-T base pairing. Primers are usually provided in lyophilized form and are resuspended in a buffer containing 10 mM Tris-HCl (pH 8.0) and 1 mM EDTA, desalted by separation on Sephadex G-25 *(16)*, and stored in aliquots at –20°C.

4.2. Reaction Buffer and Taq Polymerase

Taq polymerase is provided from the supplier at 5 U/µL and is stored at –20°C. A reaction buffer is usually included with the commercially available enzyme (Perkin-Elmer Cetus [Emeryville, CA], Gibco-BRL [Gaithersburg, MD], and so forth). An adequate 10X buffer for most PCR conditions is 500 mM KCl, 100 mM Tris-HCl (pH 8.3), 15 mM MgCl$_2$, and 0.1% gelatin *(16)*. Glycerol (10%) or formamide (5%), if used in the place of gelatin, was found to enhance the efficiency of PCR by lowering the effective temperature for template denaturation *(17)*. By carrying out denaturation at 90°C in the presence of these cosolvents, the activity of *Taq* polymerase was extended when compared to unwinding incubations at higher temperatures *(17)*.

4.3. Deoxynucleotide Triphosphates

The final concentration of dNTPs is 200 µM for a typical PCR. Higher concentrations of dNTPs (or MgCl$_2$) can result in misincorporation by *Taq* polymerase *(16)*. Ten-millimolar dNTP stocks can be purchased commercially (Perkin-Elmer Cetus, Pharmacia Biotech [Piscataway, NJ], Gibco-BRL) and are typically adjusted to pH 7.0. dNTPs should be aliquoted and stored at –20°C.

4.4. Recent Developments: AmpErase

Recently, Roche Laboratories (Branchburg, NJ) developed a PCR system that included a component, termed AmpErase (dUTP-uracil-N-glycosylase or UNG), designed to eliminate crosscontamination. With the Roche system, the PCR was carried out in the presence of dUTP instead of dTTP. The amplified DNA contained U, whereas the target molecules still contained T. The AmpErase component degrades U-containing PCR products that have been inadvertently carried over to a new reaction on the same sample, but does not affect target DNA templates that contain T instead of U *(18)*. Thus, AmpErase destroys carryover U-substituted PCR products prior to the initiation of a new amplification reaction *(18)*. AmpErase does not alter the recovery of PCR products, since it is quickly denatured at high temperatures *(18)*.

4.5. PCR Analysis of Genomic DNA Target Sequences

Good protocol for a pilot PCR analysis of a single-copy gene is to start with a crude lysate from 10^4 human cells or 0.05 µg purified DNA as template *(19)*. Mix together components in an estimated final volume of 100 µL, but leave out the polymerase enzyme. Heat at 95°C for 5 min, cool to approx 85°C, and add 2.5 U *Taq* polymerase and a small drop of mineral oil. Set the thermocycler parameters for a three-step amplification cycle, including:

1. A denaturation step at 94°C for 1 min;
2. A primer annealing step at 60°C (or 10–20°C below the melting temperature values for the particular primer/template hybrids) for 1 min; and
3. An extension step at 72°C for 2 min.

A typical PCR will include 30–35 cycles of amplification, with a final extension cycle for 10 min at 72°C, followed by a 4°C incubation. Subsequent to the completion of the PCR, amplified DNA products should be analyzed by an appropriate gel electrophoresis method. These are suggested parameters, and they may need to be modified. For example, it may be necessary to increase the amount of template or to adjust the annealing and extension cycles.

5. PCR APPLICATIONS

5.1. RT-PCR (Reverse Transcription-PCR)

PCR technology has been extended to the quantitation of low levels of gene expression by using RNA as template. In RT-PCR, RNA is isolated and reverse transcribed into cDNA by using oligo-dT, random primers, or a gene-specific primer and reverse transcriptase. This cDNA serves as substrate for the PCR with a new set of gene-specific forward and reverse primers. Products are evaluated by gel electrophoresis and Southern hybridization.

5.2. In Situ *PCR*

Clinical samples can be tested *in situ* for the presence of infectious organisms, such as HIV, by a PCR analysis performed on a histological tissue section *(20)*. Components are added to special chambers covering the slide and the cycling reactions are carried out. The PCR product is then detected by colorimetric methods. Microscopic inspection will determine the fraction of cells and the identity of cells positive for a particular target sequence.

5.3. Mutational Analysis

The discovery of the PCR has led to efficient, reliable detection of gene mutations that predispose individuals to common diseases, such as cystic fibrosis and cancer *(5,21)*. The reverse dot-blot method for analysis of mutations exploits the high product yield characteristic of the PCR. Wild-type or mutagenic primers are chemically attached to hybridization membranes. These blots are mixed with a biotin-modified PCR product and hybridized under stringent conditions designed for complete hybridization to the gene containing the characteristic mutation but not to the wild type alleles. The hybridization signal can be detected by a chemiluminescent or colorimetric reaction.

6. LIGASE CHAIN REACTION

In the ligase chain reaction technique, gene sequences are amplified by a thermo-stable DNA ligase. This method was originally shown to be an useful alternative to the PCR for the detection of gene mutations *(22)*, and has recently been successfully applied to diagnostic tests for the presence of chlamydia *(23)*, gonorrhea *(24)*, listeria *(25)*, and HPV (reviewed in ref. *26*).

The ligase chain reaction is described schematically in Fig. 2. Two sets of primers are designed to anneal at immediately adjacent regions of the target template. One pair of primers is designed to anneal to the top strand. The second set of primers is comple-mentary to the first pair and will anneal to the opposite target strand. Interprimer hybridization is prevented by including carrier DNA and including a 3'-tail on opposite primers. These primers are mixed with template and thermostable ligase and incubated at 95°C for 1 min for denaturation, and subsequently at 65°C for 4 min for primer annealing and ligation. The denaturation and annealing/ligation steps are repeated for 10–20 cycles. Amplification will occur only after ligation of the adjacent oligonucle-otides. The downstream primer must be phosphorylated at the 5'-end because DNA ligase requires a free $5'-PO_4$ and 3'-OH as substrate. The 5'-primer is end-labeled with ^{32}P, and the amplified products are visualized after gel electrophoresis and auto-radiography. Alternatively, primers are designed to carry biotin groups for nonradio-active detection of the amplified products *(25)*.

The experiment shown in Fig. 2 was designed both for the detection of a target gene (left panel) and for the analysis of gene mutations (right panel). Also, primer sets can be designed to identify sequence variation in the genome of infectious organisms, such as HIV. One advantage of the ligase chain reaction when compared to PCR is the abil-ity to identify single-base mutations (Fig. 2, right panel). In analyzing mutations by the ligase chain reaction, the 5'-oligonucleotide is engineered to contain the predicted mutation at its 3'-end. As a result, this altered base cannot hybridize to the wild-type target allele, and ligase cannot join the adjacent primers. No signal is detected in the ligase chain reaction unless the mutated base is present in the template. In contrast, the char-acterization of mutations after the PCR requires additional time-consuming steps, such as oligonucleotide hybridization, single-strand conformational polymorphism (SSCP) gel electrophoresis, or DNA sequencing.

7. NUCLEIC ACID SEQUENCE BASED AMPLIFICATION (NASBA)

NASBA is a recently developed sequence amplification technique that is particu-larly suited for RNA detection and has proven effective in analysis of transforming genes for chronic myelogenous leukemia, HIV-1, mycobacteria, and hepatitis C virus *(27–29)*. This method is a descendant of the transcription-based amplification system *(28)*. One of the major differences when compared to the PCR is that the NASBA reaction is isothermal (41°C), thereby obviating the need for an expensive thermocycler and facilitating manual processing of many samples. NASBA is also very fast, since a typical reaction is completed in approx 90 min.

Reagent kits that include all of the components necessary to perform the NASBA reaction for detection of HIV-1 RNA, as well as rigorous internal controls, have been developed by Organon-Teknica (Durham, NC) *(27)*. A related technique, termed tran-

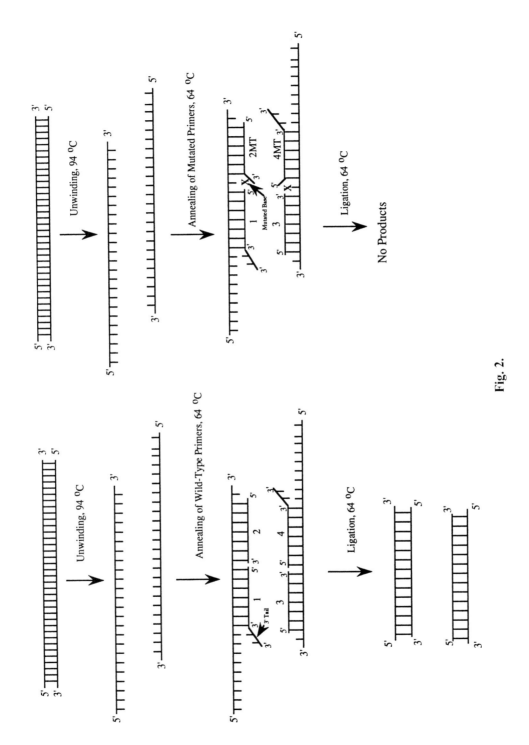

Fig. 2.

96

scription-mediated amplification *(29)*, has been successfully consolidated into a test kit specifically designed for the detection of *Mycobacterium tuberculosis* rRNA (Gen-Probe Chugai Pharmaceuticals, San Diego, CA). The Gen-Probe transcription-mediated amplification kit for mycobacteria testing is currently under expedited FDA review.

A schematic representation of NASBA is illustrated in Fig. 3. The target RNA molecule is first incubated with a primer complementary to target sequences. If DNA is the substrate, it must be denatured to a single-stranded template before primer hybridization. This primer (T7P) has a 5'-extension composed of T7 RNA polymerase promoter sequences. After extension of the T7P/target hybrid with reverse transcriptase, the RNA template is degraded by RNase H, and a second primer P2 hybridizes to the 3'-end of the cDNA and is extended by reverse transcriptase to create a double-stranded DNA molecule. This double-stranded DNA intermediate is required for recognition of the T7 promoter by RNA polymerase. Several RNA molecules are synthesized by RNA polymerase from the double-stranded DNA template. These RNA molecules are converted to DNA templates in self-generating amplification cycles every time the T7P primer hybridizes to a new RNA molecule.

An advantage to NASBA compared with PCR is that the reverse transcription reaction can be performed with thermolabile enzyme, such as AMV reverse transcriptase. Unlike AMV RT, the thermostable reverse transcriptase employed in RT-PCR (*Tth* polymerase) requires manganese instead of magnesium for activity. Manganese decreases the fidelity of subsequent *Taq* polymerase amplification cycles during the RT-PCR *(28)*.

8. BRANCHED DNA DETECTION

All of the above-mentioned techniques exploit the exponential nature of synthetic chain reactions to increase the concentration of target nucleic acid. Branched DNA (bDNA) methodology is a clear deviation from these amplification technologies *(31,32)*. The target nucleic acid is not replicated. Instead, the sensitivity of the reaction is provided by amplification of signal.

In bDNA analysis (*see* Fig. 4), several 50-mer probes (spanning 350 bases for hepatitis C virus *[32]*) containing sequences homologous to the gene of interest are incubated with the sample nucleic acid *(31,32)*. There are two types of gene-specific

---

Fig. 2. *(previous page)* The ligase chain reaction *(22)*. Genomic DNA is shown schematically at the top of both panels. Similar to the PCR, double-stranded DNA is unwound during a 94°C unwinding incubation. Four primers are designed to hybridize at adjacent sequences in the target. During the annealing reaction (64°C), wild-type (left panel) primers 1–2 anneal to the top strand and 3–4 hybridize to the complementary sequence in the bottom strand. A 3'-tail is included on primers 1 and 4 to help prevent duplex formation between complementary primers 1 and 3, or 2 and 4. The gap between primers is sealed by thermostable DNA ligase (64°C). Two copies of target sequence are products of the first ligase chain reaction cycle. Amplification of the target gene is accomplished by performing 10–20 cycles of 94°C for 1 min (unwinding) and 64°C for 2 min (annealing and ligation). In the right panel, mutagenic primers 2MT and 4MT contain an altered base at their 3'- and 5'-ends, respectively. Ligation of primer sets 1 and 2MT or 3 and 4MT is not possible, unless the altered base is also present in the genomic sequence. In the example shown, no products are formed in the ligase chain reaction with mutated primers, because only wild-type alleles are present in the genome.

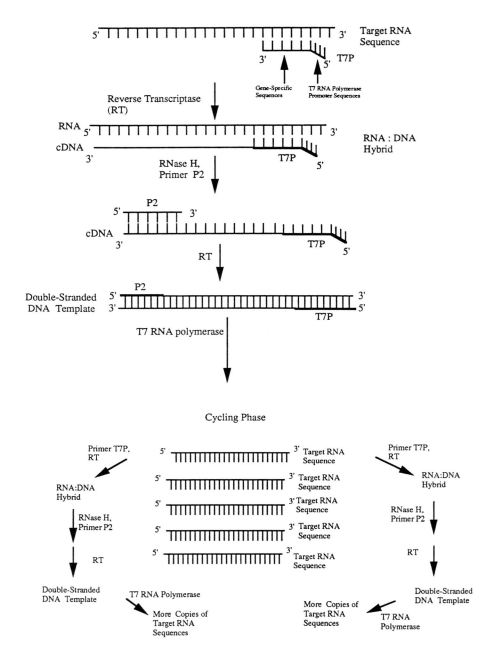

Fig. 3. NASBA *(28)*. Gene-specific sequences in primer T7P hybridize to complementary sequences in the target RNA molecule. T7P contains sequences homologous to the target and a 5'-extension containing the promoter for T7 RNA polymerase. Reverse transcriptase synthesizes a cDNA strand beginning at the 3'-end of T7P. The RNA component of the RNA/DNA hybrid is then degraded by RNase H. Primer P2 anneals to the 5'-end of the cDNA. A double-stranded DNA template is created after extension from P2 by the activity of reverse transcriptase. This template is recognized at promoter sequences by T7 RNA polymerase, and several copies of the target RNA sequence are transcribed. The cycling phase of NASBA commences, since each of the RNA copies is a substrate for another amplification cycle beginning with hybridization to primer T7P. Nonspecific annealing of T7P is reduced by a preliminary 5-min incubation at 65°C. All subsequent reactions are performed at 41°C and typically require 90 min for completion.

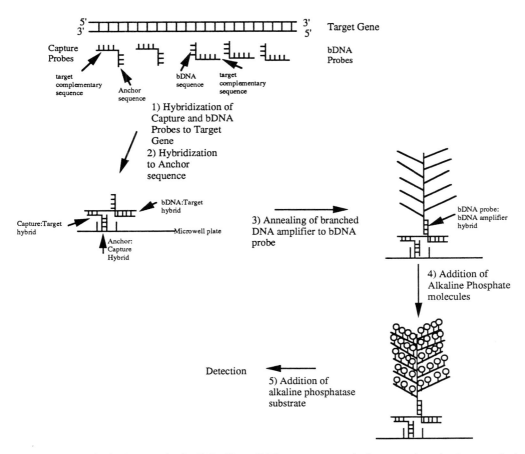

Fig. 4. Branched DNA analysis *(31)*. (Step 1) The target gene is denatured to single-stranded DNA to allow hybridization at separate gene-specific sequences on the capture and bDNA probes. The remainder of the capture and bDNA probes are free for hybridization to anchor and bDNA amplifier sequences, respectively. (Step 2) To immobilize the capture/target hybrid, anchor sequences on the capture probe anneal to their complementary DNA, which is attached to a microtiter plate. (Step 3) To facilitate signal amplification, the branched DNA amplifier recognizes its complementary sequence adjacent to the bDNA/target hybrid. (Step 4) Alkaline phosphatase molecules are attached to arms of the bDNA amplifier and signal is detected after addition of colorimetric substrate.

probes for bDNA detection: "capture probes" and "bDNA probes." One region (20–40 bases) on the capture probe is designed to hybridize with the target gene, and a separate region (20 bases) anneals to DNA covalently attached to wells in a microtiter plate. Several different bDNA primers hybridize to sequences (20–40 bases) within the target gene that are not occupied by the capture probe. Adjacent sequences (20 bases) in the bDNA primer are designed to anneal to a bDNA amplifier. This branched DNA molecule contains up to 45 sites for binding alkaline phosphatase molecules. After addition of the alkaline phosphatase probes, as many as 1755 enzyme molecules are bound by each target molecule. The alkaline phosphatase substrate, Dioxetane, is added for chemiluminescent signal detection.

The synthesis of oligonucleotide primers for the PCR is simple, automated and inexpensive. One possible drawback of the bDNA technique is that the chemical modifications of primers required for this method are not available at most nucleic acid facilities. Therefore, it is not possible for individual researchers to modify and design new tests quickly based on the bDNA methodology. This minor drawback will most certainly be corrected as more laboratories apply bDNA techniques to molecular diagnostics.

Since there are no synthetic cycles involved in bDNA analysis, the consequence of crosscontamination between samples is reduced when compared to PCR. By dramatically reducing crosscontamination artifacts, the bDNA detection system may prove to be a highly sensitive detection system with greater specificity than the PCR. The bDNA technique is currently being applied to evaluation of infectious diseases, and reagent kits designed to detect and quantify HIV-1, hepatitis C virus, and hepatitis B virus have been successfully developed (Chiron Corporation, Emeryville, CA).

ACKNOWLEDGMENTS

The author was supported by NIH grants RO1CA19492 and R29CA67156.

REFERENCES

1. Saiki, R. K., Scharf, S., Faloona, F., Mullis, K., Horn, G., Erlich, H., and Arnheim, N. Enzymatic amplification of β-globin genomic sequences and restriction site analysis of sickle cell anemia. *Science* **230:**1350–1354, 1985.
2. Mullis, K. B. and Faloona, F. A. Specific synthesis of DNA in vitro via a polymerase-catalyzed chain reaction. *Methods Enzymol.* **155:**335–350, 1987.
3. Saiki, R. K., Gelfand, D. H., Stoffel, S., Scharf, S. J., Higuchi, R., Horn, G. T., Mullis, K. B., and Erlich, H. A. Primer-directed enzymatic amplification of DNA with a thermostable DNA polymerase *Science* **239:**487–491, 1988.
4. Liu, E., Thor, A., He, M., Barcos, M., Ljung, B. M., and Benz, C. The Her2 (c-*erb*B-2) oncogene is frequently amplified in *in situ* carcinomas of the breast. *Oncogene* **7:**1027–1032, 1992.
5. Kawasaki, E., Saiki, R., and Erlich, H. Genetic analysis using polymerase chain reaction-amplified DNA and immobilized oligonucleotide probes: reverse dot-blot typing. *Methods Enzymol.* **218:**369–381, 1993.
6. Castilla, L. H., Couch, F. J., Erdos, M. R., Hoskins, K. F., Calzone, K., Garber, J. E., Boyd, J., Lubin, M. B., Deshano, M. L., Brody, L. D., et al. Mutations in the BRCA1 gene in families with early-onset breast and ovarian cancer. *Nature Genet.* **8:**387–391, 1994.
7. Mills, N. E., Fishman, C. L., Rom, W. N., Dubin, N., and Jacobson, D. R. Increased prevalence of K-*ras* oncogene mutations in lung adenocarcinoma. *Cancer Res.* **55:**1444–1447, 1995.
8. Tada, M., Omata, M., Kawai, S., Saisho, H., Ohto, M., Saiki, R. K., and Sninsky, J. J. Detection of ras gene mutations in pancreatic juice and peripheral blood of patients with pancreatic adenocarcinoma. *Cancer Res.* **53:**2472–2474, 1993.
9. Bertram, S., Hufert, F. T., Neumann-Haefelin, D., and von Laer, D. Detection of DNA in single cells using an automated cell deposition unit and PCR. *Biotechniques* **19:**616–620, 1995.
10. Kristjansson, K., Chong, S. S., Van den Veyver, I. B., Subramanian, S., Snabes, M. C., and Hughes, M. R. Preimplantation single cell analyses of Dystrophin gene deletions using whole genome amplification. *Nature Genet.* **6:**19–23, 1994.
11. Chien, A., Edgar, D. B., and Trela, J. M. Deoxyribonucleic acid polymerase from the extreme thermophile *Thermus Aquaticus*. *J. Bacteriol.* **127:**1550–1557, 1976.

12. Guyer, R. L. and Koshland, D. E. The molecule of the year. *Science* **246:**1543–1544, 1989.
13. Barnes, W. M. PCR amplification of up to 35 kb DNA with high fidelity and high yield from λ bacteriophage templates. *Proc. Natl. Acad. Sci. USA* **91:**2216–2220, 1994.
14. Cheng, S., Fockler, C., Barnes, W. M., and Higuchi, R. Effective amplification of long targets from cloned inserts and human genomic DNA. *Proc. Natl. Acad. Sci. USA* **91:**5695–5699, 1994.
15. Eckert, K. A. and Kunkel, T. A. DNA polymerase fidelity and the polymerase chain reaction. *PCR Methods Appl.* **1:**17–24, 1991.
16. Sambrook, J., Fritsch, E. F., and Maniatis, T. (Eds). *Molecular Cloning: A Laboratory Manual.* Cold Spring Harbor Laboratory, Cold Spring Harbor, NY, 1989.
17. Landre, P. A., Gelfand, D. H., and Watson, R. M. The use of cosolvents to enhance amplification by the polymerase chain reaction, in *PCR Strategies,* Innis, M. A. and Gelfand, D. H., eds., Academic, San Diego, CA, pp. 3–16, 1995.
18. Madonna, J. *PCR Laboratory*, Roche Diagnostic Systems, Branchburg, NJ, pp. 1–8, 1993.
19. Saiki, R. K. Amplification of genomic DNA, in *PCR Protocols*, Innis, M. A., Gelfand, D. H., Sninsky, J. J., and White, T. J., eds., Academic, San Diego, CA, pp. 13–20, 1990.
20. Retzel, E., Staskus, K. A., Embretson, J. E., and Haase, A. T. The *in situ* PCR: amplification and detection of DNA in a cellular context, in *PCR Strategies*, Innis, M. A. and Gelfand, D. H., eds., Academic, San Diego, CA, pp. 199–212, 1995.
21. Chehab, F. F., Wall, J., and Cai, S.-P. Analysis of PCR products by covalent reverse dot blot hybridization, in *PCR Strategies*, Innis, M. A. and Gelfand, D. H., eds., Academic, San Diego, CA, pp. 130–139, 1995.
22. Barany, F. (1991) Genetic disease detection and DNA amplification using cloned thermostable ligase. *Proc. Natl. Acad. Sci. USA* **88:**189–193, 1991.
23. Bassiri, M., Hu, H. Y., Domeika, M. A., Burczak, J., Svensson, L. O., Lee, H. H., and Mardh, P. A. Detection of *Chlamydia trachomatis* in urine specimens from women by ligase chain reaction. *J. Clin. Microbiol.* **33:**898–900, 1995.
24. Smith, K. R., Ching, S., Lee, H., Ohhashi, Y., Hu, H. Y., Fisher, H. C., and Hook, E. W. Evaluation of ligase chain reaction for use with urine for identification of *Neisseria gonorrhoeae* in females attending a sexually transmitted disease clinic. *J. Clin. Microbiol.* **33:**455–457, 1995.
25. Weidmann, M., Barany, F., and Batt, C. A. Detection of *Listeria* monocytogenes by PCR-coupled ligase chain reaction, in *PCR Strategies*, Innis, M. A. and Gelfand, D. H., eds., Academic, San Diego, CA, pp. 347–361, 1995.
26. Quinn, T. C. Recent advances in diagnosis of sexually transmitted diseases. *Sexually Transmitted Dis.* **21:**S19–S27, 1994.
27. van Gemen, B., Wiel, P. V. D., van Beuningen, R., Sillekens, P., Kirroaams. S., Dries, C., Schoones, R., and Kievits, T. The one-tube quantitative HIV-1 RNA NASBA: precision, accuracy, and application. *PCR Methods Appl.* **4:**S177–S184, 1995.
28. Kwoh, D. Y., Davis, G. R., Whitfield, K. M., Chappelle, H. L., DiMichelle, L. J., and Gingeras, T. R. Transcription-based amplification system and detection of amplified human immunodeficiency virus type 1 with a bead-based sandwich hybridization format. *Proc. Natl. Acad. Sci. USA* **86:**1173–1177, 1989.
29. Carlowicz, M. Rapid tuberculosis assay under expedited FDA review. *Clin. Lab. News* July 1–4, 1995.
30. Urdea, M. S. Branched DNA signal amplification. Does bDNA represent post-PCR amplification technology? *Biotechnology* **12:**926–927, 1994.
31. Wilber, J. C. Direct quantification of viral nucleic acids using branched DNA (bDNA) signal amplification: methodology and studies on monitoring chronic viral infections. *Clin. Immunol. Newsletter* **15:**57–61, 1995.

6

RT-PCR

Quantitative and Diagnostic PCR in the Analysis of Gene Expression

Robert B. Sisk

1. INTRODUCTION

The ability to measure RNA levels quantitatively is crucial to the study of gene expression. Northern blots, dot/slot blots, and nuclease protection assays are methods traditionally used for analysis of mRNA expression. These methods, however, require large quantities of RNA and often lack the needed sensitivity. Northern blotting, probably the most widely used method for characterizing RNA, requires 5–10 µg of purified poly(A)-mRNA and has a detection limit of approx 10^6–10^7 mRNA copies. Similarly, solution assays, such as RNase protection or S1 nuclease, require 0.1–1 µg of purified poly(A)-mRNA and have detection limits of approx 10^5–10^6 mRNA copies *(1)*. Thus, the required quantities of purified RNA make these methods impractical for many investigators because of the nature of the systems under investigation. For measuring low-abundance transcripts or working with limited amounts of material, the RT-PCR* technique is an excellent alternative to classical blotting and solution hybridization assays *(2)*. RT-PCR couples the tremendous DNA amplification powers of the PCR technique with the ability of RT to reverse transcribe small quantities of total RNA (1 ng or less) into cDNA. Using total cellular RNA rather that purified poly(A)-mRNA reduces the possibility of losing messages during the purification process and allows the use of very small quantities of starting material. For example, methods already exist for performing PCR on a single cell *(3,4)*. Other advantages of this technique are its versatility, sensitivity, rapid turnaround time, and the ability to compare multiple samples simultaneously. Although RT-PCR techniques are mostly semiquantitative, progress is being made in the development of several quantitative methods *(5)*.

RT-PCR is basically a four step process:

1. RNA isolation;
2. Reverse transcription;
3. PCR amplification; and
4. Product analysis (Fig. 1).

*See p. 119 for list of abbreviations used in this chapter.

From: Molecular Diagnostics: For the Clinical Laboratorian
Edited by: W. B. Coleman and G. J. Tsongalis Humana Press Inc., Totowa, NJ

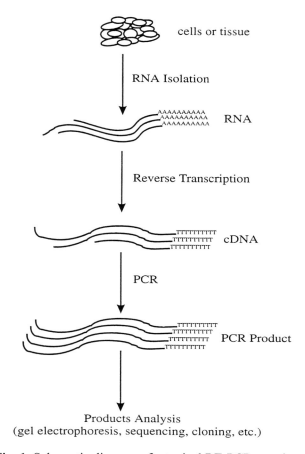

cells or tissue

RNA Isolation

RNA

Reverse Transcription

cDNA

PCR

PCR Product

Products Analysis
(gel electrophoresis, sequencing, cloning, etc.)

Fig. 1. Schematic diagram of a typical RT-PCR reaction.

RNA is isolated from cells or tissue and used as a template in a reverse transcription reaction that produces cDNA. The cDNA serves as a template for the PCR reaction. Using a set of specially designed primers, the PCR reaction amplifies a specific cDNA sequence. Following amplification, the quantity and size of a product are determined by running a small sample of the reaction on an agarose gel. Subsequent analysis usually takes the form of restriction analysis, hybridization, or nucleotide sequencing. In addition, PCR amplification products may also be used for subcloning or to generate DNA probes or expression vectors.

2. RT-PCR: THE BASIC METHOD

1 Working with RNA

 important factors in generating high-quality full-length cDNA, the sequent PCR products, is the purity and integrity of the total RNA iterial. RNases, enzymes that digest RNA, are among the hardiest of even boiling. Procedures for creating an RNase-free laboratory envi-n described in detail *(6)*. Of major importance is that one should never assume that anything is RNase-free, especially human hands. Always wear latex gloves when performing laboratory procedures involving RNA (including isolation) or preparing RNase-free solutions and materials. Sterile disposable plasticware, such as centrifuge tubes, culture tubes, pipets, pipet tips, or similar labware, should be used when possible in place of common laboratory glassware. Most microcentrifuge tubes may be removed from a previously unopened box or bag, placed in RNase-free containers, autoclaved, and used for all RNA procedures. If glassware must be used, it should be rendered RNase-free by rinsing with 0.5M sodium hydroxide followed by copious rinses with sterilized, distilled water. Alternatively, glassware may be baked at 150°C for 4 h. All solutions used with RNA need to be RNase free and should be manipulated only with RNase-free pipets and tips. If prepared in RNase-free labware, solutions for use with RNA may be made from reagent-grade materials and distilled water followed by autoclaving. As an alternative to autoclaving, solutions may be filter-sterilized with a 0.2-μm disposable sterile filter unit. Water and other solutions for use with RNA can be rendered free of RNase by overnight treatment with 0.05% DEPC at room temperature followed by autoclaving for 30 min to remove trace DEPC *(7)*. Buffers containing Tris-hydroxymethyl-aminomethane or other primary amines cannot be treated with DEPC, and some laboratories have found that RNA isolated with DEPC-treated solutions do not behave identically to RNA isolated without DEPC in enzymatic reactions.

Chaotropic agents, such as guanidinium chloride and guanidinium isothiocyanate, are capable of dissolving cellular structures and proteins, causing nucleoproteins to dissociate rapidly from nucleic acids and inactivating RNase. Several procedures using chaotropic and reducing agents for the isolation of RNA from cells and tissues have been reported in the literature. One procedure commonly used to isolate intact RNA from all types of tissues, even those rich in RNases, such as the pancreas, was first reported by Chirgwin et al. *(8)*. Improvements to this method that allow sufficient amounts of RNA to be isolated from a number of samples in several hours have been published *(9)*. Using the method of Chomcznski and Sacchi *(9)*, it is possible to isolate sufficient RNA for reverse transcription from as little as 10^3 cells. RNA isolation kits that employ these and other improvements are available from several commercial sources (Pharmacia Biotech, Invitrogen).

After purification, if there is ample material, it is advisable to check a sample of the total RNA by electrophoresis on a denaturing agarose gel containing ethidium bromide *(7)*. Undegraded total RNA run on a denaturing gel typically gives bright 28S and 18S ribosomal RNA band, at approx 4.5 and 1.9 kb, respectively. The intensity ratio of these two bands (28S/18S) should be about 1.5–2.5:1. If the 28S and 18S bands are not visible, check the reagents and glassware used for purification for RNase or other impurities and repeat the procedure.

Polyadenylated mRNA can be isolated by oligo(dT)-selection if the total RNA is undegraded and sufficient quantities exist. This step is not typically necessary in RT-PCR reactions, but may help simplify subsequent first-strand synthesis and amplification steps by removing genomic DNA contamination that can amplify along with the target cDNA during PCR, sometimes causing problems depending on the specific RT-PCR application. As a control experiment, a sample of the total RNA may be used as a template for PCR amplification (without having first been reverse transcribed). Products generated in the absence of reverse transcribed cDNA are genomic in origin. DNA can be removed from the RNA preparation by oligo(dT) purification or by DNase I treatment *(7)*. A number of kits are commercially available for the purification of mRNA from total RNA (Pharmacia Biotech, InVitrogen).

2.2. Storage of Purified RNA Samples

Total RNA and mRNA may be protected from degradation for long periods of time if stored as a precipitate in ethanol. Efficient precipitation requires the presence of salt. Therefore, $3M$ sodium acetate should be added to the RNA solution to give a final concentration of $0.3M$ prior to the addition of ethanol to a final concentration of 70%. Precipitated RNA samples should be stored at $-20°C$. When needed, the RNA precipitate can be collected by centrifugation for 30 min at 4°C. Remove as much of the ethanol as possible using a sterile RNase-free pipet tip and allow the RNA pellet to dry at room temperature for about 10 min. When dry, resuspend the pellet in the appropriate RNase-free buffer. Under optimal conditions, RNA suspended in an RNase-free buffer can be stored for several weeks at 4°C without appreciable degradation. Repeated freezing and thawing of RNA in an aqueous buffer may cause degradation. For both ethanol precipitate and aqueous storage of RNA, it is advisable to divide the pool into many small aliquots.

3. SYNTHESIS OF cDNA

3.1. Overview

Reverse transcription is the process of copying RNA into a single-stranded complementary DNA molecule. In the laboratory, this process is known as first-strand synthesis, and the cDNA that is generated is the antisense strand ("antisense" is the term generally used to describe a sequence of DNA or RNA that is complementary to mRNA). A general outline for first-strand synthesis is shown in Fig. 2 and a typical RT-PCR procedure is given in Table 1. Basically, the reaction consists of five components:

1. cDNA synthesis primer;
2. First-strand buffer;
3. The four nucleotide triphosphates;
4. Source of RNA template (either total RNA or purified mRNA); and
5. RT enzyme.

3.2. Reverse Transcriptase

Retroviral RNA-directed DNA polymerase, or RT, is the enzyme used to catalyze first-strand cDNA synthesis. Originally, RT was purified from AMV RT. Subsequently, the MMLV RT was cloned, overexpressed, and purified *(10)*. After the optimal conditions for use of this enzyme in first-strand cDNA synthesis reactions were published, it replaced AMV RT as the enzyme of choice, since commercial preparations of AMV RT tend to possess some RNase activity *(11)*. MMLV RT has an inherent RNase H activity that reduces efficient synthesis of full-length cDNA. However, a modified version of MMLV RT lacking RNase H activity became available in 1988 *(12)*. This enzyme is designated MMLV H⁻ RT *(13)*. Either of these enzyme preparations may be used for first-strand cDNA synthesis, but MMLV H⁻ tends to produce a greater yield of cDNA product and a higher percentage of full-length transcripts. Thus, MMLV H⁻ RT

FIRST-STRAND SYNTHESIS

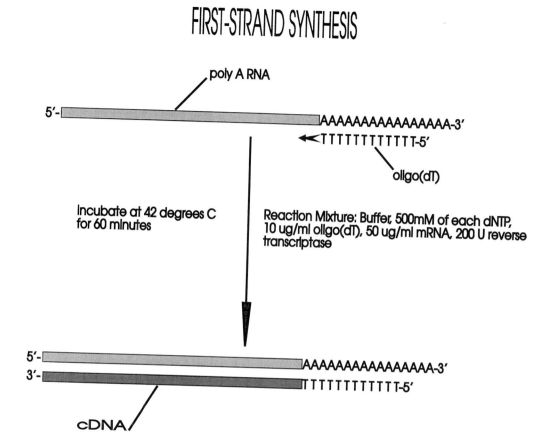

Fig. 2. Reverse transcription of RNA in first-strand synthesis reaction.

is rapidly becoming the more commonly used enzyme. High-quality preparations of AMV, MMLV, and MMLV H⁻ RT enzymes are commercially available and are usually supplied with a protocol and the appropriate buffer for optimal enzyme activity. A detailed review on RT enzymes has appeared *(14)*.

3.3. Priming First-Strand cDNA Synthesis

cDNA synthesis catalyzed by RT requires an RNA template and hybridized DNA primer with an available 3'-hydroxyl group. The mRNA is copied from the 3'-end to the 5'-end, resulting in cDNA synthesis proceeding in the 5'- to 3'-direction. To produce full-length copies of the transcript, priming must begin at the 3'-end of the mRNA. To this end, there are three types of primers generally used in cDNA synthesis: oligo(dT), random hexamers, and sequence-specific primers. Selection of the actual primer type depends on the particular RT-PCR application.

Random hexamers and oligo(dT) primers are used to convert an entire population of mRNA molecules into cDNA. Hexamers are the most common size of random primer used to prime cDNA synthesis. Random primers represent all possible nucleotide combinations for each position and anneal along the length of the mRNA molecules. Since

Table 1
Standard RT-PCR Method

1. Reverse transcription reaction:
   a. To a 0.5-mL microcentrifuge tube, add 1–5 μg of poly(A) mRNA sample in a volume of 7 μL or less, 2 μL 50 μg/mL oligo(dT) primer stock, and RNase-free H_2O to give a final volume of 9 μL. Mix the contents and spin briefly in a microcentrifuge.
   b. Incubate the tube at 70°C for 2–5 min. Then cool on ice for 2–5 min followed by a brief microcentrifugation to collect contents at the bottom.
   c. Add the remaining components of the reaction: 4 μL of 5X reverse transcription buffer stock (250 m*M* Tris-HCl, pH 8.3, 375 m*M* KCl and 125 m*M* $MgCl_2$), 2 μL 10 m*M* Dithiothreitol, 4 μL dNTP mix (consisting of 2.5 m*M* of each dNTP), 1 μL reverse transcriptase enzyme (200 U/μL). Then gently mix the contents by pipeting, followed by a brief microcentrifugation to collect contents at the bottom.
   d. Incubate at 42°C for 60 min.
   e. Denature reverse transcriptase enzyme by heating at 85°C for 10 min.
2. PCR amplification:
   a. Prepare enough PCR master mix for all of the PCR reactions plus one extra. For each reaction (50 μL total volume), mix the following reagents: 5 μL 10X PCR buffer, 36 μL sterile H_2O, 1 μL dNTP stock (containing 10 m*M* of each nucleotide), 1 μL of each gene specific primer (10 μ*M* stock), and 1 μL Taq polymerase (final concentration 50 U/mL), to a final volume of 45 μL. Mix and briefly microcentrifuge to collect contents.
   b. For each PCR reaction add 45 μL of the master mix and 2–5 μL of the cDNA synthesis. Mix and briefly microcentrifuge to collect contents. Add a drop of sterile mineral oil to each tube.
   c. PCR cycling parameters: an initial denaturation step at 95°C for 5 min, then 30 cycles of denaturation at 95°C for 60 s, annealing at 55°C (or the appropriate annealing temperature for the primers used) for 60 s, and extension at 72°C for 60 s, followed by a final extension step at 72°C for 10 min.

reverse transcription starts at many points along the mRNA molecule, this type of synthesis results in a variety of different-length cDNA molecules. The population of cDNA synthesized in this manner will be composed largely of fragments rather than full-length cDNA sequences with respect to the 3'-end of the mRNA target. When priming with random hexamers, the concentration of primer to mRNA is critical to generating the desired average length and mass yield of the product. Using MMLV H⁻ RT, a primer to mRNA molar ratio of approx 10:1 gives a satisfactory yield without sacrificing product length *(14)*. Because primers of random sequence are not specific to the RNA template, they will anneal to genomic DNA or any RNA in the sample (including ribosomal and free RNA), generating products that may lead to an increased background.

Oligo(dT) primers used in the synthesis of cDNA range in size from 12 to about 30 bases in length. This type of primer is designed to bind specifically to the poly(A) tail of the mRNA; thus, transcripts begin their synthesis at the 3'-end of the mRNA. Oligo(dT) primers are used to generate a representative population of full-length cDNAs. Although these primers are designed to target the poly(A) tail, they can also bind long stretches of adenosine within mRNA sequences. Oligo(dT) primers can be modified by adding guanosine, adenosine, or thymidine nucleotides to the 3'-end. These modified oligo(dT) primers bind to the 5' end of the poly(A), adding specificity by eliminating the homogeneity inherent with conventional oligo(dT) priming *(15)*. This method of priming often generates a cDNA population in which the 3'-ends of the mRNAs are overrepresented. Truncated transcripts can occur because of the tendency of RT enzymes to pause and terminate transcription, or because of termination of transcription as a result of secondary structure in the RNA template. However, in an optimized reaction, the combination of oligo(dT) priming with MMLV H⁻ RT will consistently yield excellent results.

Sequence-specific primers are used to reverse transcribe a fragment of a specific mRNA sequence of interest. These primers are designed such that they anneal to a region of known exonic sequence. Often a sequence-specific primer is simply the 3'-primer of the primer pair that will be used for PCR amplification. Sequence-specific primers are typically 21 nucleotides or greater in length, have a G/C content of about 50–70%, and a melting temperature >45°C. The melting temperature of a primer is defined as the midpoint of a temperature range over which a double-stranded duplex separates into single strands. Sequence-specific primers are used to prime cDNA synthesis when parts of the sequence other than the 3'-end are needed, and when mRNA secondary structure obstructs cDNA synthesis using oligo(dT). Certain specific RT-PCR protocols, such as RACE *(16)*, require the use of a sequence-specific primer. More information on sequence-specific primers may be found in Innis et al. *(16)*.

3.4. Modifications of Typical Primer Design

Choice and design of primers for cDNA synthesis depend on the overall strategy of the RT-PCR experiment and the type of application. Oligo(dT) primers can be modified by adding nucleotides to the 3'-end and 5'-end of the oligo(dT) strand. Modifications to the 3'-end are discussed in the previous section. Modifications to the 5'-end of the primer may include addition of sequences that code for restriction sites or nested primer targets. Ideally, these additions do not change the target sequence to which the primer anneals, but facilitate subsequent PCR and cloning reactions. Oligo(dT) primers with different 5'-modifications, referred to as primer-adapters, are available from many biotech companies (Stratagene, Promega, New England Biolabs). Design of sequence-specific primers should follow the same empirical rules used for standard PCR primers. These rules will be discussed later in this chapter in Section 4.1. Strict attention should be given to sequence-specific primer and mRNA primer sense. When choosing a gene-specific primer for cDNA synthesis, the primer should be antisense to the mRNA target sequence. Remember that cDNA synthesis proceeds in the 5' to 3' direction and the mRNA is copied in the reverse direction (3' to 5').

3.5. Reaction Parameters for cDNA Synthesis

The optimal reaction temperature for using MMLV H⁻ RT to synthesize first-strand cDNA is 37°C *(14)*. However, incubation temperatures as high as 50°C can be used successfully. Many of the commercial RT-PCR kits recommend performing RT reactions at 42°C. This higher reaction temperature helps to alleviate mRNA secondary structure that can impede enzyme processivity. Alternatively, RNA secondary structure can be eliminated by heating the mRNA and the synthesis primer at 70°C for 3–5 min. Heat-denatured RNA is then cooled on ice for several min, and the rest of the reaction components are added while keeping the tube on ice prior to proceeding with the standard reaction protocol. Reverse transcription reaction times vary from 30–60 min, with 60 min being the most common. Termination of the reaction is usually performed by denaturing the RT at 75–94°C for 10 min. At this point, some protocols call for an mRNA digestion step in which RNase H is added and the mixture is heated at 55°C for 10 min. This step is more common in protocols where second strand synthesis will be performed.

4. AMPLIFICATION OF cDNA BY PCR

The basic components of a PCR reaction are:

1. Reaction buffer;
2. dNTPs;
3. Primers;
4. cDNA template; and
5. *Taq* DNA polymerase.

A typical PCR amplification method is detailed in Table 1. Buffer composition varies and depends on the type of enzyme being used. Most, if not all, of the commercially available *Taq* DNA polymerases are provided with an optimal buffer. A general outline for the PCR segment of RT-PCR is shown in Fig. 3.

4.1. PCR Primer Design

In RT-PCR reactions, the selection of primers is of primary importance. Effective primers are highly specific, free of secondary structure, and form stable duplexes with target sequences. Basically, four parameters need to be considered when designing a set of primers:

1. Size of the region being amplified;
2. The location of the target region within the cDNA sequence;
3. Potential secondary structure within the region; and
4. Specificity of amplification.

The size of the region being amplified should be chosen such that PCR products produced range from 400–2000 bp in length. Products <400 bp in length are difficult to resolve well using standard argarose gel techniques, and may be obscured by unconsumed primers or PCR artifacts. Products larger than 2000 bp may be amplified less efficiently owing to the limited processivity of *Taq* polymerase under standard reaction conditions *(17)*.

The location of the region to be amplified within the gene sequence needs to be considered when designing PCR primers. Since priming with an oligo(dT) often fails to generate full-length cDNA transcripts, amplification of regions located several kilobases from the 3'-end of the mRNA are often difficult if using an oligo(dT) primer. If it is necessary to obtain sequence in the 5'-region of a gene where that sequence is not known, this can usually be accomplished using 5'-RACE techniques *(16)*. Secondary structure in the mRNA template is another reason for the failure of RT to synthesize full length cDNA transcripts, so regions known to have bulky secondary structure should be avoided if possible. RNA folding algorithms capable of predicting secondary structure within regions of known sequence are available *(18)*. If primers can be positioned so that they are located on separate exons, products resulting from the

Polymerase Chain Reaction (PCR)

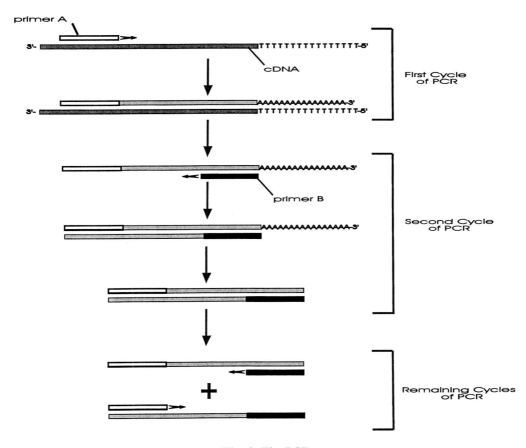

Fig. 3. The PCR.

amplification of contaminating genomic DNA can be detected. Using this technique, PCR products derived from genomic DNA will be longer than those generated from a cDNA template.

Amplification specificity depends on the primer sequence. Average primers range from 20–24 nucleotides in length. Primers of this size are usually selective enough to specify a single site in a genome of high complexity and are relatively inexpensive to synthesize. Longer primers allow higher annealing temperatures and, thus, increase the selectivity of the PCR reaction. The melting temperature of a 40-mer is estimated to be 15°C higher than that of a 20-mer of similar G:C base composition *(7)*. Using 45-mers would allow annealing to proceed at 72°C, which is the optimal temperature for *Taq* DNA polymerase. Primer annealing may be further optimized by maintaining G:C content at about 50–70%. It is also important that the 3'-ends of the primers not be complementary to each other; this will help reduce the amount of primer sequestered as primer dimers *(19)*. Some investigators suggest always including at least 2 G:C bases on the 3'-end of primers to anchor the primer at the recognition site, since G:C hydrogen binding is stronger that A:T binding. Finally, primer sequences should not share homology with sequences other than the target sequence. This will reduce the amount of nonspecific PCR products generated. Most PCR reactions require a pair of primers to amplify products. To amplify a sequence efficiently, both primers need to have similar melting temperatures. If the primers are chosen so that they are of the same approximate length and have similar G:C content, the probability that their melting temperatures will be similar is increased. Several computer algorithms and programs have been developed to facilitate the design of primers *(20,21)*.

4.2. PCR Cycle Parameters

In general, a PCR reaction consist of three cycles:

1. Denaturation;
2. Annealing; and
3. Extension.

Each cycle has a specific time and temperature that must be determined experimentally for a specific application. Optimal cycle times and temperatures may vary depending on the type and performance of the thermocycler used. The denaturation cycle usually lasts for 1 min or less at a temperature of 94°C, although time values for this cycle may vary from 30 s to 5 min. Usually the time spent at 94°C is reduced to the minimum value needed to achieve the denaturation of the template, because *Taq* has a limited half-life directly related to its exposure to high temperatures. Although 1 min does not seem long, remember that the actual exposure of *Taq* to 94°C is 1 min times the total number of cycles plus ramping time at high temperatures. The extension cycle is usually performed at 72°C for 2 min or less; 72°C is the optimal temperature for *Taq* polymerase primer extension. At this temperature, *Taq* extends the template at a rate of about 60 bases/s *(22)*.

Probably the most critical parameters of a PCR reaction are the annealing time and temperature. The maximum annealing temperature is determined by the primer with the lowest melting temperature. Exceeding this melting temperature by more than several degrees will reduce the efficiency of priming and may result in the failure to produce the product of interest. If an annealing temperature equal to the lowest primer melting temperature fails to produce a product, then it may be necessary to lower the annealing temperature. If the desired product is produced, but the number and quantities of coamplified nonspecific reaction products is unacceptable, then the annealing temperature should be raised. Optimization of the reaction conditions may require several adjustments to the annealing time and temperature. This may seem tedious, but when the power of PCR amplification is considered, reaction efficiency is crucial for product quantification. Salt concentrations also affect DNA:DNA interactions. Optimization kits, which provide *Taq* buffers with several different salts and salt concentrations, are also commercially available.

5. VISUALIZATION AND VERIFICATION OF PCR PRODUCTS

The most common method for analyzing PCR products is by gel electrophoresis followed by staining with the fluorescent dye ethidium bromide *(7)*, as shown in Fig. 4.

1 2 3 4

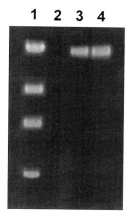

Fig. 4. Agarose gel electrophoresis of an RT-PCR product. RNA from three different rat liver epithelial cell lines were reverse transcribed and PCR was performed using gene-specific primers directed against the MOK-2 zinc-finger protein-encoding gene transcript. Lane 1, DNA size standards (2 kb, 1.2 kb, 0.8 kb, and 400 bp, descending order). Lanes 2–4, RT-PCR products from WB-F344, GN6TF, and GP7TB rat liver epithelial cell lines, respectively. Lanes 3 and 4 show the 1.9 kb MOK-2 RT-PCR amplification product.

PCR products from 200–2000 bp can be resolved quickly and efficiently on a 1.6% agarose gel. Ethidium bromide may be added to the gel before casting, or the gel may be soaked in a 0.5 µg/mL solution after electrophoretic separation of DNA products. Once the ethidium bromide has intercalated into the DNA, the DNA product can be visualized by UV illumination. Another method often used to quantify products is the incorporation of radioactive, fluorescent, or biotinylated precursor dNTPs. PCR products may be labeled by incorporating labeled nucleotides or through the use of labeled primers. Labeled products are separated by electrophoresis on either agarose or poly-acrylamide gels and visualized by the appropriate techniques (i.e., autoradiography for radioactively labeled products).

The generation of DNA products of the expected size on an agarose gel is an encouraging sign that the PCR reaction worked as expected. However, the identity of the DNA product should be verified by a secondary method while establishing a PCR procedure. Verification can be accomplished by a variety of methods, such as nucle-otide sequencing, restriction mapping, or sequence-specific probe hybridization. DNA sequencing of PCR products represents the most informative method for product veri-fication. Typically, the product DNA is cloned and sequence determined using stan-dard methods. However, with the advent of microsequencing techniques, purified PCR products can be sequenced without having to be cloned (23,24). This approach signifi-cantly shortens the time required to verify a product by eliminating the cloning step and subsequent production of false positives. In addition, it is to the advantage of the investigator to sequence a pool of PCR products rather than an individual cloned DNA because of the relatively high error rate of the *Taq* enzyme under standard PCR condi-tions. Restriction mapping of PCR products is probably the most simple verification method. To use this method, the amplified sequence must contain one or more known unique restriction sites. Thus, products may be verified by digestion with the appropriate restriction endonuclease with subsequent visualization of restriction fragments after gel electrophoresis. Sequence-specific hybridization may also be used to verify PCR products. In this method, a synthetic oligonucleotide that recognizes a unique sequence within the amplified region is hybridized to the PCR product, which is immobilized on a hybridization membrane. Successful hybridization is measured by autoradiography, and the resulting autoradiogram may be used to quantitate the amount of product produced. This method also has the added advantage that stringent hybridization and washing conditions may be used along with other probes to differentiate between related gene transcripts that are similar in size.

6. CONSIDERATIONS FOR QUANTITIVE RT-PCR

Because amplification is initially an exponential process, small differences, such as priming efficiency, can dramatically influence the final concentration of products. Even when these parameters are controlled precisely, there are often sample-to-sample and day-to-day variations that are difficult to control. This makes accurate quantitation of the initial amount of mRNA in sample by RT-PCR difficult. However, measuring the relative quantities or comparing the levels of mRNA in different samples is possible, but requires that certain standards be followed. When using PCR to compare the abundance of different cDNAs, they must be amplified with identical efficiencies. Several methods exist for measuring the efficiency of an RT-PCR reaction. In the first method, an internal mRNA standard is coreverse transcribed and coamplified with the transcript under investigation to help overcome nonspecific variations inherent in each sample. This standard is typically a synthetic RNA molecule, and for more precise measurement, may be a slightly modified version of the molecule under study *(25)*. Another method is dilution analysis, in which the RNA under analysis is serially diluted and an RT-PCR reaction is performed on each dilution. The results of the PCR reaction for each dilution are quantitated and then compared for a consistent increase in amplification. This information can then be used to calculate the concentration of the target prior to dilution. Although this discussion on the use of RT-PCR to quantify mRNA levels has centered around PCR, the complete process is composed of two steps, reverse transcription and PCR. When attempting to quantify mRNA levels, both steps must be considered. A complete analysis of all the factors involved in both steps is beyond the scope of this chapter, but has been reviewed in detail *(26)*.

7. DNA TEMPLATE CONTAMINATION: PROBLEMS AND CONCERNS

When performing RT-PCR, it is always important to be aware of potential sources of DNA contamination. The power to amplify very small amounts of DNA to detectable levels demands that special care be taken to prevent crosscontamination between different samples. This is especially true for PCR targets expected to be present in low numbers, because greater efforts are usually required to amplify these sequences. Sources of contamination include genomic DNA contamination of RNA, crosscontamination among different samples processed simultaneously, laboratory contamination of cloned targets, and carryover of PCR products. In general, the likelihood of contamination may be reduced by working in a clean laboratory, wearing clean gloves at all times, and practicing good sterile techniques when preparing reagents and performing RT-PCR experiments. Carryover products from other PCR reactions may be controlled by maintaining separate areas to handle pre- and post-PCR solutions and by using separate, dedicated pipeters with aerosol-free pipet tips and dedicated PCR solutions. In addition, when making up PCR solutions, aliquot each component into 5 or 10 reaction aliquots, so that each tube is used only once. Adherence to these guidelines will enable sources of contamination to be identified more rapidly with less expense to the investigator should contamination problems occur. A more detailed discussion of how to prevent PCR contamination can be found in recent reviews *(27,28)*.

8. POSITIVE AND NEGATIVE CONTROLS IN RT-PCR

Proper positive and negative controls must be performed throughout RT-PCR experiments. Positive controls for RT-PCR reactions should include a well-characterized RNA template source that has been proven to contain a high level of the transcript under investigation. Negative control reactions can be performed by including template RNA that is known not to contain the target transcript. Total RNA or mRNA that is not reverse transcribed can be used in control reactions to detect contamination from an outside source, such as genomic DNA or previously amplified cDNA. RT-PCR reactions containing all of the necessary components except a template source should also be performed to eliminate possible systematic contamination of buffers, dNTPs, enzyme, or water by template RNA or DNA.

9. SPECIALIZED APPLICATION OF RT-PCR

Since its introduction, RT-PCR has seen many applications in research and diagnostic laboratories. Most of these applications take advantage of the small amounts of RNA needed to perform the RT-PCR reactions. In some situations, the expression of a gene is so low that RT-PCR may be the only method by which it can be studied. Also, since RT-PCR is relatively rapid and simple to perform, the methodology is ideal when the volume of samples to be analyzed is large or when the results of such analyses must be obtained rapidly.

RT-PCR applications fall into several groups. The most common uses are detection, comparison, and quantitation of expressed genes as discussed above. In this type of application, the sequence of the transcript being studied must be known. A second type of RT-PCR application, RACE, requires sequence knowledge of only a small fragment of the 3' or 5'-end of the gene. With this information, RT-PCR can be used to clone a larger fragment of the gene quickly. A third technique, differential display, exploits RT-PCR to compare patterns of gene expression between two or more mRNA populations. Differential display RT-PCR requires no prior knowledge of mRNA sequences. In general, these applications differ by the type of primer used (Fig. 5), as discussed in the following sections.

9.1. RT-PCR Applications in the Quantitation of Specific mRNA Targets

Measuring gene expression within a single cell is an excellent example of how the RT-PCR technique can be applied to study samples of limited size. In this method, RT-PCR is coupled with the patch-clamp recording technique, allowing the collection and comparison of both electrophysiological and mRNA expression data. Electrophysical measurements are performed on a whole cell. When the recording is complete, the cell contents are aspirated through the tip of the electrode and expelled into a microcentrifuge tube. Reagents for first-strand synthesis are added to the tube and

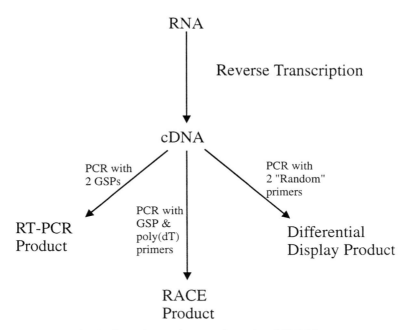

Fig. 5. Experimental strategies using RT-PCR.

reverse transcription is performed. Once cDNA synthesis is complete, PCR can be used to amplify the transcript under investigation. This type of comparison is used to correlate cell responses with their molecular counterpart. For example, in a recent paper, neuronal sodium current expression was shown to be correlated with expression of specific alternatively spliced sodium channel mRNAs in single neurons *(29)*. Single-cell RT-PCR is becoming very popular, and several recent papers are available to describe the method and its application in more detail *(3,4)*.

In some cases, the gene transcript of interest is present in such small amounts that RT-PCR may be the only method that can detect it. For example, the defective gene in patients with Duchenne and Becker Muscular Dystrophy is expressed at very low levels (0.01–0.001% of total muscle mRNA), and the mRNA is difficult to study in both normal and pathological tissue specimens because it is large (14 kb). Chelly and coworkers have successfully used RT-PCR to obtain a quantitative estimate of the dystrophin gene transcript in clinical samples by coamplifying the mRNAs of the dystrophin gene and a reporter gene, aldolase A *(30)*.

Another evolving RT-PCR application is in the quantification of gene expression. When using RT-PCR to quantify mRNA, careful attention must be given to differences in RNA loading, reverse transcription, and PCR amplification efficiencies. Considerable effort is being expended by researchers to perfect protocols that allow efficient and representative measuring of mRNA levels. For example, Dostal and coworkers have developed the multiplex RT-PCR titration assay that permits the simultaneous amplification of renin, angiotensinogen, and elongation factor-1α (EF-1α) mRNAs *(31)*. In this method, the abundant and ubiquitously expressed EF-1α mRNA is used as a control to correct for unequal RNA loading. Tube-to-tube variability in the efficiencies of reverse transcription and PCR amplification is measured by competition between endogenous target mRNAs and deletion-mutant com-

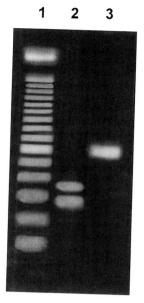

Fig. 6. Agarose gel electrophoresis of RACE RT-PCR amplification products. Lane 1, DNA size standards (100 bp ladder). Lane 2, 3'-RACE product (260 bp) generated using a gene specific primer for WDNM1 and oligo(dT). Lane 3, 5'-RACE product (600 bp) generated using a gene specific primer for WDNM1 and a primer directed against a linker sequence that was ligated to the 5'-terminus of the WDNM1 cDNA.

petitor RNA. Differences in PCR amplification efficiencies of homologous templates are corrected by titration of target mRNAs with range of concentrations of competitor RNAs.

9.2. RACE

RACE, a modification of the RT-PCR technique, is used to amplify nucleic acid sequences from an mRNA template between a defined internal site and unknown sequences at either the 3'- or the 5'-end of the mRNA *(32)*. Several different approaches to performing RACE have been described in the literature *(16,33,34)*. The method described by Chenchik and coworkers *(35)* allows both 5'- and 3'-RACE to be performed from the same cDNA template. In general, double-stranded cDNA is made by performing a first- and second-strand cDNA synthesis reaction using either total RNA or purified mRNA. The primer used to perform the first-strand synthesis is about 50 nucleotides in length, recognizes the polyA tail of the mRNA, and has a unique primer target sequence on its 5'-end. An adapter containing a second unique primer target site is ligated to both ends of the double stranded cDNA. This generates a library of double-stranded cDNAs each having a 3'-target site that differs from its 5'-target site. A specific cDNA may be amplified from this library using a gene-specific primer and a primer for either the 3' or 5' unique target site added to the cDNA sequence during synthesis. The gene-specific primer is designed from sequence information of the fragment of interest. For example, to obtain more of the 3'-sequence of a gene fragment, a PCR reaction would be performed with a gene-specific primer (designed from fragment sequence information) and a primer that matches the target added to the 3'-end of the cDNA during first-strand synthesis (Fig. 6).

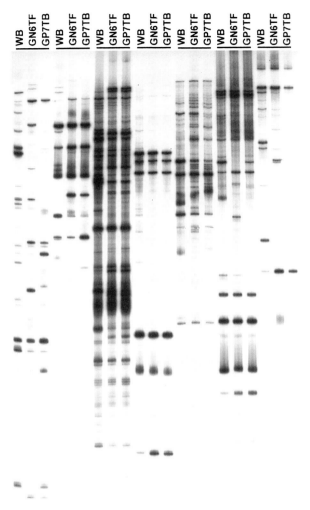

Fig. 7. RNA fingerprint gel of reaction products generated by differential display RT-PCR. The differential display RT-PCR reactions were performed on mRNA samples from WB-F344, GN6TF, and GP7TB rat liver epithelial cell lines. Each three-way comparison (indicated by bars) represents a different combination of primers consisting of oligo(dT) and random hexamers.

In an analogous manner, the 5'-sequence of a particular fragment may be obtained using a gene-specific primer and the primer that matches the target included on the adapter. RACE is an excellent method for obtaining the 3'- or 5'-sequence of a gene quickly, because very little sequence information about the target mRNA is needed. It is possible to design gene-specific primers for either 3'- or 5'-prime RACE reactions with as little as 21 nucleotides of sequence information. Race procedures are also useful for amplifying and cloning rare mRNAs that are difficult to study using conventional cloning methodologies.

9.3. Differential Display RT-PCR: RNA Fingerprint Analysis

Differential display, also referred to as RNA fingerprinting, is a modification of the basic RT-PCR method that permits the isolation and identification of RNAs that are differentially expressed in two or more RNA populations *(36)*. Like simple RT-PCR, the protocol for differential display consists of two steps, cDNA synthesis followed by PCR amplification. The two methods differ, however, in the type of primers used for the amplification reaction. The reverse transcription reaction for differential display uses a poly(dT) primer that targets the poly(A) tail of the mRNA producing a population of cDNAs with a poly(T) region located on their 5'-ends. In the PCR step, this same poly(dT) primer is used for amplification along with a short primer, usually 10 nucleotides in length, of arbitrary sequence. The short primer anneals at different positions on the cDNAs relative to the 5'-poly(T) region of the cDNA. Amplification produces a subpopulation of the cDNAs that are defined by this pair of primers. This subpopulation consists of a variety of sequences ranging in size from approx 100–700 bp in length that can be resolved on an acrylamide sequencing gel (Fig. 7). A given pair of primers produces a reproducible banding pattern on the gel referred to as an RNA fingerprint. Different primer sets provide different RNA fingerprints. Bands that are expressed in one RNA sample, but absent from another are eluted from the gel, reamplified, cloned, confirmed by Northern blot analysis, and sequenced. A number of improvements have been made to the differential display technique since it was first published *(37–39)*.

ABBREVIATIONS

RT-PCR, reverse transcription polymerase chain reaction; RT, reverse transcriptase; cDNA, complementary DNA; DEPC, diethyl pyrocarbonate; AMV RT, avian myeloblastosis virus reverse transcriptase; MMLV RT, Moloney murine leukemia virus reverse transcriptase; RACE, rapid amplification of cDNA ends.

REFERENCES

1. Shuldiner, A. R. and Huang, Z. Reducing false positives with RNA template-specific PCR (RS-PCR), in *Reverse Transcriptase PCR*, Larrick, J. W. and Siebert, P. S., eds., Ellis Horwood, London, pp. 50–60, 1995.
2. Saiki, R., Scharf S., Faloona F., Mullis, K., Horn, G., Erlich, H., and Arnheim, N. Enzymatic amplification of beta-globin genomic sequences and restriction site analysis for diagnosis of sickle cell anemia *Science* **230**:1350–1354, 1985.
3. Lambolez, B., Audinat, E., Bochet, P., and Rossier, J. RT-PCR on single cell after patch-clamp recording, in *Reverse Transcriptase PCR*, Larrick, J. W. and Siebert, P. S., eds., Ellis Horwood, London, pp. 21–49, 1995.
4. Tong, J., Bendahhou, S., Chen, H., and Agnew, W. S. A simplified method for single-cell RT-PCR that can detect and distinguish genomic DNA and mRNA transcripts. *Nucleic Acids Res.* **22**:3253–3254, 1994.
5. Ferre, F., Marchese, A., Pezzoli, P., Griffin, S., Buxton, E., and Boyer, V. Quantitative PCR: An overview, in *The Polymerase Chain Reaction*, Mullis, K. B., Ferre, F., and Gibbs, R. A., eds., Birkhauser, Boston, pp. 67–88, 1994.
6. Blumberg, D. D. Equipping a laboratory. *Methods Enzymol.* **152**:3–20, 1987.
7. Sambrook J., Fritsch E. F., and Maniatis T., eds. *Molecular Cloning: A Laboratory Manual,* 2nd ed. Cold Spring Harbor Laboratory, Cold Spring Harbor, 1989.
8. Chirgwin, J. M., Przybyla, A. E., MacDonald, R. J., and Rutter, W. J. Isolation of biologically active ribonucleic acid from sources enriched in ribonucleases. *Biochemistry* **18**:5294–5299, 1979.
9. Chomcznski, P. and Sacchi, N. Single-step method of RNA isolation by acid quanidinium thiocyanate-phenol-chloroform extraction. *Anal. Biochem.* **162**:156–159, 1987.

10. Kotewicz, M. L., D'Alessio, J. M., Driftmier, K. M., Blodgett, K. P., and Gerard, G. F. Cloning and overexpression of Maloney murine leukemia virus reverse transcriptase in *Escherichia coli*. *Gene* **35**:249–258, 1985.

11. Gerard, G. F. Comparison of cDNA synthesis by avian and cloned murine reverse transcriptase. *Focus* **7**:1–3, 1985.

12. Kotewocz, M. L., Sampson, C. M., D'Alessio, J. M., and Gerard, G. F. Isolation of cloned Moloney murine leukemia virus reverse transcriptase lacking ribonuclease H activity. *Nucleic Acids Res.* **16**:265–277, 1988.

13. Gerard, G. F., D'Alessio, J. M., and Kotewiz, M. L. cDNA synthesis by cloned Moloney murine leukemia virus reverse transcriptase lacking RNAase H activity. *Focus* **11**:66–69, 1989.

14. Gerard, G. F. and D'Alessio, J. M. Reverse transcriptase (EC 2.7.7.49). The use of cloned Moloney leukemia virus reverse transcriptase to synthesize DNA from RNA, in *Enzymes of Molecular Biology*, *Methods in Molecular Biology*, vol. 16, Burrell, M. M., ed., Humana, Totowa, NJ, pp. 73–92, 1993.

15. Borson, N. D., Sato, W. L., and Drewes, L. R. A lock–docking oligo(dT) primer for 5' and 3' RACE PCR. *PCR Methods Appl.* **2**:144–148, 1992.

16. Innis, M. A., Gelfand, D. H., Snisky, J. J., White, T. J., eds. *PCR Protocols: A Guide to Methods and Applications*. Academic, San Diego, 1990.

17. Block, W. A Biochemical perspective of the polymerase chain reaction. *Biochemistry* **30**:2735–2747, 1991.

18. Pallansch, L., Beswick, H., Talian, J., and Zelenka, O. Use of an RNA folding algorithm to choose regions for amplification by the polymerase chain reaction. *Anal. Biochem.* **185**:57–62, 1990.

19. Wu, D. Y., Ugozzoli, L., Pal, B. K., Qian, J., and Wallace, R. B. Laboratory methods: the effect of temperature and oligo nucleotide primer length on the specificity and efficiency of amplification by the polymerase chain reaction. *DNA Cell Biol.* **10**:233–238, 1991.

20. Lowe, T., Sharefkin, J., Yang, S. Q., and Diffenbach, C. W. A computer program for selection of oligonucleotide primers for polymerase chain reactions. *Nucleic Acids Res.* **18**:1757–1761, 1990.

21. Sakuma, Y. and Nishigaki, K. Computer prediction of general PCR products based on dynamical solution structures of DNA. *J. Biochem.* **116**:736–741, 1994.

22. Innis, M. A., Myambo, K. B., Gelfand, D. H., and Brow, M. A. DNA sequencing with Thermus aquaticus DNA polymerase and direct sequencing of polymerase chain reaction-amplified DNA. *Proc. Natl. Acad. Sci. USA* **85**:9436–9440, 1988.

23. Casanova, J. L., Pannetier, C., Jaulin, C., and Kourilsky, P. Optimal conditions for directly sequencing double-stranded PCR products with Sequenase. *Nucleic Acids Res.* **18**:4028, 1990.

24. Bachman, B., Luke, W., and Hunsmann, G. Improvement of PCR amplified DNA sequencing with the aid of detergents. *Nucleic Acids Res.* **18**:1309, 1990.

25. Becker-Andre, M. Evaluation of absolute mRNA levels by polymerase chain reaction-aided transcript titration assay (PATTY), in *Reverse Transcriptase PCR*, Larrick, J. W. and Siebert, P. S., eds., Ellis Horwood, London, pp. 121–149, 1995.

26. Larrick, J. W. and Siebert, P. S., eds. *Reverse Transcriptase PCR*. Ellis Horwood, London, 1995.

27. Kwok, S. and Higuchi, R. Avoiding false positives with PCR. *Nature* **339**:237–238, 1989.

28. Sarkar, G. and Sommer, S. S. Shedding light on PCR contamination. *Nature* **343**:27, 1990.

29. O'Dowd, D. K., Gee, J. R., and Smith, M. A. Sodium current density correlates with expression of specific alternatively spliced sodium channel mRNAs in single neurons. *J. Neurosci.* **15**:4005–4012, 1995.

30. Chelly, J., Kaplan, J. C., Maire, P., Gautron, S., and Kahn, A. Transcription of the dystrophin gene in human muscle and non-muscle tissue. *Nature* **333**:858–860, 1988.

31. Dostal, D. E., Rothblum, K. N., and Baker, K. M. An improved method for absolute quantification of mRNA using multiplex polymerase chain reaction: determination of renin and angiotensinogen mRNA levels in various tissues. *Anal. Biochem.* **223**:239–250, 1994.

32. Frohman, M. A., Dush, M. K., and Martin, G. R. Rapid production of full-length cDNAs from rare transcripts: amplification using a single gene-specific oligonucleotide primer. *Proc. Natl. Acad. Sci. USA* **85**:8998–9002, 1988.

33. Ohara, O. Dorit, R. L., and Gilbert, W. Direct genomic sequencing of bacterial DNA: the pyruvate kinase I gene of Escherichia coli. *Proc. Natl. Acad. Sci. USA* **86**:6883–6887, 1989.

34. Loh, E. Y., Elliott, J. F., Cwirla, S., Lanier, L. L., and Davis, M. M. Polymerase chain reaction with single-sided specificity: analysis of T cell receptor delta chain. *Science* **243**:217–220, 1989.

35. Chenchik, A., Moqadam, F., and Siebert, P. Marathon cDNA amplification: a new method for cloning full-length cDNAs. *CLONTECHniques* **X**:5–8, 1995.

36. Liang, P. and Pardee, A. Differential display of eukaryotic messenger RNA by means of the polymerase chain reaction. *Science* **257**:967–970, 1992.

37. Liang, P., Averboukh, L., and Pardee A. B. Distribution and cloning of eukaryotic mRNAs by means of differential display: refinements and optimization. *Nucleic Acids Res.* **21**:3269–3275, 1993.

38. Hadman, M., Adam, B. L., Wright, G. L., and Bos, T. J. Modifications to the differential display technique reduce background and increase sensitivity. *Anal. Biochem.* **226**:383–386, 1995.

39. Guimaraes, M. J., Lee, F., Zlotnik, A., and McClanahan, T. Differential display by PCR: novel findings and applications. *Nucleic Acids Res.* **23**:1832,1833, 1995.

PCR-Based Methods for Mutation Detection

Elizabeth M. Rohlfs and W. Edward Highsmith, Jr.

1. INTRODUCTION

Since its development in 1985 the polymerase chain reaction (PCR) has revolutionized basic and applied research *(1,2)*. With DNA or cDNA as a template, millions of copies of a target sequence are generated during the reaction. Introduction of the thermophilic *Thermus aquaticus* polymerase increased the specificity of the reaction and made automation and routine use possible *(3–5)*. The ability of PCR to produce multiple copies of a discrete portion of the genome has resulted in its incorporation into techniques used in a wide variety of research and clinical applications. Clinical applications include diagnosis of inherited disease, HLA typing, identity testing, infectious disease diagnosis, and management, hematologic disease diagnosis and staging and susceptibility testing for cancer.

The development of technically simple and reliable methods to detect sequence variations in specific genes is becoming more important as the number of genes associated with specific diseases grows. DNA sequencing is considered the "gold standard" for characterization of specific nucleotide alterations that result in genetic disease. Although sequencing technology has improved substantially over the past decade, the technique is still too cumbersome for use in screening large numbers of patient samples in a clinical setting. However, as the technology improves, sequencing may yet become fast, simple, and reproducible enough to play a role in the clinical laboratory. Until that time, there are a number of PCR-based mutation detection strategies that can be used to identify both characterized and uncharacterized mutations and sequence variations.

The degree of genetic heterogeneity, or the number of different mutations in a single gene (each of which cause a specific disorder) influences the method used for mutation detection. For diseases that exhibit no or limited heterogeneity (e.g., sickle cell anemia), assay systems designed to detect specific mutations are appropriate. For disorders in which the mutational spectrum is wide (e.g., Duchenne/Becker Muscular Dystrophy or Marfan syndrome), a scanning method is needed. A scanning method is also appropriate for analysis of newly identified disease genes, for which there is little or no information regarding the number of disease-causing mutations (e.g., the *BRCA2* gene in breast cancer).

From: Molecular Diagnostics: For the Clinical Laboratorian
Edited by: W. B. Coleman and G. J. Tsongalis Humana Press Inc., Totowa, NJ

In most applications, PCR is used to amplify specific regions of DNA known to carry or suspected of carrying a mutation. The specific DNA sequence, whether normal or mutated, is then identified by hybridization or electrophoretic separation of the PCR products. In a few techniques the PCR itself is designed to identify specifically the normal and mutant DNA sequence. In this chapter, we will discuss PCR-based techniques for the analysis of DNA and RNA in the clinical laboratory.

2. THE POLYMERASE CHAIN REACTION

The standard PCR reaction takes place in a closed tube that is subject to a series of temperature changes or cycles. The initial phase of a cycle involves heating the reaction mixture, including template, primers, polymerase, and free deoxynucleotides, to 92–96°C to denature the double-stranded template and, in subsequent cycles, the double-stranded reaction products. When the reaction mixture is cooled during the second phase of the cycle, oligonucleotide primers anneal to opposite strands of the template flanking the target sequence. The optimal annealing temperature ranges from 45–72°C and is related to the melting temperature of the primers, which is determined by their length and guanine (G) + cytosine (C) content, and the concentration of monovalent cations. In the final stage, at 72°C, the polymerase extends the primers from the 3'-ends toward each other along the template strands. The entire cycle is ordinarily repeated 25–40 times, and because the products are also used as template in subsequent reactions, there is an exponential increase in the number of copies resulting in the generation of a discrete portion of DNA which is defined by the 5'-ends of the primers.

3. FUNDAMENTALS OF HYBRIDIZATION

Hybridization is the process in which complementary nucleic acids are paired to produce DNA–DNA or DNA–RNA hybrids. The target sequence is an area of a gene that may contain a sequence variant or mutation of interest. The target sequence is probed with a fragment of DNA or RNA that is complementary to the target sequence. Binding is achieved through hydrogen bonding of complementary bases: two hydrogen bonds between adenine (A) and thymine (T) (or uracil if RNA); three hydrogen bonds between guanine (G) and cytosine (C). Hybridization can take place when both nucleic acids are in solution or when one is bound to a solid support (e.g., nylon membrane) and the other is in solution. To detect binding between the nucleic acids, one is labeled with radioactivity, digoxigenin, or biotin, and is called the "probe." The signal from a radioactively labeled probe is visualized by exposing the hybridization membrane to X-ray film, whereas other labels either fluoresce or require a subsequent colorimetric reaction for detection. The colorimetric approach is most often employed in clinical laboratories because of issues involving disposal of radioactive waste and worker safety.

Hybridization conditions are optimized for each application in order to achieve acceptable sensitivity and specificity of duplex formation (6). The efficiency of hybridization is affected by a number of factors, including:

1. Blocking reagents used;
2. The time of hybridization;
3. The volume of hybridization solution;
4. The presence of dextran sulfate or other polymer in the hybridization solution;
5. The salt concentration of the hybridization solution;

6. The solvent concentration of the hybridization solution;
7. The hybridization temperature; and
8. The washing conditions employed.

Nonspecific binding of the probe to nontarget DNA in the sample increases the background signal, but can be reduced by use of blocking agents. Typically these include Denhardt's reagent *(7)* or nonfat dried milk in combination with fragmented salmon sperm DNA and a detergent, such as SDS. The blocking agent is included in the prehybridization solution and the hybridization solution, which also includes the probe. Limiting the duration of hybridization, which can vary significantly between techniques, also reduces the background signal. Southern and northern blot hybridization can require overnight incubation, whereas hybridization with very short DNA fragments, called oligonucleotides, for dot blot and reverse dot blot analysis, can be completed in approx 1 h. The washing conditions should also be sufficiently stringent (i.e., high temperature and ionic strength and the presence of detergents, such as SDS) to remove all unbound probe and nonspecific hybridization.

In general, the volume of the hybridization solution should be kept to a minimum, but be sufficient to keep the membrane wet. The smaller the volume, the more concentrated the probe, which will increase the kinetics of duplex formation. The hybridization reaction can also be increased by addition of a polymer, such as sodium dextran sulfate. The rate of hybridization between a radiolabeled probe and genomic DNA is increased 100 times in the presence of 10% sodium dextran sulfate *(8)*; however, it is much less effective when short oligonucleotide probes are used. The increased rate of hybridization is attributed to an increase in the effective concentration of the probe by occupation of the solution volume by the polymer.

The temperature chosen for optimal hybridization is based on the melting temperature of the duplex molecule (T_m). T_m is defined as the temperature at which one-half of the probe and target strands are annealed and one-half are denatured. The T_m for a DNA:DNA duplex can be calculated using an equation that takes into consideration the salt (Na^+) and solvent (formamide) concentration of the hybridization solution and the length of the probe, as shown in Eq. (1) (Table 1) *(9)*. To optimize annealing, the actual incubation temperature is lowered 20–25°C below the calculated T_m. This usually works out to approx 42–68°C, depending on the concentration of formamide. The addition of formamide to the hybridization solution reduces the T_m by destabilizing hydrogen bonding *(10)*. There are similar equations for both RNA:RNA and RNA:DNA duplex formation.

Oligonucleotide probes are usually 19–22 bases long and designed to be specific for a particular region of DNA. The hybridization is carried out at temperatures 5–10°C below the T_m to allow perfect matches to anneal, but reduce the number of mismatches formed between sequences that differ by only one base. The presence of one mismatched base, 5 bases from the end of an oligonucleotide, reduces the T_m by 11.6°C *(11)*. Location of the mismatch at the end of the oligonucleotide does not affect the T_m as significantly as those located in the middle of the probe. Equation (2) (Table 1) can be used to calculate the T_m for oligonucleotides from 14 to approx 70 bases long *(6)*. Because of the short length of oligonucleotide probes, they form duplexes that are less stable than those of large DNA probes. Therefore, the stringency of the post-hybridization washing should be more moderate and of a shorter duration.

Table 1
Equations Related to Nucleic Acid Hybridization and Electrophoresis

Eq. (1) Determination of the melting temperature of a DNA:DNA duplex:

$$T_m = 81.5°C - 16.6 \, (\log_{10}[Na^+]) + 0.41\% \, (\%G + C) - 0.63 \, (\%formamide) - (600/l)$$

l = length of probe in base pairs

Eq. (2) Determination of the melting temperature for oligonucleotides (14–70 bases in length):

$$T_m = 81.5 - 16.6 \, (\log_{10}[Na^+] + 0.41 \, (\%G + C) - (600/l)$$

l = length of probe in base pairs

Eq. (3) Electrophoretic driving force:

$$F = (X) \, (Q) = (V) \, (Q)/l$$

F = the force driving the ion forward
X = the electric field strength or voltage drop
Q = the charge on the analyte molecule
V = the applied voltage
l = the length of the gel

Eq. (4) Stokes' Law:

$$F' = 6 \, \pi \, r \, \eta \, v$$

F' = the counterforce
π = a constant (3.14159)
r = the radius of the analyte
η = the viscosity of the matrix
v = the velocity of the analyte movement (l/t)

Eq. (5) Derivations from Stokes' Law and the driving force equation (when F = F'):

$$(X) \, (Q) = 6 \, \pi \, r \, \eta \, v$$

or

$$v/X = Q/6 \, \pi \, r \, \eta = \mu$$

v/X = analyte velocity through the gel matrix (cm/s) per unit field strength (V/cm)
μ = electrophoretic mobility (cm^2/V · s)

The use of a calculated T_m to predict the optimal hybridization temperature is complicated by differences in G + C content when more than one oligonucleotide is included in a hybridization solution. Pools of oligonucleotides are often used to detect mutant and/or wild-type sequence for disease diagnosis. To eliminate the effect of G + C content on the T_m, TMAC1* can be substituted for sodium chloride in the hybridization solution *(12)*. TMAC1 binds to A + T to prevent their preferential melting, making the melting temperature (and the incubation temperature) dependent on the length of the oligonucleotide. Since the melting temperature of A + T is shifted to that of G + C by TMACl, the melting profile is also significantly sharpened. For example, a duplex that melts over a 5–10°C range in the presence of Na$^+$ will melt within 1°C in a TMACl solution. The optimal hybridization temperature is usually set at 5°C less than the dissociation temperature or T_d. The T_d for an 18-bp oligonucleotide in 3.0M TMACl has been estimated to be 57–58°C *(12)*.

*See p. 157 for list of abbreviations used in this chapter.

4. APPLICATIONS OF HYBRIDIZATION TECHNIQUES IN THE DNA DIAGNOSTIC LABORATORY

4.1. Detection of Known Mutations and Sequence Variants by ASO Hybridization or Dot Blot

Alternative forms of genes exist owing to normal genetic variation or mutation. Each form of a gene is referred to as an allele. For example, an individual who is a carrier of CF can be described as having one wild-type (normal) CF allele and one mutant CF allele. ASO hybridization detects specific alleles through hybridization with complementary (and therefore specific) nucleic acid probes. The procedure originally utilized relatively large quantities of genomic DNA and required enzymatic and electrophoretic purification of the target sequence prior to hybridization *(13)*. PCR has improved and simplified this technique by greatly increasing the quantity of DNA target sequence *(14)*. A sufficient quantity of target sequence can be amplified by PCR from as little as 1 ng of genomic DNA and produce a signal when spotted on a nylon membrane and probed. The labeled ASO probes are approx 20 bases long and hybridize to the area in which the mutation or sequence variant is located. A mismatch between the probe and the target DNA destabilizes the hybridization and, under the proper conditions, prevents annealing. To analyze various alleles that only differ by one base, very specific and stringent conditions are required to prevent crosshybridization. If two alleles are to be typed, the DNA of interest and control DNA are both spotted on two separate membranes and probed with the individual oligonucleotides. Therefore, if an individual is heterozygous for the base change, a signal will be present on both membranes. Genotyping CF patients and their carrier parents by this method demonstrated the high frequency of the 3-bp deletion, $\Delta F508$ *(15)*. ASO hybridization has been used to screen for *RAS* gene mutations in acute myeloid leukemia *(16)*, identify mutations in platelet glycoproteins, *(17)* and identify the α_1-antitrypsin variant, α_1-AT Pittsburgh *(18)*.

Deletions account for approx 65% of the known mutations in DMD and Becker Muscular Dystrophy *(19)*. The location of the deletion in the proband can be determined by multiplex PCR, but carrier status of female relatives cannot be assigned by this method. Dosage analysis by densitometric evaluation of an ASO signal intensity can be used to determine carrier status *(20)*. Amplification of the target sequence must be limited to the exponential phase of the PCR reaction for accurate quantification of the product. A nondeleted exon is also amplified, and the ratio of the signal intensities from a control individual and the individual in question is compared. The signal intensity ratio of a carrier is approximately half that of a control individual.

When developing an ASO procedure, both sense and antisense oligonucleotides should be evaluated. A significant difference in signal intensity was observed when differentiating between the β^A and β^S alleles of the β-globin gene using sense or antisense oligonucleotide probes *(21)*. It was determined that more sense strand formed during amplification, resulting in a stronger signal from the antisense probe. This asymmetric amplification of PCR products was most likely the result of differences in primer annealing temperature.

Modification of the oligonucleotide probes by covalent attachment of horseradish peroxidase has made ASO hybridization more clinically useful, since use of radioactivity in clinical laboratories is frequently discouraged *(22)*. The signal is visualized

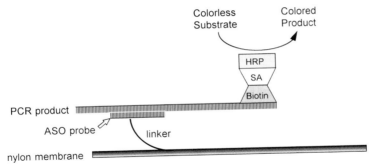

Fig. 1. Schematic representation of reverse dot blot technique. An ASO probe is joined to a nylon membrane by either a deoxyribothymidine tail or an amine group (linker). The biotin-labeled complementary PCR product hybridizes to the membrane-bound probe and is detected by a colorimetric reaction catalyzed by horseradish peroxidase (HRP). The HRP is attached to streptavidin (SA), which binds with the biotin of the PCR product.

as a blue precipitate, but is less intense than that seen with radioactive probes. However, the enzymatic probes are stable for up to 1 yr, and with good amplification of the target DNA, they produce an easily visualized signal.

4.2. Detection of Known Mutations and Sequence Variants by Reverse Dot Blot

Although the ASO/PCR method is a powerful technique for the detection of sequence variants, screening individual samples for multiple allelic variants requires multiple hybridization reactions. The reverse dot blot method eliminates this disadvantage by bonding multiple ASOs to a nylon membrane as individual spots *(23,24)*. Both the mutant and wild-type oligonucleotides are immobilized on the solid support, which is then hybridized with the target PCR product (Fig. 1). Each sample produces at least one signal indicating homozygosity (two identical alleles) or two signals for heterozygosity (two different alleles).

The oligonucleotides may be bound to the membrane by adding long 3'-deoxyribothymidine tails (poly[dT]) using terminal deoxyribonucleotidyltransferase. The poly(dT) tails bind the oligonucleotides to the membrane by forming crosslinks to the nylon when exposed to UV light. However, variable sensitivity of the signal owing to variable length of the poly(dT) tail has been reported *(25)*. Alternatively, a primary reactive amine group with a linker that can be covalently attached to the membrane is added to the 5'-end of the oligonucleotide *(24,26)*. Although multiple ASOs are attached to a single membrane and hybridized in one reaction with the target DNA, to maintain the efficiency of the assay, the oligonucleotides must be designed to hybridize under the same temperature and salt conditions. Factors affecting hybridization stability include length of the oligonucleotide, the type of mismatch, and the position of the mismatch. Better discrimination is achieved with shorter probes, when the mismatch is in the middle of the probe, and by avoiding G · T mismatches. It is also possible to pool several probes in one spot when screening for many possible alleles *(26)*.

Detection of probe–target duplexes is accomplished using biotinylated primers or biotinylated dUTP in the PCR reaction *(25)*. When hybridization of the PCR product

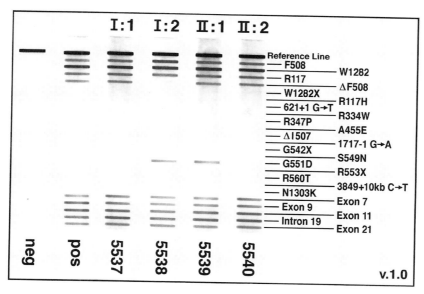

Fig. 2. Reverse dot blot analysis for 16 CF mutations. The father (I:1, 5537) is a carrier of the ΔF508 mutation, the mother (I:2,5538) is a carrier of the G551D mutation, and the affected child (II:1, 5539) carries both the ΔF508 and G551D mutations. The unaffected child (II:2, 5540) carries only the ΔF508 mutation. Pos indicates the positive control; neg indicates the negative control (courtesy of Sarah Adkins, Molecular Genetics Laboratory, University of North Carolina Hospitals).

has occurred, the biotin binds streptavidin–horseradish peroxidase, which converts a colorless substrate, tetramethylbenzidine, to a visible chromagen. Biotin will also bind avidin–alkaline phosphatase, which converts nitroblue tetrazolium salt to a blue precipitate or reacts with adamantyl 1,2-dioxetane phosphate to produce light *(25)*.

The reverse dot blot is particularly suited for diagnostic screening when many different mutations produce disease, each at a relatively low frequency, as in CF and β-thalassemia. Cuppens et al. amplified six *CFTR* exons in one multiplex PCR reaction and hybridized the products to 21 different oligonucleotides representing 11 different mutations *(27)*. Using this analysis, they were able to detect 85% of all the CF mutations in the Belgian population. A reverse dot blot in a strip format has been developed by Roche Molecular Systems (Somerville, NJ) and is under evaluation at the University of North Carolina Hospitals Molecular Genetics Laboratory. Eight different regions of the *CFTR* gene are amplified in a single PCR reaction and then hybridized to 16 CF mutation ASOs, which are bound to a nylon membrane. Figure 2 shows results from a family with one child who is affected with CF and one who is a carrier. The father (I:1) carries the ΔF508 mutation and the mother (I:2) the G551D mutation. The affected child (II:1) has received one mutation from each parent. (Two mutated alleles are necessary in order to be affected with CF). The unaffected brother (II:2) has only the ΔF508 mutation and is a carrier. Similarly, 95% of the β-thalassemia mutations worldwide can be detected by amplifying four regions of the β-globin gene followed by reverse dot blot analysis of the products using probes specific for 42 mutations *(28,29)*. Furthermore, in addition to diagnosis of inherited disease, the reverse dot blot technique has proven sensitive and specific enough to detect fewer than 100 mycobacteria in a clinical sample and to differentiate five different mycobacterial species *(30)*.

Allele-specific hybridization techniques are useful for the identification of previously characterized mutations and sequence variants. Other techniques for the identification of specific alleles utilize electrophoretic separation of PCR products. Many electrophoretic applications have also been developed to scan entire genes for previously uncharacterized mutations and sequence variants.

5. FUNDAMENTALS OF ELECTROPHORESIS

Electrophoresis refers to the migration of charged molecules through a liquid or gel medium under the influence of an electric field. Zone electrophoresis, or the migration of macromolecules through a porous support medium or gel, is almost universally used in molecular biology laboratories today. Electrophoresis (all discussion in this chapter will involve zone electrophoresis, but will be referred to as electrophoresis for brevity) is a powerful separation tool, being able to detect the differential migration of macromolecules with only subtly different structures.

The rate of migration of a macromolecule through a gel matrix is dependent on several factors, including:

1. The net charge on the molecule at the pH at which the assay is conducted;
2. The size and shape of the molecule;
3. The electric field strength or voltage drop;
4. The pore size of the gel; and
5. Temperature.

The forces acting on the analyte to drive it through the gel are the charge on the molecule and the electric field strength. Equation (3) describes the electrophoretic driving force (Table 1). The forces acting to retard the movement of the molecule are the frictional forces, determined by the velocity of the analyte, the pore size of the gel, and the size and shape of the molecule. The opposition of the acceleration of the analyte by the frictional forces is described by Stokes' Law, as shown in Eq. (4) (Table 1). When the electrophoretic driving force equals the frictional force (F = F'), the result is a constant velocity of the analyte molecule through the gel matrix (Eq. [5], Table 1). The term v/X describes the velocity of the analyte through the gel matrix (cm/s) per unit field strength (V/cm) under constant conditions (i.e., the same buffer conditions and the same gel viscosity). This term (given by the symbol μ) is defined as the electrophoretic mobility of the analyte (expressed as $cm^2/V \cdot s$). From the units of the electrophoretic mobility, it can be seen that if the gel is run under constant voltage conditions (V/cm constant) for a given period of time (seconds), then $(cm^2/V \cdot s)(V \cdot s/cm)$ = distance of migration (in cm). Thus, if gels are run such that the product of the voltage and the time are constant, the same analyte will migrate the same distance into the gel. For convenience, this is typically expressed as volt-hours. For example, if one gel is run at 50 V for 10 h (500 Vh) and an identical gel (constant length, viscosity, and buffer concentration) is run at 100 V for 5 h (500 Vh), the same analyte will appear at the same position on both gels. This ability to reproduce gel profiles is one of the principal reasons that constant voltage run conditions are preferred for DNA analysis. An exception to this is the pre-

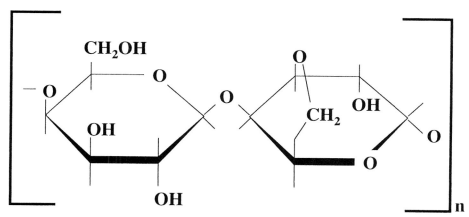

Fig. 3. Agarbiose molecule. Structure of agarbiose, the repeating subunit of agarose.

ferred conditions for DNA sequencing. Although a full discussion of sequencing technology is beyond the scope of this chapter, it should be pointed out that sequencing gels are run at elevated temperature to ensure the adequate denaturation of the single-stranded DNA molecules; in this case, running the gel at constant watts is helpful in maintaining an even heating of the gel.

In protein analysis, the pH of the electrophoresis buffer can be a powerful tool in optimizing specific separations. This is because the type (acidic or basic) and number of ionizable groups found on proteins are variable. However, for DNA analysis, it is the charge of the phosphate backbone that is dominant. Therefore, DNA electrophoresis is typically performed at a slightly alkaline pH to ensure full ionization of the phosphate residues.

5.1. The Gel Matrix: Agarose

There are two types of gel matrix in common use in DNA laboratories: agarose and polyacrylamide. Agarose is a polysaccharide commercially derived from seaweed. The agarose polymer consists of multiple agarbiose molecules linked together into linear chains with an average mol wt of 120 kDa. The agarbiose subunit is a disaccharide consisting of β-D-galactose and 3,6-anhydro-α-L-galactose. (Fig. 3) *(31)*. The partially purified material, agar, consists of noncharged polymer chains, agarose, and negatively charged chains. The negative charges are typically owing to sulfate (SO_4) residues. In general, the more highly purified the agarose, the lower the sulfate concentration, the higher the quality of the separation, and the higher the price. Agarose is supplied as a white, nonhydroscopic powder. A gel is prepared by mixing agarose powder with buffer, boiling the mixture, pouring the molten gel into a casting tray, and cooling. During this process, the agarose chains shift from existing in solution as random coils to a structure in which the chains are bundled into double helices. The average pore size for agarose gels is typically in the range of 100–300 nm³. Agarose gels are used at concentrations near 1% (w/v) for separating DNA fragments in the 1–20 kb size range. Examples of applications common in the DNA diagnostic laboratory include restriction digestion analysis of large plasmids and Southern transfer analysis of genomic DNA.

Recently, a series of chemically modified agaroses with smaller pore sizes have been developed by scientists at FMC BioProducts (Rockland, ME). These modified gel matrices are prepared by melting and casting similarly to unmodified agarose, but owing to the smaller pore sizes, are very useful for DNA separations in the 100–1000-bp size range. These products are marketed under the trade names NuSieve and MetaPhor Agaroses (FMC BioProducts).

5.2. The Gel Matrix: Polyacrylamide

The advent of PCR has had profound effects on the clinical laboratory's ability to use the tools of molecular biology for clinical diagnostic testing. However, it is important to understand the effect that PCR technology has had on the availability and choice of electrophoretic techniques in the clinical laboratory. The principal effect of PCR on the practice of electrophoresis has been to shift the size of the analytes from large fragments of DNA, as used in the Southern transfer, to small fragments of DNA, typically from 100–1000 bp in length. The chemically modified agaroses (which have been optimized for the separation of low-mol-wt DNA fragments) are the most commonly used matrices for the analysis of PCR products. For very high resolution, it is necessary to use polyacrylamide gels.

Polyacrylamide gels are prepared from a monomer, acrylamide, and a crosslinker, typically bis-acrylamide. (**Note:** Acrylamide is a potent neurotoxin and is readily absorbed through the skin. When using acrylamide in aqueous solution, wear gloves and a lab coat. When weighing powdered acrylamide, wear goggles and perform the weighing operation in a chemical hood.) The first step in preparing a polyacrylamide gel is to add a free radical initiator to a solution of monomer and crosslinker. The most commonly used initiator system is TEMED and APS (Fig. 4). APS reacts with the TEMED to form a TEMED derivative with a free, or unpaired electron. This type of molecule is termed a free radical and is highly reactive. The TEMED radical reacts with an acrylamide molecule, forming a TEMED–acrylamide radical. This first step of the polymerization process is termed chain initiation. The next step is chain elongation, in which the polymer chain grows by repetitive addition of acrylamide monomers to the growing chain with the free radical terminus. Chain branching occurs when a bis-acrylamide molecule is added to the end of the chain. Chain termination occurs when two free radicals react, giving a stable compound with paired electrons. In order to achieve complete polymerization, it is important that compounds that quench free radical reactions, such as alcohols or oxygen, be excluded from the reaction mixture. Oxygen is typically removed from the acrylamide/bis-acrylamide solution by degassing under vacuum for 15–30 min prior to the addition of the initiators. To avoid oxygen contact during the polymerization process, the gel is generally cast between two glass plates. After polymerization, the gel is run in a vertical format.

The pore size of the final polyacrylamide gel is determined by the concentration of the acrylamide monomer and the ratio of the crosslinker to monomer. These parameters are referred to as %T and %C, respectively, and are defined as follows: %T = mass of all monomers and crosslinkers/100 mL vol, and %C = mass of the crosslinker/mass of all monomers and crosslinkers/100 mL volume. The pore sizes in polyacrylamide gels are typically much smaller than those in agarose gels. Thus, they are used for DNA fragments of smaller size. Gels with %C of approx 3–5% and %T ranging from 5–15%

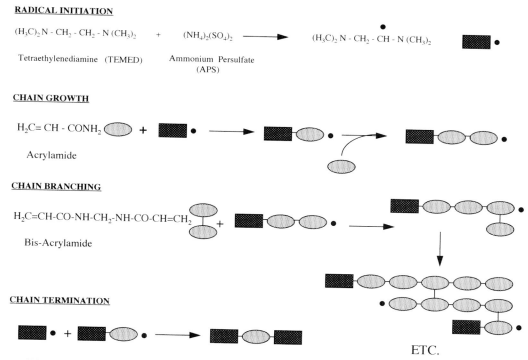

Fig. 4. Schematic demonstrating the polymerization of acrylamide and bis-acrylamide monomers. TEMED is represented by ■; acrylamide is represented by ⬭; bis-acrylamide monomer is represented by ⬯; and the unpaired electron in free radicals is represented by •.

are the most often used gels in the DNA laboratory, giving superior separations in the 100–1000 bp size range.

A series of gel products with improved performance for specific applications were developed by scientists at AT Biochem (Malvern, PA). These materials use acrylamide as a monomer, but incorporate proprietary co-monomers and novel crosslinkers. Recently, this line of products has been acquired by FMC BioProducts. A gel matrix offering longer reads for DNA sequencing and a matrix optimized for the detection of conformational changes in single-strand conformation polymorphism or heteroduplex analysis are currently marketed under the trade names Long Ranger and Mutation Detection Enhancement Gel (or MDE gel), respectively.

6. APPLICATIONS OF ELECTROPHORESIS IN THE DNA DIAGNOSTIC LABORATORY

There are two general types of problems that are readily solved by electrophoretic techniques in the molecular laboratory. The first is the need to assess the size of DNA fragments accurately; the second is the need to identify both characterized and uncharacterized mutations or sequence variants.

6.1. Sizing of DNA Fragments by Electrophoresis

The need to determine the size of DNA fragments is a common occurrence in the molecular laboratory. Examples include verification of the identity of cloned DNA fragments by restriction enzyme digestion, determination of the size of a band detected by Southern transfer, and verification of the size of a PCR product.

The size range of DNA fragments separable by any gel system is a function of the pore size of the matrix (this parameter is related to the viscosity of the matrix shown in Eq. [4], Table 1). The pore size is primarily a function of concentration in agarose gels and %T and %C in acrylamide gels. Even though the optimum separation ranges for different gels vary widely, they all have the same general profile. For all gels, there will be a region of optimal separation that is proportional to the log of the size of the DNA fragment. Similarly, there will be a point at which all DNA fragments are smaller than the effective pore size and will be not be retarded by the gel matrix, and a point at which all DNA fragments are too large for any of the gel pores. At these two points, mobility is independent of molecular size and all DNA fragments above or below these limits comigrate. In the laboratory, size determinations are typically made by comparison to a size marker that has been run on the same gel as the unknown sample. A variety of size markers containing DNA fragments of known length are commercially available. A standard curve is prepared by plotting the log of the migration distance of each band in the size marker vs its size in base pairs. The migration distance of the unknown band is plotted and the size of the fragment read off the graph.

6.2. Single-Stranded Conformational Polymorphism (SSCP) Analysis for Detection of Mutations and Sequence Variants

SSCP analysis is one of the most widely used mutation scanning systems. The reasons for its popularity are its high sensitivity to the presence of sequence variations and its technical simplicity. The technique, developed in Hayashi's laboratory and first reported in 1989, involves PCR amplification of the region of the gene to be studied, denaturation of the double-stranded PCR product by heat, and electrophoresis on a nondenaturing polyacrylamide gel *(32)*. During the electrophoresis, the single-stranded DNA fragments fold into a three-dimensional shape according to their primary sequence. The separation then becomes a function of the shape of the single-stranded molecules. If wild-type and mutant PCR products differ in their sequence, even by only a single nucleotide, they will likely adopt different three-dimensional structures and exhibit different electrophoretic mobilities (Fig. 5). Figure 6 shows SSCP analysis of three breast tumor cell lines with mutations in exon 8 of the *p53* gene *(33,34)*.

In order to prevent the two single strands from reannealing to form double-stranded DNA, the concentration of DNA in the loading buffer is kept very low. Thus, in order to visualize the bands, radioactive labeling of the DNA is typically required. However, as an alternative, silver staining seems to give adequate sensitivity and is increasing in popularity.

The issue of sensitivity of mutation scanning methods is a difficult one. Sensitivity is likely to be influenced by many factors, including, but not limited to, type of base substitution, length of the fragment examined, the local base sequences, the G + C content of the DNA fragment, and the location of the sequence variation relative to the ends of the fragment. For each of the mutation scanning methods, with the sole exception of denaturing gradient gel electrophoresis, there is no precise theory that can be used to predict whether a given method will detect a particular mutation. Thus, the only determinations of sensitivity of mutation scanning methods have been empirical. Typi-

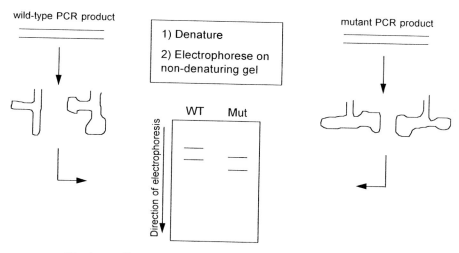

structure = f(sequence) and electrophoretic mobility = f(structure)

Fig. 5. Schematic representation of SSCP analysis. In SSCP analysis, the electrophoretic mobilities of the single-stranded DNA species are a function of their three-dimensional conformation. This conformation is determined by the most thermodynamically favored intrastrand base-pairing, which, in turn, is directly determined by the primary sequence. Thus, if two DNA fragments differ in sequence, they will fold into different conformations and exhibit different electrophoretic mobilities.

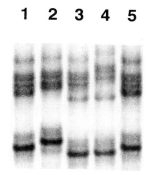

Fig. 6. Detection of *p53* sequence variants by SSCP analysis. A 183-bp fragment of exon 8 of the *p53* gene was amplified from DNA extracted from four different breast tumor cell lines and human placenta (wild-type control). ^{32}P labeled dATP was included in the PCR to label the products that were separated by electrophoresis through a 0.5X MDE gel at room temperature. Lane 1, wild-type control; lane 2, MDA-MB-231 cells; lane 3, MDA-MB-468 cells; lane 4, Bt-474 cells; lane 5 SkBr3 cells. The cell lines in lanes 2–4 contain mutations in exon 8 resulting in aberrant migration of the PCR products (courtesy of Lori Terry and J. Carl Barrett, Laboratory of Molecular Carcinogenesis, NIEHS).

cally, studies of sensitivity have used a set of previously characterized mutations found in the gene that the author is studying. Few of the variables listed above are addressed in most studies, and no study to date has addressed them all.

The reported sensitivity of SSCP has ranged from 35 to near 100%. Sheffield and colleagues used a set of artificial mutants originally created by Myers et al. to study the effect of sequence variation on the promoter region of the mouse β-globin gene *(35,36)*. They demonstrated a pronounced effect of fragment length on sensitivity. At low fragment sizes (100–150 bp), SSCP had a sensitivity approaching 100%; however, when the length increased to 500 bp, the sensitivity dropped to approx 50%. Running the SSCP gels under different conditions has been reported to increase sensitivity, as has running the gels on specialty matrices, such as MDE *(37)*. Approximately 20% of recent SSCP reports have used MDE instead of standard formulations of acrylamide. Currently, many large laboratories run SSCP gels under several electrophoretic conditions (e.g., at room temperature and at 4°C, and with gels containing zero or 10% glycerol) The use of multiple run conditions can raise the sensitivity of the technique to virtually 100% *(38)*.

6.3. Heteroduplex Analysis (HA) in Mutation Detection

HA is a mutation scanning method based on the electrophoretic resolution of wild-type double-stranded DNA fragments from fragments of identical length and sequence, but having one base-pair mismatch. The mismatch is formed when a wild-type DNA fragment is mixed with a mutant DNA fragment. When the mixture is heated to denature the double-stranded material and allowed to cool and reanneal the single-stranded molecules, four types of molecules result:

1. Wild-type DNA—formed when the Watson strand of the wild-type reanneals with the Crick strand of the wild-type;
2. Mutant DNA—formed when the Watson strand of the mutant reanneals with the Crick strand of the mutant; and
3. Two heteroduplex species, formed when the Watson strand of the wild-type reanneals with the Crick strand of the mutant and when the Watson strand of the mutant reanneals with the Crick strand of the wild-type (Fig. 7).

Two types of heteroduplexes exist, the structures of which have been predicted by Bhattacharyya and Lilley *(39)*. The first type is formed when the sequence difference between the two DNA fragments is one or more point mutations; the resulting heteroduplex is termed a "bubble" type heteroduplex. The second type is formed when the sequence difference between the two fragments is a small insertion or deletion; the resulting heteroduplex is termed a "bulge" type heteroduplex. Although "bulges" result in a large structural perturbation from the double-stranded homoduplex and are readily resolvable on polyacrylamide gels, the change in overall structure owing to a "bubble" is much more subtle, and these heteroduplexes typically are not resolvable from the homoduplexes on agarose or polyacrylamide gels.

In 1991, a communication from Bhattacharyya's laboratory reported the superior separation of heteroduplex species on Hydrolink D-5000 (AT Biochem) *(40)*. (**Note:** This gel matrix is no longer commercially available). Since the proprietary formulation of D-5000 had not been developed for increased resolution of heteroduplexes, the results were a surprise to the scientists at AT Biochem who developed it. However, they quickly responded to the challenge of reformulating the material for optimum heteroduplex resolution. The resulting product, MDE, has made HA a viable technique for mutation detection. The development and properties of the Hydrolink series of gel matrixes have been described *(41)*. Figure 8 shows HA of exon 10 of the *CFTR* gene.

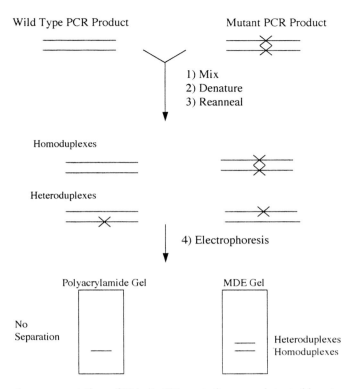

Fig. 7. Schematic representation of HA. In HA mutations are detected by structural perturbations in the double-stranded DNA duplex owing to the presence of one or more mismatches. Heteroduplexes owing to single-base mismatches are not detected with high sensitivity on agarose or polyacrylamide, but are typically resolved on specialty matricies, such as MDE (FMC BioProducts).

The samples with mutations and sequence variants are characterized by the presence of extra bands with aberrant migration.

Although no comprehensive analysis of the sensitivity of the technique has been published, a recent study by Pignatti's laboratory is typical *(42)*. In this study, the authors compared the rate of detection of SSCP and HA using a set of known mutations. Although neither technique was 100% sensitive, HA detected slightly more mutations (14 of 15) than did SSCP (10 of 15 using two electrophoretic conditions) using the same templates. The authors note that the combination of SSCP and HA detected all of the known mutations. Thus, these authors suggest using both techniques for maximum sensitivity. A bibliography of HA and SSCP analysis using MDE gels is available from FMC BioProducts.

6.4. Mutation Detection Using Denaturing Gradient Gel Electrophoresis (DGGE)

DGGE was one of the first scanning methods used for the identification of mutations in DNA *(43)*. The method is based on the principle that the denaturation, or melting, of double-stranded DNA, by heat or denaturants, such as hydroxide ion, urea, or by formamide, does not occur in a single step. Rather, DNA melts in domains. As the temperature or the denaturant concentration rises, the region or domain with the high-

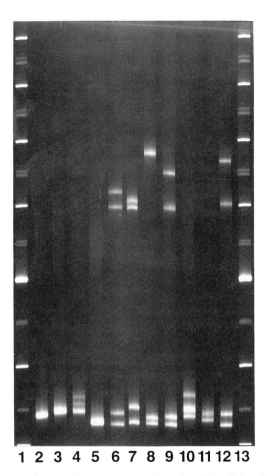

1 2 3 4 5 6 7 8 9 10 11 12 13

Fig. 8. Detection of mutations and sequence variants by HA of the *CFTR* gene. Exon 10 of the *CFTR* gene was amplified by PCR for HA. The gel is 1.5 mm thick by 40 cm long, 1X MDE (FMC BioProducts) containing 15% urea. The gel was run for 21,000 Vh in 0.6X Tris-borate-EDTA buffer and stained with ethidium bromide. Lanes 1 and 13 are size markers (100 bp ladder); lane 2 is an MM homozygote at position 470; lane 3 is a VV homozygote at position 470; lane 4 is a heterozygote for the M470V polymorphism; lane 5 is a homozygote for the ΔF508 mutation; lane 6 is a ΔI507/wild-type heterozygote; lane 7 is a compound heterozygote for ΔF508 and I506V; lane 8 is compound heterozygote for ΔF508 and F508C; lane 9 is a compound heterozygote for ΔF508 and Q493X; lane 10 is an I506V/wild-type heterozygote; lane 11 is a F508C/wild-type heterozygote; lane 12 is a ΔF508/wild-type heterozygote.

est A + T content will melt first. If the temperature or the denaturant concentration is kept constant, the DNA structure composed of double-stranded DNA and a single region of single-stranded character will be stable. If the temperature is increased again, the region with the next highest A + T content will melt next. This melting by domain continues until the region with the highest G + C content is melted and the character of the DNA is completely single-stranded. Since the identity of the melting domains is a function of the base sequence, a change in the base sequence (i.e., a mutation) will likely change the melting profile (Fig. 9). If the mutation does not alter the melting

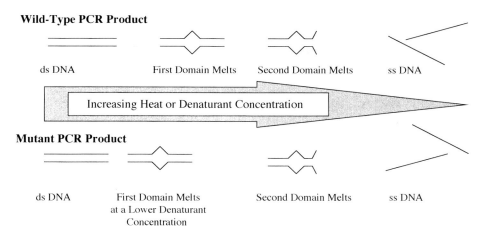

Fig. 9. DNA melts in domains. When treated with heat or chemical denaturants (urea or formamide), double-stranded DNA does not melt all at once; rather it melts in domains.

profile, it will not be detected. However, if a heteroduplex is formed and then subjected to melting analysis, a change in melting profile will almost certainly be seen. Thus, for maximum sensitivity, DNA heteroduplexes are formed between a control DNA fragment of known sequence and the test DNA.

The melting profile of heteroduplex DNA is observed by electrophoresis on a transverse denaturing gradient gel. In this system, a polyacrylamide gel is poured containing a gradient of denaturant, typically urea and formamide. After polymerization, the gel is rotated 90°, the DNA heteroduplex sample is applied to a single trough-like well, and the electrophoresis is carried out. The DNA migrating through the region of the gel with the lowest denaturant concentration migrates as typical double-stranded (DNA); the DNA migrating through the denaturant concentration corresponding to the first melting domain will migrate with significantly lower mobility; the DNA migrating through the region corresponding to the next melting domain will migrate more slowly still. This step function of decreasing mobility continues until the highest melting-point domain denatures, yielding rapidly moving single-stranded DNA. After visualization of the DNA with ethidium bromide or silver, a stair-step pattern is seen. In the case of a heteroduplex sample, the domain containing the mismatch will melt early, yielding a characteristic doublet pattern. (Fig. 10).

Clearly, pouring gradient gels and analyzing samples one at a time is labor-intensive and time consuming. Fortunately, the melting profile of any DNA fragment can be modeled mathematically. Computer programs are commercially available that calculate the melting profile for PCR-amplified DNA *(44)*. Using this tool, gradients can be optimized for each piece of DNA. Using optimized gradients, gels can be run in a more conventional manner, i.e., with the electrophoresis driving the DNA into ever higher denaturant concentrations. In this format, a sample bearing a low melting domain, such as a heteroduplex, will exhibit a band of slower mobility (Fig. 11).

In theory, mutations in the highest melting domain will not be detected by DGGE because it is difficult to determine electrophoretically the exact point at which the transition from the slow migrating species (with the last melting domain intact) to the rapidly

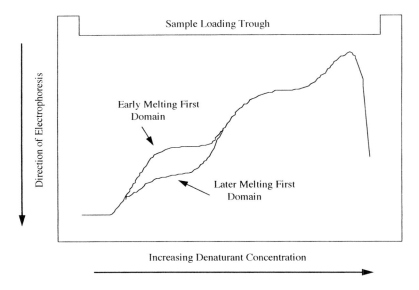

Sample Loading Trough

Direction of Electrophoresis

Early Melting First
Domain

Later Melting First
Domain

Increasing Denaturant Concentration

Fig. 10. Schematic representation of a transverse denaturing gradient gel experiment. The direction of electrophoresis is from top to bottom and the denaturant concentration increases from left to right. Shown is the melting profile of the DNA fragments represented in Fig. 9. The first domain in the mutant PCR product melts at a lower denaturant concentration than the first domain of the wild-type product. Thus, the mobility transition occurs further to the left (lower denaturant concentration) for the mutant product, giving the characteristic "cat's eye" pattern.

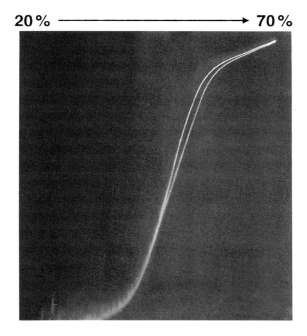

20% ⟶ 70%

Fig. 11. Example of an actual DGGE analysis.

migrating single-stranded species occurs. In order to eliminate this caveat to the technique, a "GC clamp" is typically added to the amplified product by preparing one of the PCR primers with a 5'-tail of 30–50 nucleotides of 100% G + C content. Thus, the artificial "GC clamp" becomes the highest melting domain, and mutations in all of the original domains can be detected *(45)*. Although the sensitivity of DGGE for the detection of unknown mutations approaches 100%, the popularity of the method seems to be decreasing because of the expense of PCR primers that are 70–80 nucleotides in length, the difficulty in amplification with primers of such high melting temperatures, and the difficulties associated with the need to prepare reproducible gradient gels freshly.

6.5. Mutation Detection by Chemical Cleavage of Mismatched Nucleotides (CCM)

The CCM technique, described by Cotton et al. in 1988, takes advantage of the differential reactivity of perfectly paired and mismatched bases to chemical-modifying reagents *(46)*. In heteroduplex species in which a thymine nucleotide is mismatched, the T-residue is hypersusceptible to chemical modification by osmium tetroxide (OSO_4, a commonly used shadowing reagent for electron microscopy) *(46)*. Similarly, mismatched cytosine nucleotides are hypersusceptible to attack by hydroxylamine ($HONH_2$). DNA strands containing either a modified T- or C-nucleotide are then cleaved with piperidine ($C_5H_{11}N$). In practice, the DNA to be screened for mutations is amplified then mixed with a 5 to 10-fold molar excess of wild-type amplicon. This control DNA, referred to as the probe, is typically labeled on one strand with ^{32}P. After mixing, melting, and reannealing, the resultant heteroduplexes are divided into two aliquots. One aliquot is treated with osmium tetroxide and the other with hydroxylamine. After treatment with these reagents, the samples are treated with piperidine and separated by electrophoresis on a sequencing-type polyacrylamide gel. If a mutation is present, it will be detected as an extra band after autoradiography. If the sample is tested twice, once with each strand of the probe DNA labeled, virtually 100% of all mutations will be detected. Furthermore, the exact position of the mutation can be defined by sizing the cleavage product. Although the sensitivity of CCM for the detection of mutations is very high, 95–100%, the toxicity of the reagents, the large number of steps and manipulations, and the high background seen with many templates has limited the number of laboratories that have used this technique (reviewed in refs. *47,48*).

6.6. Mutation Detection by Ribonuclease Cleavage of Mismatched RNA:DNA Duplexes

Mutation detection based on ribonuclease cleavage was developed when it was recognized that ribonucleases could cleave single-stranded RNA and that it was possible to synthesize radioactive RNA probes *(49)*. RNA probes, or riboprobes, are synthesized using wild type genomic DNA as a template with ^{32}P incorporated as a label. The probe is hybridized to denatured target DNA to produce RNA:DNA hybrids. When there is a mismatch between the wild type RNA probe and the DNA owing to a mutation, the base or bases that have not annealed to the DNA are cleaved by RNase A. The products of the digestion are denatured and separated by gel electrophoresis. A mutation is indicated by the presence of cleavage fragments of lower molecular weight than the full length-probe. The size of the cleavage products is used to determine the location of the specific mutation. Although this technique has been used to detect mutations in the hypoxanthine phosphoribosyltransferase,

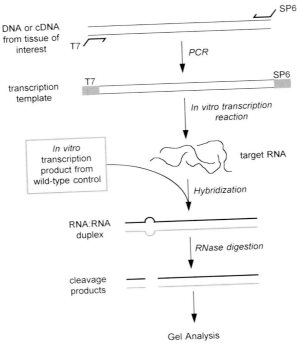

Fig. 12. Schematic representation of NICRA. The DNA or cDNA is amplified using primers with 5' T7 or SP6 promoter sequence to generate a template for in vitro transcription. The template, or target RNA, is hybridized with wild-type RNA to produce RNA:RNA duplexes. When a mismatch is present because of a mutation in the target RNA, the duplexes are cleaved by RNase. The digested products are separated by gel electrophoresis and visualized by staining with ethidium bromide (courtesy of Ambion, Inc., Austin, TX).

type I collagen, and K-*ras* genes, it has not been widely employed partly because of the inability of RNase A to cleave completely all mismatches *(50–52)*. Single-stranded RNA resulting from mismatches involving the purines adenine and guanine are not efficiently recognized by RNase A. However, mismatches involving the pyrimidines cytosine and uracil or larger areas of single-stranded RNA (owing to two mismatched sites in close proximity, a deletion, or an insertion) are effectively cleaved. Modification and improvement of this method was made by incorporating PCR amplification of the target sequence and use of RNase I *(53)*. The starting template is either mRNA or genomic DNA. It is advantageous to use mRNA as a template, since there are no intron sequences present. RNase I recognizes all four bases when they are present at the site of a mismatch. However, like the original RNase cleavage mismatch protocols, incomplete digestion of the hybrid molecules makes it difficult to distinguish between homozygotes and heterozygotes.

A nonisotopic RNase cleavage assay (NIRCA) for mutation detection has recently been developed by Ambion, Inc. (Austin, TX) *(54)*. Beginning with DNA or cDNA, the sequence to be screened is amplified using a forward primer with a T7 bacterial promoter sequence and a reverse primer with an SP6 bacterial promoter sequence (Fig. 12). Target segments up to 1.0 kb long may be amplified and screened in one reaction. The added bacterial promoter sequences allow the PCR products to be tran-

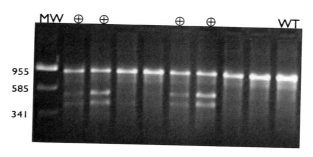

950bp exon II.

Fig. 13. Detection of mutations in the *BRCA1* gene using NIRCA. Target regions of the *BRCA1* gene were amplified by nested PCR from genomic DNA from at-risk relatives of a familial breast cancer patient and from a normal control. The primers had promoter (T7 and SP6) sequences on the 5'-ends. Crude PCR products (2 μL) were transcribed with T7 and SP6 RNA polymerase. Complementary normal and test transcripts were mixed, heated briefly, and cooled to make double-stranded RNA targets. Targets were treated with RNase for 45 min at 37°C, separated by electrophoresis through a 2% agarose gel, and then stained with ethidum bromide. Samples in lanes marked ⊕ were scored as positive for a putative mutation. WT lane shows wild-type control sample. DNA size markers are indicated at the left margin (courtesy of Marianna M. Goldrick, Ambion, Inc. Austin TX).

scribed in an in vitro system to produce large quantities of target RNA. The target RNA is hybridized with wild-type RNA to form RNA:RNA duplexes. Since both template strands are transcribed, reciprocal mismatches (i.e., A · C and G · U) are created when each strand hybridizes to the wild-type RNA. This increases the likelihood that a mismatch will be cleaved since all sites are not cleaved with equal efficiency.

The hybrids are treated with RNase and any unpaired mismatched residues accessible to the enzyme are cleaved. The cleavage products are stained with ethidium bromide, separated by gel electrophoresis, and compared to the wild type homoduplex, which was also treated with enzyme. The wild-type homoduplex should be a single band of the highest molecular weight, since it is resistant to cleavage. Although it is not possible to determine if the cleavage is at the 5'- or 3'-end of the target segment without rescreening, the size of the cleavage product does give a good estimation of the position of the mutation. A significant advantage of this method is the visualization of the cleavage products without radioactive probes. As shown in Fig. 13 this method can be used to screen for germline mutations in the breast and ovarian cancer susceptibility gene *BRCA1*. In addition to the detection of mutations, NIRCA can also identify the genotype of a sample by hybridization of the sample to its own RNA transcripts. If a sample is heterozygous for a mutation, self-hybridization results in mismatched hybrids, which are cleaved. However, if a sample is homozygous, self-hybridization results in completely matched duplexes that are resistant to cleavage.

7. TECHNIQUES FOR DETECTION OF KNOWN MUTATIONS AND SEQUENCE VARIANTS

Restriction endonucleases have proven to be extremely useful in the analysis and characterization of PCR products. Digestion of PCR products with endonucleases can be used to confirm the amplification of desired sequences when the size of the fragments can be predicted from known restriction sites. In addition, it can be used to identify sequence variants and provide linkage information for pedigree analysis when a mutation has not been identified or before a gene is cloned *(55,56)*.

Restriction endonucleases protect bacteria from invasion by foreign DNA by recognizing and cleaving specific sequences in double stranded DNA *(57)*. The bacteria's own DNA is protected from digestion through methylation or modification of the restriction sites, so they are not recognized by the enzyme. There are three classes of endonucleases with different cofactor requirements and different DNA recognition abilities. The class II enzymes are most commonly used in molecular biology applications. They require only the presence of Mg^{2+}, recognize DNA sequences approx 4–8 bases long, and cleave at or near the recognition site. Many of these sites are palindromic and when cleaved result in "blunt" or "sticky" ends. These new ends are extremely advantageous for ligation of the fragment into vectors for further manipulation. The appropriate digestion conditions and buffer for each enzyme are usually supplied by the manufacturer. Since most enzymes are active at 37°C, several can be combined in one reaction if a single product is to be cut at several sites or if a multiplex reaction contains several different products with different restriction sites. The resulting fragments are separated on an agarose or acrylamide gel, depending on the required resolution and stained with ethidium bromide for visualization.

There are numerous restriction sites throughout any region of DNA. Some of these sites are polymorphic in that on a given allele, the site may be present or absent. This may be part of normal variation and not cause disease. The presence or absence of the site affects whether the DNA fragment is cleaved by an endonuclease. If the polymorphism is closely linked to a disease locus, in some families it may be used as a marker to follow inheritance of the mutant (disease-producing) allele. Prior to the development of direct detection methods to identify CF mutations, analysis of linked RFLPs was used for prenatal diagnosis *(56)* and is still useful when both mutations in the parents have not been determined. This type of analysis requires that an affected individual and both parents are available for testing to ascertain which parental alleles carry the mutant genes. DNA obtained from chorionic villus sampling or amniocentesis is the template for PCR amplification of the region encompassing the polymorphism. Based on the restriction fragment patterns resulting from digestion of the PCR products, the genotype of the fetus is determined. Linkage marker analysis for prenatal diagnosis is not 100% accurate owing to the possibility of recombination between the alleles during meiosis. Therefore, it is desirable to analyze several markers to increase the certainty of the diagnosis.

Once a mutation has been detected and characterized by methods that screen for novel mutations, RFLP analysis may be used to screen samples for the same mutation if it creates or destroys a restriction site. The sequence flanking the mutation is amplified, digested with the appropriate enzyme, and the fragments are resolved by gel electrophoresis. For example, the CF mutation 2789 + 5G>A creates an *Ssp*I cutting site. When a 305-bp region of the gene that encompasses this mutation is amplified and digested, three fragments result. (One additional fragment results from a constitutive site present in both alleles). The wild-type allele is cut only once at the constitutive site to produce two fragments (Fig. 14) *(58)*. Mutations and sequence variants that alter restriction sites have been identified in all genes studied. A short list includes genes coding for low-density lipoprotein receptor *(59)*, fumarylacetoacetase *(60)*, cystic fibrosis transmembrane receptor *(61)*, apolipoprotein E *(62)*, and phenylalanine hydroxylase *(63)*.

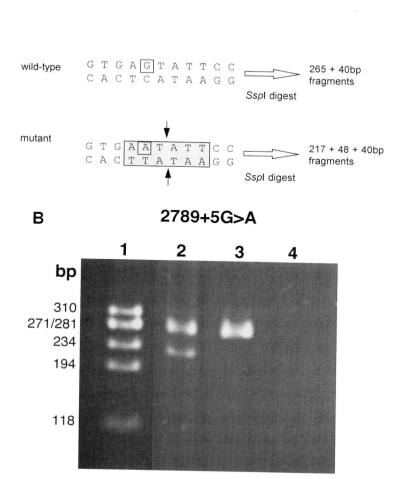

Fig. 14. RFLP analysis of the CF mutation 2789 + 5G >A. **(A)** The wild-type PCR product is digested with *Ssp*I to two fragments owing to the presence of a constitutive restriction site not associated with the mutation. When the G (surrounded by a small box) is mutated to an A, an additional *Ssp*I site is created to yield three fragments. The *Ssp*I site is indicated by the shaded box and the cutting site is indicated by the arrows. **(B)** A 305-bp region of the *CFTR* gene that flanks the 2789 + 5G >A mutation was amplified and digested with *Ssp*I. The PCR products were separated by electrophoresis through a 4% agarose gel and then stained with ethidum bromide. Lane 1, φX174 DNA size markers; lane 2, individual heterozygous for the 2789 + 5G >A mutation (265- and 217-bp fragments); lane 3, normal individual (265-bp fragment); lane 4, water blank. The 40- and 48-bp fragments migrate quickly through the gel and are not visible (courtesy of Michelle L. Blalock, Molecular Genetics Laboratory, University of North Carolina Hospitals).

Unfortunately, it is only occasionally that a sequence variant changes a restriction site. Therefore, in order to preserve the simplicity of mutation detection by PCR/ restriction digestion, PCR-mediated site-directed mutagenesis can be applied *(64)*. This technique creates or destroys restriction sites in the PCR product by introduction of a base substitution near the mutation by modifying the primers. This allows the detection of point mutations as well as small insertions and deletions that cannot be resolved through gel fractionation of the PCR products. A polymerase must be used that does not have exonuclease activity, or the mismatched primer will be corrected. The mismatched base may be several bases from the 3'-end of the primer to stabilize the primer-template hybrid without decreasing the efficiency of the polymerase or the specificity of the amplification. Several CF mutations can be detected by introduced restriction sites with mismatches 1, 2, or 3 bases from the 3'-end *(65,66)*.

Failure of the endonuclease to digest a PCR product can lead to misleading results. Control samples, homozygous and heterozygous for both alleles, should be amplified and digested at the same time as the unknown. Additional endogenous or engineered restriction sites within the PCR product can act as an internal control for complete digestion. When an 87-bp PCR product that spans the IVS-1-110 mutation in the β-globin gene is digested with *Mbo*I, two fragments are produced. When the same product from a wild-type allele is digested with *Mbo*I, three fragments are generated. In this protocol, a primer with three mismatched bases creates only one *Mbo*I site in the mutant allele, but two in the wild-type allele acting as an internal control for digestion efficiency *(67)*. In some instances, such as the G542X and 2789 + 5G>A CF mutations, an additional constitutive site will be present within the PCR product, which will also act as an internal control for digestion *(65)* (Fig. 15).

Although the previous examples have described analysis of missense mutations, the PSM method can also be applied to detect small insertions and deletions. The CF insertion mutation 2869insG and the ΔF508 deletion mutation can be detected by PSM *(65,66)*. The ΔF508 mutation is detected by creating a *Dpn*II site in the wild-type allele. When an individual is heterozygous for this mutation, pairing of the single-stranded wild-type and mutant products occurs following PCR. This hybrid molecule or heteroduplex produces a third band characteristic of heterozygosity after gel electrophoresis (Fig. 16). The decision to introduce a restriction site into either allele is usually based on the location of the mismatch from the 3'-end of the primer and the commercial availability of the enzyme. However, the assay is more specific for a particular mutation when the primers are designed to introduce a cutting site into the mutant allele *(66,67)*. If the restriction site is introduced in the wild-type allele, any mutation in that region can prevent the digestion of the PCR product and therefore is more sensitive, but not as specific.

8. OTHER PCR-BASED MUTATION DETECTION TECHNIQUES

8.1. Allele-Specific PCR

Allele-specific PCR *(68)*, also referred to as amplification refractory mutation system *(69)* or PCR amplification of specific alleles *(70)*, is based on the observation that under certain conditions when there is mismatch between the 3'-end of a primer and the DNA template, elongation by *Taq* polymerase will not occur. Therefore, when a single base change, small deletion, or insertion results in a 3'-mismatch, absence of amplification indicates the presence of a mutation. This method was first used to detect the A to T transversion in the human β-globin gene, which is responsible for sickle cell anemia *(68)*. Two different primers, one specific for the wild-type allele and one specific for the mutant allele, are used in combination with the same second primer (Fig. 17). Each sample is analyzed using both sets of primers to distinguish heterozygotes from

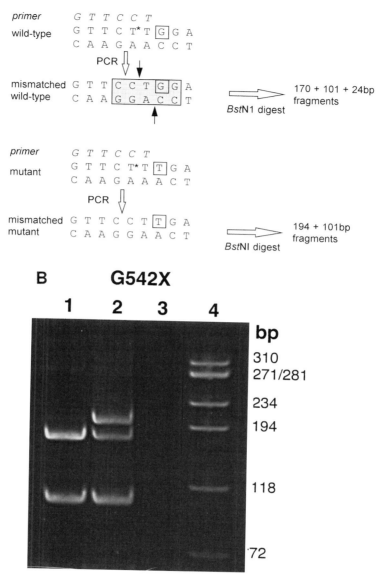

Fig. 15. PSM analysis of the CF mutation G542X. **(A)** A *Bst*NI site is introduced into the wild-type PCR product by changing the T (indicated by an asterisk) to a C during PCR amplification using mismatched primers. The new BstNI site is indicated by the shaded box and the cutting site is indicated by the arrows. *Bst*NI digestion produces three fragments owing to the presence of the introduced restriction site and a constitutive restriction site not associated with the mutation. When the wild-type G (surrounded by a small box) is mutated to a T, a *Bst*NI site is not created by the mismatched primers. The PCR product with the mutation is cut only once at the constitutive restriction site to produce two fragments. **(B)** A 295-bp region of the *CFTR* gene that flanks the G542X mutation was amplified and digested with *Bst*NI. The PCR products were separated by electrophoresis through a 10% acrylamide gel and then stained with ethidium bromide. Lane 1, normal individual (170- and 101-bp fragments); lane 2, individual heterozygous for the G542X mutation (195-, 170-, and 101-bp fragments); lane 3, water blank; lane 4, φX174 DNA size markers. The 24-bp fragment migrates quickly through the gel and is not visible (courtesy of William G. Learning, Molecular Genetics Laboratory, University of North Carolina Hospitals).

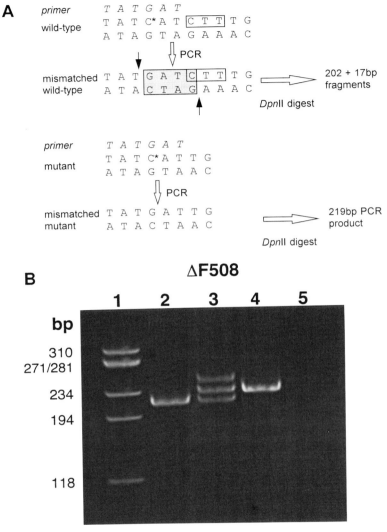

Fig. 16. PSM analysis of the CF mutation ΔF508. **(A)** A *Dpn*II site is introduced into the wild-type PCR product by changing the C (indicated by an asterisk) to a G during PCR amplification using mismatched primers. The *Dpn*II site is indicated by the shaded box and the cutting site is indicated by the arrows. *Dpn*II digestion produces two fragments from the wild-type PCR product. When the CTT is deleted in the mutant, a *Dpn*II site is not created by the mismatched primers. **(B)** A 219-bp region of the *CFTR* gene that flanks the ΔF508 mutation was amplified and digested with *Dpn*II. The PCR products were separated by electrophoresis through a 10% acrylamide gel and then stained with ethidum bromide. Lane 1, φX174 DNA size markers; lane 2, normal individual (202-bp fragment); lane 3, individual heterozygous for the ΔF508 mutation (219-bp, heteroduplex, and 202-bp fragments); lane 4, individual homozygous for the ΔF508 mutation (219-bp fragment); lane 5, water blank. The 17-bp fragment migrates quickly through the gel and is not visible (courtesy of William G. Learning, Molecular Genetics Laboratory, University of North Carolina Hospitals).

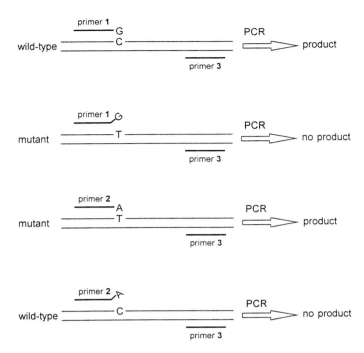

Fig. 17. Schematic representation of allele-specific PCR. Primers 1 and 2 differ by only the 3'-base and are specific for either the wild-type or mutant allele. When the primer binds to the complementary target sequence, amplification occurs. Amplification cannot result from non-specific binding of the primers, since the 3'-base does not hybridize to the target preventing elongation by *Taq* polymerase. The third common primer is not allele-specific.

homozygotes of either the wild-type or mutant allele. The primer design and reaction conditions are critical to prevent amplification from the mismatched primer. Wu et al. obtained discrimination between alleles using 14 base primers with A · A and T · T mismatches that were annealed at a relatively high temperature of 55°C *(68)*. However, any combination of mismatched primers and template will work with a mismatch at, or one base from, the 3'-end *(70,71)*. When primer destabilization is not achieved with the terminal mismatched base, an additional mismatch can be added three bases from the 3'-end *(69)*. Standard magnesium and oligonucleotide titrations determine appropriate conditions for amplification. Specificity can also be increased by decreasing the concentration of DNA, deoxynucleotides, *Taq* polymerase, and the number of PCR cycles, and by increasing the annealing temperature and length of the primers *(71,72)*. An internal control, which may or may not be from the gene of interest, should be coamplified along with the target sequence to demonstrate that the lack of product is not the result of a technical error. The PCR products are fractionated on an agarose gel followed by ethidium bromide staining to visualize the bands. No isotopes or restriction enzyme digestion is required. It is absolutely necessary that the polymerase, such as *Taq* polymerase, lack 3' to 5' exonuclease activity otherwise the mismatched base will be corrected *(4)*. The two allele-specific primers and one common primer can be used in the same reaction when one allele-specific primer is longer than the other *(73)*.

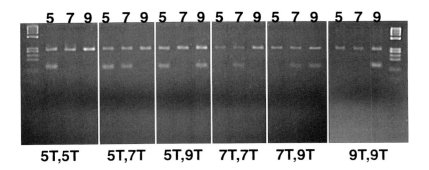

Fig. 18. Analysis of the *CFTR* intron 8 polythymidine tract by allele-specific PCR. A 136–140 bp region of the *CFTR* gene was amplified using forward primers specific for each polythymidine tract of 5, 7, or 9 T's. A 290-bp region of the dystrophin gene was coamplified as a control. The PCR products were separated by electrophoresis through a 4% agarose gel and then stained with ethidum bromide. The first and last lanes are φX174 DNA size markers. The numbers along the top indicate the allele-specific primer used in the PCR reaction. The numbers along the bottom indicate the genotype (courtesy of Kenneth J. Friedman, Molecular Genetics Laboratory, University of North Carolina Hospitals).

The alleles are then distinguished based on the size of the product after electrophoresis. This modification eliminates the need for an internal control and eliminates decreased specificity of the reaction from higher concentrations of DNA template.

An allele-specific PCR protocol has been designed to detect variable numbers of thymidines present in intron 8 of the *CFTR* gene *(74)* (Fig. 18). The primers are specific for each polythymidine tract of 5, 7, or 9 Ts. They are identical except for the number of As that are located at the 3'-end of the primer followed by a single C. Each sample to be analyzed is amplified in three separate reactions using each allele-specific primer and a common forward primer. At a relatively high annealing temperature of 66.5°C, the primers only anneal to the complementary allele. The 7A and 9A primers will not anneal to a 5T allele, presumably because of a looping out of the extra two or four As, respectively, resulting in primer destabilization. Because of the 3'-terminal C, the 5A primer will not anneal to either a 7A or 9T allele.

Allele-specific amplification has been applied to detection of single base changes and small deletions and insertions in a number of clinically applicable situations. It is used to detect mutations in genes that are associated with inherited disease, including α_1-antitrypsin *(69)*, phenylalanine hydroxylase *(70)*, factor IX *(71)*, and steroid 21-hydroxylase *(75)*. It has also been employed in human platelet alloantigen typing by discriminating between alleles that encode the six major human platelet alloantigens *(76)*.

8.2. COP

COP is based on competition between primers in which one primer is completely complementary to the DNA template and the other is not *(77)*. Unlike allele-specific PCR, the mismatch is located in the middle of the primer and both primers are present in the same reaction. However, under the appropriate conditions, only the perfect match will anneal and, along with a common reverse primer, produce a PCR product. The competition between primers increases with increasing primer concentration and

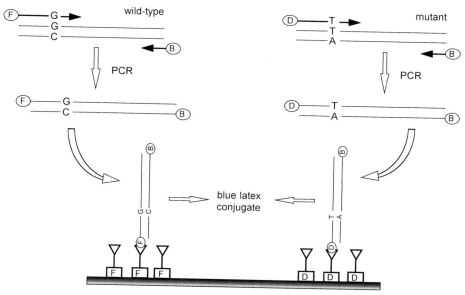

Fig. 19. Schematic representation of COP. Allele-specific primers are labeled with either fluorescein-5-isothiocyanate (F) or dansylchloride (D) and the common reverse primer is labeled with biotin. All three primers are present during the PCR in order to amplify the two possible alleles. To determine which allele-specific PCR products have been amplified, the reactions are immunochromatographed across a membrane that has bound antifluorscein and antidansyl antibodies. The bound products are visualized by addition of a blue latex conjugate that binds biotin (B).

decreasing primer length *(77)*. In addition, the most effective competition that produces correct primer matching occurs with small primers (12–16-mers) present in excess of the template and when the stringency of the annealing is low. In the initial report, COP was shown to discriminate between the normal human hypoxanthine phosphoribosyltransferase allele and the G to A transition mutant *(77)*. The amplification was visualized by autoradiography using one labeled and one unlabeled primer in the same reaction. Two reactions were needed in order to detect both alleles.

Modification of the COP system was made to detect five mutations in the β-globin gene that account for 90% of the β-thalassemia cases in Greece. A fluorescein-5-isothiocyanate label was attached to the wild-type allele-specific primer and a dansylchloride label to the mutant allele-specific primer *(78)* (Fig. 19). The common reverse primer was labeled with biotin to provide colorimetric detection of the PCR products. All three primers were included in the reaction to amplify the two possible alleles. The PCR products were immunochromatographed across a membrane with antifluorescein and antidansyl antibodies attached at discrete locations. The products, with their allele-specific labels, bound to the appropriate antibody and then were detected by addition of a blue latex conjugate that binds biotin. Therefore, the genotype was determined by the presence of a blue color in which a single spot indicated homozygosity and two spots indicated heterozygosity. A similar color complementation assay using allele-specific fluorescent oligonucleotide primers has been used to

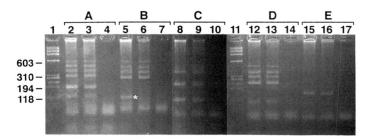

Fig. 20. DMD/Becker Muscular Dystrophy multiplex to detect deletions in the dystrophin gene. Nineteen exons of the dystrophin gene were analyzed for deletions in five multiplex PCR reactions **(A–E)**. The exons amplified in each multiplex and the size of PCR products are listed in Table 2. The PCR products were separated by electrophoresis through a 4% agarose gel and then stained with ethidium bromide. Lanes 1 and 11, φX174 DNA size markers; lanes 2, 5, 8, 12, and 15, normal male; lanes 3, 6, 9, 13, and 16, affected male; lanes 4, 7, 10, 14, and 17, water blanks. The affected male has a deletion of exon 52, indicated by the asterisk. This is diagnostic of DMD (courtesy of Kenneth. J. Friedman, Molecular Genetics Laboratory, University of North Carolina Hospitals).

detect a 4-bp deletion and a missense mutation in the β-globin gene *(79)*. The two allele-specific forward primers were conjugated to different dyes and the common reverse primer was unlabeled. Once the unincorporated primers were removed from the reaction mixture by centrifugation, the color of the PCR products indicated the genotype. The heterozygote genotype produces a color complementary to the individual fluorescent dyes.

8.3. Multiplex PCR

Multiplex PCR is the simultaneous amplification of multiple loci in one reaction using several primer pairs. This technique was initially developed to identify deletions in the dystrophin gene *(80)*, but has been expanded to include any PCR reaction involving amplification of multiple loci whether for ASO *(81)*, reverse dot blot (27), PSM or restriction digestion *(82)*, sequencing *(83,84)*, or allele-specific PCR *(85)*. As a result, it has been employed in a multitude of clinical and research investigations in which multiple sequence variations exist at a single locus.

Multiplex PCR analysis is particularly suited for analysis of the dystrophin gene since deletions account for approx 65% of the mutations in DMD and Becker Muscular Dystrophy *(19)*. The multiple PCR products produced in a single reaction serve as internal controls for amplification when an exon or exons are deleted. Chamberlain et al. used nine primer sets in one multiplex reaction to amplify nine commonly deleted exons to detect approx 80% of the deletions in DMD *(86)*. The combination of this multiplex with one that amplifies eight exons plus the muscle promoter of the dystrophin gene detects 98% of the deletions found in patients with DMD or Becker Muscular Dystrophy *(87)*. Figure 20 shows five multiplex PCR reactions for 19 dystrophin exons. The size of the products range from 100–547 bp, which allow them to be individually resolved on a single agarose gel (Table 2). This patient has a deletion of exon 52. When combining multiple primer sets in one reaction, the primers should be designed to anneal at a similar temperature and the reaction conditions,

Table 2
Multiplex PCR for Detection of Deletions in the Dystrophin Gene

Multiplex reaction									
A		B		C		D		E	
Exon	bp	Exon	bp	Exon	bp	Exon	bp	Exon	bp
45	547	Pr/1	535	51	388	19	459	42	155
49	439	17	416	54	329	8	360		
43	357	12	331	6	202	55	303		
16	290	50	271	53	100	13	238		
47	181	52	113						

including extension time, free nucleotide concentration, and polymerase concentration should be carefully adjusted to amplify all areas of interest successfully (*80*, reviewed in ref. *88*).

Numerous mutations in the *CFTR* gene cause CF, which encourages its frequent analysis using multiplex systems. For example, a multiplex reverse dot blot detects 11 mutations *(27)*, a 10-mutation multiplex uses naturally occurring restriction sites, PCR-generated restriction sites, and differences in product size to differentiate wild-type and mutant alleles *(82)*, and a 12-mutation multiplex reaction is followed by ASO analysis *(81)*. Genes associated with carcinogenesis are also typically mutated in many locations with many different types of mutations. Amplification of all or part of the *p53* gene in a multiplex format screens for insertions or deletions *(89)*, followed by direct sequencing of the PCR products to detect other less apparent changes, such as point mutations *(84)*. The *APC* gene, which is frequently mutated in individuals with familial adenomatous polyposis coli, can also be analyzed for deletions by multiplex allele-specific PCR *(85)*.

8.4. Protein Truncation Test

The PrTT is a multifaceted methodology with three components: cDNA synthesis by reverse transcription, PCR, and protein synthesis (Fig. 21). This assay is relatively complex and most useful as a tool for screening genes that have been shown to contain primarily nonsense or frameshift mutations. As a group, these types of mutations are referred to as truncating or translation terminating mutations. Proteins synthesized from such mutant alleles are abnormally shortened or truncated, if they are produced at all. PrTT has the distinct advantage of analyzing only coding sequence, which is particularly important for large genes with numerous exons. In addition, larger PCR products than those used for SSCP can be used; hence, fewer reactions are required for analysis of the entire gene. Since the end point of the assay is a protein product, silent changes or polymorphisms will not be detected, yet at the same time neither will missense mutations. PrTT was first applied to analysis of mutations in the dystrophin gene *(90)* and in the *APC* gene in families with familial adenomatous polyposis (FAP) *(91)*.

The PrTT method is based on RAWTS as described by Sarkar and Sommer *(92)* for rapid and sensitive direct sequencing from RNA. For the RAWTS technique, which is not commonly used today, RNA was purified from white blood cells or tissues and

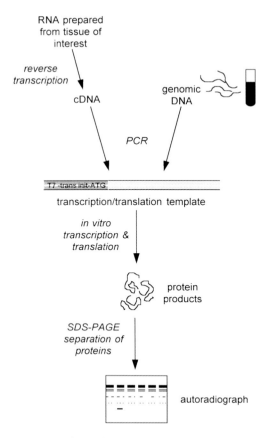

Fig. 21. Schematic representation of PrTT. RNA or DNA (prepared from tissue such as lymphocytes) is the starting material for PrTT. RNA is reverse transcribed into cDNA prior to PCR. The PCR reaction generates the template for in vitro transcription and translation (*see* Fig. 22) and the protein products that are produced are separated by SDS-PAGE and visualized by autoradiography.

reverse transcribed using an oligo(dT) primer to generate nonspecific cDNA. The cDNA was then amplified using a gene-specific primer with a T7 bacterial promoter sequence on the 5'-end. This assay was designed to obtain sequence information, but it was also observed that the PCR products could be used to generate protein products by in vitro translation (or insertion into an expression vector) when the primer also contained a translation initiation signal and an initiation codon (ATG). Like RAWTS, PrTT begins with total RNA prepared from any source, such as peripheral blood lymphocytes, and is followed by cDNA synthesis using an oligo(dT) primer or random hexamer primers. PCR products are amplified from the cDNA using overlapping primer sets specific for the gene of interest. A gene that is expressed at very low levels in the tissue of interest may be difficult to screen by this technique. A solution to this problem is to perform nested PCR (i.e., two rounds of PCR, the first with primers outside the target sequence).

For example, to scan the entire *APC* coding sequence the cDNA is amplified in five overlapping segments *(91)*. Approximately 24% of the coding sequence, which includes

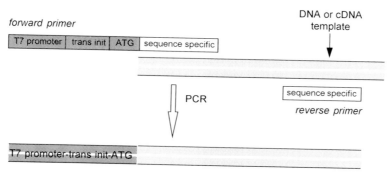

Fig. 22. Generation of in vitro transcription/translation template for PrTT using specialized forward primer. The forward primer is composed of T7 bacterial promoter sequence, a translation initiation site, an initiation codon (ATG), and target specific sequence. Only the target-specific sequence anneals to the DNA or cDNA template. However, the extra sequence is incorporated into the products in subsequent cycles when the products also serve as a template for PCR.

the mutation cluster region, can also be analyzed in one 2-kb segment directly from genomic DNA *(93,94)*. It is estimated that analysis of this region will detect up to 50% of the germline mutations in FAP and 75% of the mutations in colorectal tumors. Since the dystrophin gene coding sequence is larger, it is amplified in 10 segments. The number of segments is based on amplification efficiency and the ability to resolve the protein products by gel electrophoresis. Data indicate that PrTT can analyze products up to at least 2.5 kb *(95)*. The overlapping segments also allow truncating mutations present at either end of the segment, which are therefore more difficult to resolve, to be detected twice *(90)*.

In order to generate a template for in vitro protein synthesis, the forward primer has a T7 bacterial promoter sequence, a translation initiation site, and an ATG initiation codon on the 5'-end (Fig. 22). Although only the sequence specific portion of the primer anneals to the template DNA or cDNA, the extra sequence is fully incorporated into the products when they serve as template in subsequent cycles. The PCR products are the template for the coupled in vitro transcription and translation assay. These assays are commercially available from a number of manufacturers as a kit. The reactions contain ^{35}S-methionine to produce labeled peptides, which are separated by SDS-polyacrylamide gel electrophoresis (SDS-PAGE), dried, and autoradiographed. When a shortened or truncated protein is identified, the size of the protein is determined to provide an estimation of the location of the corresponding mutation. The indicated portion of the genomic DNA is sequenced to determine the precise mutation.

The efficiency of the assay relies on the interpretation of the protein gels. In most cases, there are several bands present of varying intensity, which may be owing to alternative splicing, internal methionines that are acting as additional start sites, or incomplete transcription or translation. Despite the need for careful interpretation of the protein gels, the PrTT assay has been used successfully to identify mutations in a number of genes with a high incidence of truncating mutations. For example, 22 DMD

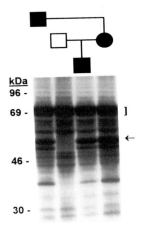

Fig. 23. Segregation of a truncated polypeptide in a family with NF1. The autoradiograph shows translation products synthesized in vitro from segment 2 of the NF1 transcript following electrophoresis through a 12.5% SDS-polyacrylamide gel. Each lane contains a sample from the individual in the pedigree above. The bracket indicates the wild-type polypeptide which is present in every lane. The arrow indicates truncated polypeptides that are seen in the proband, her affected father, and her affected son, but not her husband. The truncated protein is the result of a nonsense mutation Q1017X, which encodes a premature translation termination signal *(97)* (courtesy of Oxford University Press and Ruth A. Heim, Molecular Genetics Laboratory, University of North Carolina Hospitals).

patients who did not have a deletion in the dystrophin gene by multiplex PCR or Southern blotting were analyzed, and 12 truncated proteins were detected. The corresponding truncating mutations were confirmed by sequencing *(96)*. Five of the patients had small deletions or rearrangements that produced aberrant RT-PCR products. The coding sequence of the remaining five samples was analyzed by chemical cleavage mismatch, but no mutations were found. Based on this study, the combination of RT-PCR and PrTT detected approx 77% of the mutations in DMD patients. The *NF1* gene has also been analyzed by PrTT, with mutations identified in 14 of 21 individuals with neurofibromatosis type 1 (NF1) *(97)*. Figure 23 shows segregation of a truncated protein in family members diagnosed with NF1. PrTT analysis has the potential to be an important tool for diagnosing mildly affected NF1 patients or presymptomatic individuals. PrTT has also been used to analyze patients for germline mutations in the breast and ovarian cancer susceptibility gene *BRCA1*. Analysis of 45 affected individuals using this technique detected eight patients with germline mutations *(98)*.

9. CONCLUSION

The PCR and other molecular biology techniques have revolutionized analysis of the human genome. This is most striking in the rapid development of techniques that use PCR for the detection of mutations that cause inherited genetic disease. Advances in technology have allowed physicians to confirm difficult clinical diagnoses, and to offer prenatal diagnosis and carrier detection, as well as susceptibility testing. It is expected that with further developments in automation and technological advances, many of the techniques described in this chapter (which are still relatively costly and labor-intensive) will contribute to the routine use of molecular diagnostic testing in clinical practice.

ABBREVIATIONS

APS, ammonium persulfate; ASO, allele-specific oligonucleotide; CCM, chemical cleavage of mismatches; CF, cystic fibrosis; CFTR, cystic fibrosis transmembrane conductance regulator; COP, competitive oligonucleotide priming; DGGE, denaturing gradient gel electrophoresis; HA, heteroduplex analysis; NIRCA, nonisotopic RNase cleavage assay; MDE, mutation detection enhancement; PSM, PCR-mediated site-directed mutagenesis; PrTT, protein truncation test; RAWTS, RNA amplification with transcript sequencing; RFLP, restriction fragment length polymorphism; SDS, sodium dodecyl sulfate; SSCP, single-strand conformational polymorphism; TEMED, tetramethylethylenediamine; TMACl, tetramethyl-ammonium chloride.

ACKNOWLEDGMENTS

The authors gratefully acknowledge the suggestions and comments of Ruth A. Heim, and the generous contribution of figures from Sarah Adkins, Michelle L. Blalock, Kenneth J. Friedman, Ruth A. Heim, and William G. Learning (Molecular Genetics Laboratory, University of North Carolina Hospitals), Lori Terry and J. Carl Barrett (Laboratory of Molecular Carcinogenesis, National Institute of Environmental Health Science), and Marianna M. Goldrick (Ambion, Inc.).

REFERENCES

1. Saiki, R. K., Scharf, S., Faloona, F., Mullis, K. B., Horn, G. T., Erlich, H. A., and Arnheim, N. Enzymatic amplification of β-globin genomic sequences and restriction site analysis for diagnosis of sickle cell anemia. *Science* **230:**1350–1354, 1985.
2. Mullis, K. B. and Faloona, F. A. Specific synthesis of DNA *in vitro* via a polymerase-catalyzed chain reaction. *Methods Enzymol.* **155:**335–350, 1987.
3. Brock, T. D. and Freeze, H. *Thermus aquaticus* gen. n. and sp. n., a non-sporulating extreme thermophile. *J. Bacteriol.* **98:**289–297, 1969.
4. Chien, A., Edgar, D. B., and Trela, J. M Deoxyribonucleic acid polymerase from the extreme thermophile *Thermus aquaticus. J. Bacteriol.* **127:**1550–1557, 1976.
5. Saiki, R. K., Gelfand, D. H., Stoffel, S., Scharf, J. J., Higuchi, R., Horn, G. T., Mullis, K. B., and Erlich, H. A. Primer-directed enzymatic amplification of DNA with a thermostable DNA polymerase. *Science* **239:**487–491, 1988.
6. Sambrook, J., Fritch, E. F., and Maniatis, T, eds., *Molecular Cloning: A Laboratory Manual,* 2nd ed. Cold Spring Harbor Laboratory, Cold Spring Harbor, New York, pp. 947–957, 1989.
7. Denhardt, D. T. (1966) A membrane-filter technique for the detection of complementary DNA. *Biochem. Biophys. Res. Commun.* **23:**641–646.
8. Wahl, G. M., Stern, M., and Stark, G. R. Efficient transfer of large DNA fragments form agarose gels to diazobenzyloxymethyl-paper and rapid hybridization by using dextran sulfate. *Proc. Natl. Acad. Sci. USA* **76:**3683–3687, 1979.
9. Bolton, E. T. and McCarthy, B. J. A general method for the isolation of RNA complementary to DNA. *Proc. Natl. Acad. Sci. USA* **48:**1390–1397, 1962.
10. Casey, J. and Davidson, M. Rates of formation and thermal stabilities of RNA:DNA and DNA:DNA duplexes at high concentrations of formamide. *Nucleic Acids Res.* **4:**1539–1552, 1977.

11. Wallace, R. B., Shaffer, J., Murphy, R. F., Bonner, J., Hirose, T., and Itakura, K. Hybridization of synthetic oligodeoxynucleotides to φ χ 174 DNA: the effect of single base pair mismatch. *Nucleic Acids Res.* **6**:3543–3557, 1979.

12. Wood, W. I., Gitschier, J., Lasky, L. A., and Lawn, R. M. (1985) Base composition-independent hybridization in tetramethylammonium chloride: a method for oligonucleotide screening of highly complex gene libraries. *Proc. Natl. Acad. Sci. USA* **82**: 1585–1588.

13. Conner, B. J., Reyes, A. A., Morin, C., Itakura, K., Teplitz, R. L., and Wallace, R. B. (1983) Detection of sicke cell β^S-globin allele by hybridization with synthetic oligonucleotides. *Proc. Natl. Acad. Sci. USA* **80**:278–282.

14. Saiki, R. K., Bugawan, T. L., Horn, G. T., Mullis, K. B., and Erlich, H. A. (1986) Analysis of enzymatically amplified β-globin and HLA-DQα DNA with allele-specific oligonucleotide probes. *Nature* **324**:163–166.

15. Kerem, B., Rommens, J. M., Buchanan, J. A., Markiewicz, D., Cox, T. K., Chakravarti, A., Buchwald, M., and Tsui, L. Identification of the cystic fibrosis gene: genetic analysis. *Science* **245**:1073–1080, 1989.

16. Farr, C. J., Saiki, R. K., Erlich, H. A., McCormick, F., and Marshall, C. J. Analysis of RAS gene mutations in acute myeloid leukemia by polymerase chain reaction and oligonucleotide probes. *Proc. Natl. Acad. Sci. USA* **85**:1629–1633, 1988.

17. Kuijpers, R. W. A. M., Simsek, S., Faber, N. M., Goldschmeding, R., van Wermerkerken, R. K. V., and von dem Borne A. E. G. K. R. Single point mutation in human glycoprotein IIIa is associated with a new platelet-specific alloantigen (Mo) involved in neonatal thrombocytopenia. *Blood* **81**:70–76, 1993.

18. Vidaud, D., Emmerich, J., Alhenc-Geals, M., Yvart, J., Fiessinger, J. N., and Aiach, M. Met 358 to arg mutation of alpha$_1$-antitrypsin assoiciated with protein C deficiency in a patient with mild bleeding tendency. *J. Clin. Invest.* **89**:1537–1543, 1992.

19. Darras, B. T., Blattner, P., Harper, J. F., Spiro, A. J., Alter, S., and Francke, U. Intragenic deletions in 21 Duchenne Muscular Dystrophy (DMD)/Becker Muscular Dystrophy (BMD) families studied with the dystrophin cDNA: location of breakpoints on *Hind*III and *Bgl*II exon-containing fragment maps, meiotic and mitotic origin of the mutations. *Am. J. Hum. Genet.* **43**:620–629, 1988.

20. Prior, T. W., Papp, A. C., Snyder, P. J., Highsmith, W. E., Friedman, K. J., Perry, T. R., Silverman, L. M., and Mendell, J. R. Determination of carrier status in Duchenne and Becker muscular dystrophies by quantitative polymerase chain reaction and allele-specific oligonucleotides. *Clin. Chem.* **36**:2113–2117, 1990.

21. Skogerboe, K. J., West, S. F., Murillo, M. D., and Tait, J. F. PCR dot blots: large signal differences between sense and anti-sense probes. *Biotechniques* **9**:154–157, 1990.

22. Siaki, R. K., Chang, C., Levenson, C. H., Warren, T. C., Boehm, C. D., Kazazian, H. H., and Erlich, H. A. Diagnosis of sickle cell anemia and β-thalassemia with enzymatically amplified DNA and nonradioactive allele-specific oligonucleotides. *New Engl. J. Med.* **319**:537–541, 1988.

23. Saiki, R. K., Walsh, P. S., Levenson, C. H., and Erlich, H. A. Genetic analysis of amplified DNA with immobilized sequence-specific oligonucleotide probes. *Proc. Natl. Acad. Sci. USA* **86**:6230–6234, 1989.

24. Kawasaki, E., Saiki, R., and Erlich, H. Genetic analysis using polymerase chain rection-amplified DNA immobilized oligonucleotide probes: reverse dot-blot typing. *Methods Enzymol.* **218**:369–381, 1993.

25. Chehab, F. F. and Wall, J. Detection of multiple cystic fibrosis mutations by reverse dot blot hybridization: a technology for carrier screening. *Hum. Genet.* **89**:163–168, 1992.

26. Zhang, Y., Coyne, M. Y., Will, S. G., Levenson, C. H., and Kawasaki, E. S. Single-base mutational analysis of cancer and genetic diseases using membrane bound modified oligonucleotides. *Nucleic Acids. Res.* **19**:3929–3933, 1991.

27. Cuppens, H., Buyse, I., Baens, M., Marynen, P., and Cassiman, J. Simultaneous screening for 11 mutations in the cystic fibrosis transmembrane conductance regulator gene by multiplex amplification and reverse dot-blot. *Mol. Cell. Probes.* **6**:33–39, 1992.

28. Cai, S., Wall, J., Kan, Y. W., and Chehab, F. F. Reverse dot blot probes for the screening of β-thalassemia mutations in Asians and American blacks. *Hum. Mutat.* **3**:59–63, 1994.

29. Maggio, A., Giambona, A., Cai, S. P., Wall, J., Kan, Y. W., and Chehab, F. F. Rapid and simultaneous typing of hemoglobin S, hemoglobin C and seven Mediterranean β-thalassemia mutations by covalent reverse dot-blot analysis: application to prenatal diagnosis in Sicily. *Blood* **81**:239–242, 1993.

30. Hance, A. J., Gandchamp, B., Levy-Frebault, V., Lecossier, D., Rauzier, J., Bocart, D., and Gicquel, B. Detection and identification of mycobacteria by amplification of mycobacterial DNA. *Mol. Microbiol.* **3**:843–849, 1989.

31. FMC BioProducts Catalog 1995, Technical Applications, p. 70.

32. Orita, M., Suzuki, Y., Sekiya, T., and Hayashi, K. Rapid and sensitive detection of point mutations and DNA polymorphisms using the polymerase chain reaction. *Genomics* **5**:874–879, 1989.

33. Hollstein, M., Sidransky, D., Vogelstein, B., and Harris, C. C. p53 mutations in human cancers. *Science* **253**:49–53 1991.

34. Levine, A. J., Momand, J., and Finlay, C. A. The p53 tumor suppressor gene. *Nature* **351**:453–456, 1991.

35. Sheffield, V. C., Beck, J. S., Kwitek, A. E., Sandstrom, D. W., and Stone, E. M. The sensitivity of single-strand conformational polymorphism analysis for the detection of single base substitutions *Genomics* **16**:325–332, 1993.

36. Myers, R. M., Lerman, L. S., and Maniatis, T. Saturation mutagenesis of cloned DNA fragments. *Science* **229**:242–247, 1985.

37. Lin-Goerke, J., Ye, S., and Highsmith, W. E. Effects of gel matrix on the sensitivity of SSCP analysis: A study of the effects of novel gel matrices, fragment size, GC content, and base alteration. *Am. J. Hum. Genet.* **55(Suppl.):** A188, 1994.

38. Ravnik-Glavac, M., Glavac, D., and Dean, M. Sensitivity of SSCP and heteroduplex method for mutation detection in the cystic fibrosis gene. *Hum. Mol. Genet.* **3**:801–807, 1994.

39. Bhattacharyya, A. and Lilley, D. M. J. The contrasting structures of mismatched DNA sequences containing looped-out bases (bulges) and multiple mismatches (bubbles). *Nucleic Acids Res.* **17**:6821–6840, 1989.

40. Keen, J., Lester, D., Inglehearn, C., Curtis, A., and Bhattacharyya, S. Improved detection of heteroduplexes on Hydrolink gels. *Trends Genet.* **7**:5, 1991.

41. Molinari, R. J., Conners, M., and Shorr, R. G. Hydrolink gels for electrophoresis, in *Advances in Electrophoresis*, vol. 6, Chrambach, A., Dunn, M. J., and Radola, B. J., eds., VCH, New York, pp. 44–60, 1993.

42. Rossetti, S., Corra, S., Biasi, M. O., Turco, A. E., and Pignatti, P. F. Comparison of heteroduplex and single-strand conformation analysis, followed by ethidium fluorescence visualization for the detection of mutations in four human genes. *Mol. Cell. Probes* **9**:195–200, 1995.

43. Myers, R. M., Lumelsky, N., Lerman, L. S., and Maniatis, T. Detection of single base substitutions in total genomic DNA. *Nature* **313**:495–498, 1985.

44. Lerman, L. S. and Silverstein, K. Computational simulation of DNA melting and its application to denaturing gradient gel electrophoresis. *Methods Enzymol.* **155**:482–501, 1987.

45. Abrams, E. S., Murdaugh, S. E., Lerman, L. S. Comprehensive detection of single base changes in human genomic DNA using denaturing gradient gel electrophoresis and a GC clamp *Genomics* **7**:463–475, 1990.

46. Cotton, R. G. H., Rodrigues, N. R., and Campbell, R. D. Reactivity of cytosine and thymine in single-base-pair mismatches with hydroxylamine and osmium tetoxide and its application to the study of mutations. *Proc. Natl. Acad. Sci. USA* **85**:4397–4401, 1988.

47. Grompe, M. The rapid detection of unknown mutations in nucleic acids. *Nature Genet.* **5:**111–117, 1993.

48. Saleeba, J. A., Ramus, S. J., and Cotton, R. G. H. Complete mutation detection using unlabeled chemical cleavage. *Hum. Mutat.* **1:**63–69, 1992.

49. Myers, R. M., Larin, Z., and Maniatis, T. Detection of single base substitutions by ribonuclease cleavage at mismatches in RNA:DNA duplexes. *Science* **230:**1242–1246, 1985.

50. Gibbs, R. A. and Caskey, C. T. Identification and localization of mutations at the Lesch-Nyhan locus by ribonuclease A cleavage. *Science* **236:**303–305, 1987.

51. Marini, J. C., Lewis, M.B., Wang, Q., Chen, K. J., and Orrison, B. M. Serine for glycine substitutions in type I collagen in two cases of type IV osteogenesis imperfecta (OI). *J. Biol. Chem.* **268:**2667–2673, 1993.

52. Forrester, K., Almoguera, C., Han, K., Grizzle, W. E., and Perucho, M. Detection of high incidence of K-*ras* oncogenes during human colon tumorigenesis. *Nature* **327:**298–303, 1987.

53. Murthy, K. K., Shen, S.-H., and Banville, D. A sensitive method for detection of mutations—A PCR-based RNase Protection assay. *DNA Cell Biol.* **14:**87–94, 1995.

54. Goldrick, M. M., Kimball, G. R., Martin, L. A., Tseng, J. Y.-H., Sommers, S. S. and Lee, Q. NIRCA: a rapid robust method for screening for unknown point mutations. *Biotechniques* **21:**106–112, 1996.

55. Kogan, S. C., Doherty, M., and Gitschier, J. An improved method for prenatal diagnosis of genetic diseases by analysis of amplified DNA sequences. *New Engl. J. Med.* **317:**985–990, 1987.

56. Feldman, G. L., Williamson, R., Beaudet, A. L., and O'Brien, W. E. Prenatal diagnosis of cystic fibrosis by DNA amplification for detection of KM-19 polymorphism. *Lancet* **ii:**102, 1988.

57. Yuan, R. Structure and mechanism of multifunctional restriction endonucleases. *Ann. Rev. Biochem.* **50:**285–315, 1981.

58. Highsmith, W. E., Burch, L. H., Zhou, Z., Olsen, J. C., Strong, T. V., Smith, T., Friedman, K. J., Silverman, L. M., Boucher, R. C., Collins, F. S., and Knowles, M. R. Identification of a splice site mutation (2789 + 5G > A) associated with small amounts of normal cystic fibrosis transmembrane conductance regulator mRNA and mild cystic fibrosis. *Hum. Mutat.*, 1996, in press.

59. Vohl, M., Couture, P., Moorjani, S., Torres, A. L., Gagne, C., Despres, J., Lupien, P., Labrie, F., and Simard, J. Rapid restriction fragment analysis for screening four point mutations of the the low-density lipoprotein receptor gene in French Canadians. *Hum. Mutat.* **6:**243–246, 1995.

60. Rootwelt, H., Berger, R., Gray, G., Kelly, D. A., Coskun, T., and Kvittingen, E. A. Novel splice, missense, and nonsense mutations in the fumarylacetoacetase gene causing tyrosinemia type I. *Am. J. Hum. Genet.* **55:**653–658, 1994.

61. Cutting, G. R., Kasch, L. M., Rosenstein, B. J., Zielenski, J., Tsui, L., Antonarkis, S. E., and Kazazian, H. H. A cluster of cystic fibrosis mutations in the first nucleotide-binding fold of the cystic fibrosis conductance regulator protein. *Nature* **346:**366–369, 1990.

62. Hixson, J. E. and Vernier, D. T. Restriction isotyping of human apolipoprotein E by gene amplification and cleavage with *Hha*I. *J. Lipid Res.* **31:**545–548, 1990.

63. Eiken, H. G., Odland, E., Boman, H., Skjelkvale, L., Engebretsen, L. F., and Apold, J. Application of natural and amplification created restriction sites for the diagnosis of PKU mutations. *Nucleic Acids Res.* **19:**1427–1430, 1991.

64. Haliassos, A., Chomel, J. C., Tesson, L., Baudis, M., Kruh, J., Kaplan, J. C., and Kitzis, A. Modification of enzymatically amplified DNA for the destruction of point mutations. *Nucleic Acids Res.* **17:**3606, 1989.

65. Friedman, K. J., Highsmith, W. E., and Silverman, L. M. Detecting multiple cystic fibrosis mutations by polymerase chain reaction-mediated site-directed mutagenesis. *Clin. Chem.* **37:**753–755, 1991.

66. Gasparini, P., Bonizzato, A., Dognini, M., and Pignatti, P. F. Restriction site generating polymerase chain reaction (RG-PCR) for the probeless detection of hidden genetic variation: application to the study of some common cystic fibrosis mutations. *Mol. Cell. Probes* **6:**1–7, 1992.

67. Lindeman, R., Hu, S. P., Volpato, F., and Trent, R. J. Polymerase chain reaction (PCR) mutagenesis enabling rapid non-radioactive detection of common β-thalassaemia mutations in Mediterraneans. *Br. J. Haematol.* **78:**100–104, 1991.

68. Wu, D. Y., Ugozzoli, L., Pal, B. K., and Wallace, R. B. Allele-specific enzymatic amplification of β-globin gneomic DNA for diagnosis of sickle cell anemia. *Proc. Natl. Acad. Sci. USA* **86:**2757–2760, 1989.

69. Newton, C. R., Graham, A., Heptinstall, L. E., Powell, S. J., Summers, C., Kalsheker, N., Smith, J. C., and Markham, A. F. Analysis of any point mutation in DNA. The amplification refractory mutation system (ARMS). *Nucleic Acids Res.* **17:**2503–2516, 1989.

70. Sarkar, G., Cassady, J., Bottema, C. D. K., and Sommer, S. S. Characterization of polymerase chain reaction amplification of specific alleles. *Anal. Biochem.* **186:**64–68, 1990.

71. Sommer, S. S., Groszbach, A. R., and Bottema, C. D. K. PCR amplification of specific alleles (PASA) is a general method for rapidly detecting known single-base changes. *Biotechniques* **12:**82–87, 1992.

72. Bottema, C. D. K. and Sommer, S. S. PCR amplification of specific alleles: rapid detection of known mutations and polymorphisms. *Mutat. Res.* **288:**93–102, 1993.

73. Dutton, C. and Sommer, S. S. Simultaneous detection of multiple single-base alleles at a polymorphic site. *Biotechniques* **11:**700–702, 1991.

74. Friedman, K. J., Heim, R. A., Knowles, M. R., and Silverman, L. M. Rapid characterization of the CFTR intron 8 polythymidine tract: association with variant phenotypes. *Hum. Mutat.* 1996, in press.

75. Wilson, R. C., Wei, J., Cheng, K. C., Mercado, A. B., and New, M. I. Rapid deoxyribonucleic acid analysis by allele-specific polymerase chain reaction for detection of mutations in the steroid 21-hydroxylase gene. *J. Clin. Endocrinol. Metab.* **80:**1635–1640, 1995.

76. Skogen, B., Bellissimo, D. B., Hessner, M. J., Santoso, M. J., Aster, R. H., Newman, P. J., and McFarland, J. G. Rapid determination of platelet alloantigen genotypes by polymerase chain reaction using allele-specific primers. *Transfusion* **34:**955–960, 1994.

77. Gibbs, R. A., Nguyen, P., and Caskey, C. T. Detection of single DNA base differences by competitive oligonucleotide priming. *Nucleic Acids Res.* **17:**2437–2448, 1989.

78. Athanassiadou, A., Papachatzopoulou, A., and Gibbs, R. A. Detection and genetic analysis of β-thalassemia mutations by competitive oligopriming. *Hum. Mutat.* **6:**30–35, 1995.

79. Chehab, F. F. and Kan, Y. W. Detection of specific DNA sequences by fluorescence amplification: a color complementation assay. *Proc. Natl. Acad. Sci. USA.* **86:**9178–9182, 1989.

80. Chamberlain, J. S., Gibbs, R. A., Ranier, J. E., Nguyen, P. N., and Caskey, C. T. Deletion screening of the Duchenne muscular dystrophy locus via multiplex DNA amplification. *Nucleic Acids Res.* **16:**11,141–11,156, 1988.

81. Shuber, A. P., Skoletsky, J., Stern, R. and Handelin, B. L. Efficient 12-mutation testing in the CFTR gene: a general model for complex mutation analysis. *Hum. Mol. Genet.* **2:**153–158, 1993.

82. Axton, R. A. and Brock, D. J. H. A single-tube multiplex system for the simultaneous detection of 10 common cystic fibrosis mutations. *Hum. Mutat.* **5:**260–262, 1995.

83. Gibbs, R. A., Nguyen, P.-H., Edwards, A., Civtello, A. B., and Caskey, C. T. Multiplex DNA deletion detection and exon sequencing of the hypoxanthine phosphoribosyltransferase gene in Lesch-Nyan families. *Genomics* **7:**235–244, 1990.

84. Berg, C., Hedrum, A., Holmberg, A., Ponten, F., Uhlen, M., and Lundeberg, J. Direct solid-phase sequence analysis of the human p53 gene by use of multiplex polymerase chain reaction and α-thiotriphosphate nucleotides. *Clin. Chem.* **41:**1461–1466, 1995.

85. Cama, A., Palmirotta, R., Curia, M. C., Esposito, D. L., Ranieri, A., Ficari, F., Valanzano, R., Battista, P., Modesti, A., Tonelli, F., and Mariani-Costantini, R. Multiplex PCR analysis and genotype-phenotype correlations of frequent APC mutations. *Hum. Mutat.* **5:**144–152, 1995.

86. Chamberlian, J. S., Gibbs, R. A., Ranier, J. E., and Caskey, C. T. Multiplex PCR for the diagnosis of Duchenne muscular dystrophy, in *PCR Protocols: A Guide to Methods and Applications*, Innis, M. A., Gelfand, D. H., Sinsky, J. J., and White, T. J., eds., Academic, New York, pp. 272–281, 1990.

87. Beggs, A. H., Koenig, M., Boyce, F. M., and Kunkel, L. M. Detection of 98% of DMD/BMD gene deletions by polymerase chain reaction. *Hum. Genet.* **86:**45–48, 1990.

88. Edwards, M. C. and Gibbs, R. A. Multiplex PCR: advantages, development, and applications. *PCR Methods Appl.* **3:**S65–S75, 1994.

89. Runnebaum, I. B., Nagarajan, M., Bowman, M., Soto, D., and Sukumar, S. Mutations in p53 as potential molecular markers for human breast cancer. *Proc. Natl. Acad. Sci. USA* **88:**10,657–10,661, 1991.

90. Roest, P. A. M., Roberts, R. G., Sugino, S., van Ommen, G. B., and den Dunnen, J. T. Protein trunction test (PTT) for rapid detection of translation-terminating mutations. *Hum. Mol. Genet.* **2:**1719–1721, 1993.

91. Powell, S. M., Petersen, G. M., Krush, A. J., Booker, S. , Jen, J., Giardiello, F. M., Hamilton, S. R., Vogelstein, B., and Kinzler, K. W. Molecular diagnosis of familial adenomatous polyposis. *New Engl. J. Med.* **329:**1982–1987, 1993.

92. Sarkar, G. and Sommer, S. S. Access to a messenger RNA sequence or its protein product is not limited by tissue or species specificity. *Science* **244:**331–334, 1989.

93. Miyoshi, Y., Nagase, H., Ando, H., Horji, A., Ichii, S., Nakatsuru, S., Aoki, T., Miki, Y., Takesada, M., and Nakamura, Y. Somatic mutations of the APC gene in colorectal tumors: mutation cluster region in the APC gene. *Hum. Mol. Genet.* **1:**229–233, 1992.

94. van der Luijt, R., Khan, P. M., Vasen, H., van Leeuwen, C., Tops, C., Roest, P., den Dunnen, J., and Fodde, R. Rapid detection of translation-terminating mutations at the adenomatous polyposis coli *(APC)* gene by direct protein truncation test. *Genomics* **20:**1–4, 1994.

95. Roest, P. A. M., Roberts, R. G., van der Tuijn, A. C., Heikoop, J. C., van Ommen, G. B., and den Dunnen, J. T. Protein truncation test (PTT) to rapidly screen the DMD gene for translation terminating mutations. *Neuromusc. Disord.* **3:**391–394, 1993.

96. Gardner, R. J., Bobrow, M., and Roberts, R. G. The identification of point mutations in Duchenne muscular dystrophy patients by using reverse-transcription PCR and the protein truncation test. *Am. J. Hum. Genet.* **57:**311–320, 1995.

97. Heim, R. A., Kam-Morgan, L. N. W., Binnie, C. G., Corns, D. D., Cayouette, M. C., Farber, R. A., Aylsworth, A. S., Silverman, L. M., and Luce, M. C. Distribution of 13 truncating mutations in the neurofibromatosis 1 gene. *Hum. Mol. Genet.* **4:**975–981, 1995.

98. Hogervorst, F. B. L., Cornelis, R. S., Bout, M., van Vliet, M., Oosterwijk, J. C., Olmer, R., Bakker, B., Klijm, J. G. M., Vasen, H. F. A., Meijers-Heijboer, H., Menko, F. H., Cornelisse, C. J., den Dunnen, J. T., Devilee, P., and van Ommen, G. B. Rapid detection of *BRCA1* mutations by the protein truncation test. *Nature Genet.* **10:**208–212, 1995.

8

Nucleic Acid Hybridization and Amplification *In Situ*

Principles and Applications in Molecular Pathology

Matthew S. Cowlen

1. INTRODUCTION

The ability of pathologists to diagnose disease has been enhanced significantly by the application of nucleic acid technologies, such as Southern blot hybridization and the polymerase chain reaction (PCR). These techniques are used routinely in clinical molecular diagnostic laboratories to detect and analyze genetic alterations associated with human disease. However, the ability to associate the nucleic acid sequence of interest with histopathologic or cytogenetic abnormalities directly is lost when tissue is destroyed during the extraction of nucleic acids. The analysis of nucleic acids *in situ* overcomes this limitation. ISH* offers the combined advantages of molecular biology, analytical morphology, and cytogenetics by facilitating the analysis of DNA or RNA in tissues and chromosomes. ISA of nucleic acid sequences using PCR is a developing technology that offers increased sensitivity compared to conventional ISH for detecting low-copy sequences. *In situ* nucleic acid techniques are discussed in detail in this chapter, with emphasis on the principles and clinical relevance of each technique.

2. ISH

ISH uses labeled nucleic acid probes to detect specific DNA or RNA targets in tissue sections, intact cells, or chromosomes. ISH combines the remarkable specificity and sensitivity of nucleic acid hybridization with the ability to obtain cytogenetic and morphologic information. The basic principle underlying ISH is the intrinsic ability of single-stranded DNA or RNA to anneal specifically to a complementary sequence and form a double-stranded hybrid. The same principle is the foundation of Southern and Northern blot hybridization of extracted nucleic acids, in which a labeled probe is used to visualize target sequences bound to a membrane support. With ISH, nucleic acid targets remain localized in tissue sections, intact cells, metaphase chromosomes, or interphase nuclei attached to glass slides. Hybrids between the target sequence and

*See page 186 for list of abbreviations used in this chapter.

From: Molecular Diagnostics: For the Clinical Laboratorian
Edited by: W. B. Coleman and G. J. Tsongalis Humana Press Inc., Totowa, NJ

labeled probe are detected by microscopy and can be viewed in relation to chromosomal structure or tissue morphology.

3. FISH IN THE CYTOGENETIC ANALYSIS OF CHROMOSOMAL ABNORMALITIES

FISH uses fluorescent probes for the detection of genetic aberrations in metaphase chromosomes and interphase nuclei. The use of FISH in the detection of chromosomal abnormalities has several advantages over traditional cytogenetic techniques, including the ability to perform cytogenetic analysis on interphase cells, which eliminates the need for in vitro cell culture, thereby reducing turnaround time and facilitating the analysis of a wide range of cell types; and the ability to analyze complex rearrangements and other alterations that are difficult to assess by chromosome banding techniques. Several variations of FISH have been developed, including comparative genomic hybridization (1), the simultaneous analysis of multiple probes by digital imaging (2), and the enumeration of cells containing specific DNA sequences by flow cytometry (3). FISH has applications in the molecular diagnosis of cancer, including the detection of gene amplification, deletions, rearrangements, aneuploidy, marker chromosomes, residual disease, and recurrence, particularly in hematological malignancies (4–7). FISH provides a rapid and sensitive method for the detection of prenatal and postnatal chromosome aberrations (8), and is an important tool used in positional cloning of the human genome (9). The basic steps involved in FISH for molecular cytogenetics are:

1. Prepare metaphase chromosomes or interphase nuclei;
2. Denature target DNA and double-stranded probes;
3. Hybridize hapten-labeled or fluorescent probes to target DNA;
4. Wash to remove probe bound to nontarget sequences;
5. Incubate with fluorescent ligand for detection of hapten-labeled probes; and
6. Detect hybrids by fluorescence microscopy.

Metaphase chromosomes for FISH are isolated by blocking the progression of mitosis from metaphase to anaphase in rapidly dividing cells. This usually requires culturing cells in vitro in the presence of growth factors or other mitogens to stimulate cell growth (10). Progression from metaphase to anaphase is blocked by adding an agent, such as colchicine, that disrupts the mitotic spindle. Cells are then lysed on a microscope slide, leaving metaphase chromosomes attached to the surface. Chromosome structure is clearly visible in metaphase spreads and can be analyzed in relation to fluorescence hybridization signals. However, it is difficult to obtain metaphase spreads from cells that respond poorly to cell culture, since the isolation of metaphase chromosomes requires actively dividing cells. Obtaining high-quality metaphase chromosomes that are representative of solid tumors in vivo is particularly problematic. The need for rapidly dividing cells for FISH can be eliminated by isolating nuclei from cells in interphase. Because cell culture is not required, interphase cytogenetics offers greatly reduced turnaround times and extends the availability of FISH analysis to archived blood smears (11,12) and paraffin-embedded tissue sections, including solid tumors (13). Interphase nuclei can be isolated from cells in suspension by fixing cells in methanol:acetic acid (3:1) and lysing in hypotonic buffer on microscope slides. Slides can be used immediately for FISH or

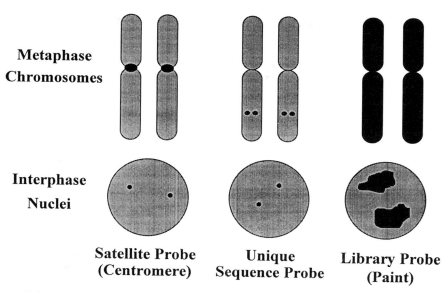

Fig. 1. Schematic representation of hybridization signals (black shading) observed with FISH probes in metaphase chromosomes and interphase nuclei. Satellite probes display two fluorescence signals in normal diploid cells near the centromeres of homologous chromosomes. In contrast, monosomy would appear as one signal, and trisomy as three signals (not shown). Unique sequence probes display two signals on each homologous chromosome in metaphase, representing individual sister chromatids that are present following DNA replication, whereas interphase nuclei display one signal for each chromosome. Chromosome-specific DNA libraries hybridized to sequences throughout the chromosome and are generally referred to as chromosome paints.

can be stored for future use after dehydration in graded alcohols. Deparaffinized tissue sections require protease treatment to increase probe accessibility.

The three general types of nucleic acid probes used for FISH are satellite probes, whole chromosome paints, and unique sequence probes (Fig. 1). Satellite probes hybridize to chromosome-specific, repetitive DNA sequences located near the centromeres in metaphase spreads or interphase nuclei. These probes are particularly useful in detecting the loss or gain of a chromosome (aneuploidy). Satellite probes are also used as controls in mixtures with other probes to ensure proper chromosome identification. This can be especially important when analyzing deletions and translocations. Chromosome-specific telomere probes can be used to detect terminal deletions and translocations. Chromosome paints contain chromosome-specific DNA libraries that hybridize to sequences throughout the entire chromosome and can be used to analyze structural rearrangements, including translocations (Figs. 2 and 3). Chromosome paints are best suited for analysis of metaphase chromosomes owing to the diffuse nature of the signal in interphase nuclei. Unique sequence probes are genomic clones that are complementary to single-copy loci and can be used with either metaphase spreads or interphase nuclei to detect translocations (Fig. 4), gene amplification (Fig. 5), and deletions (Fig. 6). FISH probes are commercially available from several commercial sources (including Oncor [Gaithersburg, MD], Boehringer-Mannheim [Indianapolis, IN]).

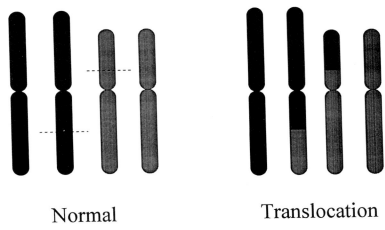

Normal   Translocation

Fig. 2. Schematic representation of the detection of a reciprocal translocation by FISH using a chromosome-specific DNA library. Chromosome translocations (breakpoint represented by dashed lines) can be detected using DNA libraries to paint (black shading) the entire chromosome. The identity of the unpainted chromosome involved in the translocation can be ascertained using either paints or satellite probes, or by chromosome banding techniques.

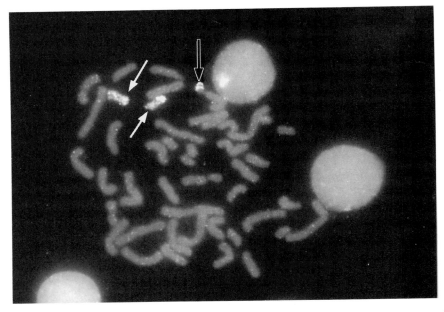

Fig. 3. Identification of a chromosome translocation by FISH using DNA library probes. A biotin-labeled DNA library specific for chromosome 18 was used with an avidin/fluorescein detection system to elucidate a translocation involving chromosome 18 and chromosome 21 in metaphase chromosomes. The translocation created a derivative chromosome, der(21)t(18;21). The translocated portion of chromosome 18 is visible on the short arm of chromosome 21 (open arrow). The normal chromosome 18, and the remainder of the translocated chromosome are also visible (closed arrows). The identity of chromosome 21 was determined in a separate hybridization using chromosome 21-specific probes (not shown) (photomicrograph contributed by Kathleen Kaiser-Rogers and Kathleen Rao, University of North Carolina at Chapel Hill).

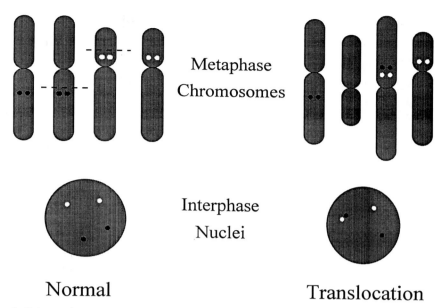

Fig. 4. Schematic representation of the detection of a reciprocal translocation by FISH using unique sequence probes. Translocations can be detected by FISH using differentially labeled probes that hybridize to unique sequences flanking the translocation breakpoint (dashed lines). The translocation results in the juxtaposition of the probes in the derivative chromosome, which is visible in both metaphase chromosomes and interphase nuclei.

Probes for FISH are usually labeled with nonfluorescent haptens that can be detected through their ability to bind fluorescent ligands (Fig. 7). The most common haptens used to label FISH probes are biotin and digoxigenin. Biotin has high affinity for avidin and streptavidin, which can be conjugated with fluorescent molecules and used to detect biotin-labeled probes. Fluorescent antidigoxigenin antibody conjugates are used to detect digoxigenin-labeled probes. Weak signals can be amplified by using a fluorescence-labeled secondary antibody. Ligands are conjugated with fluorescent dyes such as fluorescein and rhodamine. Fluorochromes with distinct excitation and emission wavelength maxima can be used in combination with different ligands to detect multiple hapten-labeled probes simultaneously *(2,14)*. The identification of multiple chromosomal aberrations by multicolor FISH analysis can be enhanced by using probes that are directly labeled with fluorescent nucleotide conjugates *(4,15)*. Probes that are directly labeled have several advantages over hapten-labeled probes, including shortened protocols and reduced number of required reagents. Moreover, the number of fluorescent labels that can be visualized simultaneously is not limited by the number of available hapten/ligand pairs. Propidium iodide or DAPI is used as a counterstain to provide contrast with probe fluorescence and to visualize chromosomes or nuclei. DAPI is particularly useful in metaphase chromosomes, because it creates a banding pattern that is identical to G-banding. Therefore, fluorescence signals from locus-specific probes can be viewed in relation to chromosome bands, which is important for positional cloning.

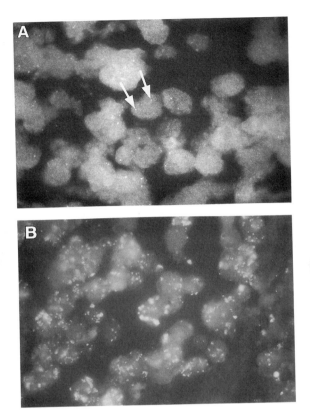

Fig. 5. Detection of N-*myc* gene amplification in a neuroblastoma by FISH. A digoxigenin-labeled N-*myc* probe was used with an anti-digoxigenin antibody/fluorescein detection system. Two copies of N-*myc* are visible (arrows) in normal cells (**A**), whereas numerous intense fluorescence signals are evident in neuroblastoma cells containing amplified N-myc sequences (**B**) (photomicrographs contributed by Peter Ferlisi and Georgette Dent, University of North Carolina at Chapel Hill).

Hybridization of FISH probes requires that double-stranded DNA be denatured to form single-stranded targets. Denaturation can be accomplished by placing slides containing metaphase spreads or interphase nuclei in a solution containing 300 mM NaCl, 30 mM sodium citrate, pH 7.0, and 70% formamide, incubating at 70°C, and dehydrating in ice-cold graded alcohols. A small volume of hybridization mixture containing labeled probe is placed on the slide and a coverslip is sealed onto the slide with rubber cement to prevent evaporation. Slides are then incubated at a temperature based on the melting temperature for the probe. Melting temperature is dependent on the salt and formamide concentrations of the hybridization buffer, and on the length and GC content of the hybrid. Posthybridization washes reduce background fluorescence by removing any probe that is bound to nontarget sequences. The stringency of the hybridization reaction and posthybridization washes can be modified by altering the temperature or the salt concentration and/or formamide concentration of the buffer. Following posthybridization washes, slides are incubated with a solution containing fluorescent ligands, washed to reduce nonspecific ligand binding, and coverslipped for fluores-

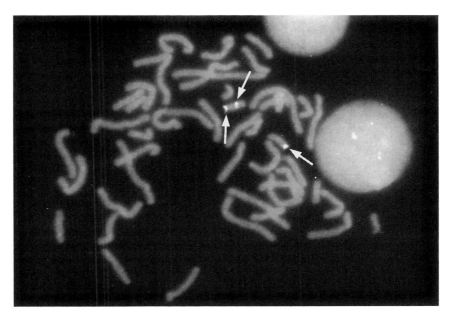

Fig. 6. Detection of a deletion in the DiGeorge region of chromosome 22 by FISH. A unique sequence probe labeled with digoxigenin was used with an antidigoxigenin antibody/fluorescein detection system in metaphase chromosomes. The normal copy of chromosome 22 exhibits two fluorescence signals. The DiGeorge probe can be seen in the central portion of the chromosome corresponding to 22q11, and a distal chromosome 22 control probe is visible in the telomeric region. The copy of chromosome 22 containing the DiGeorge deletion exhibits a signal from the control probe only (photomicrograph contributed by Kathleen Kaiser-Rogers and Kathleen Rao University of North Carolina at Chapel Hill).

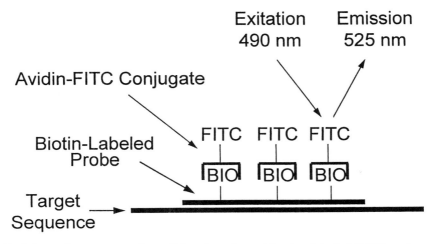

Fig. 7. Schematic representation of the detection of hapten-labeled FISH probes. In this example, a probe labeled with biotin (designated BIO) is detected with a conjugate of avidin and fluorescein isothiocyante (designated FITC). Fluorescein emits light at 525 nm during excitation by 490 nm light.

cence microscopy using an aqueous mounting medium. An antifade additive, such as phenylenediamine dihydrochloride, will reduce photobleaching during microscopy.

FISH images are obtained and analyzed using fluorescence microscopy, using either single or multiple band pass filters to obtain the appropriate excitation and emission wavelengths. A triple band pass filter can be used with some dye combinations, such as fluorescein, rhodamine, and DAPI, to view multiple fluorescent signals simultaneously. The quantification and analysis of FISH signals are enhanced substantially through the use of a digital imaging system, which is comprised of a fluorescence microscope with a cooled CCD camera interfaced with image analysis computer software. This technology provides increased sensitivity and flexibility for FISH, and has been used to analyze seven DNA probes simultaneously *(2,4)*. Chromosomes are labeled with multiple fluorescent dyes, and each dye is imaged individually. Then, a composite image is generated digitally to visualize all targets simultaneously. Fewer fluorescent dyes are required for techniques, such as ratio coding and combination coding, in which each chromosome is detected by one or more dyes *(4)*. Composite images blend the different colors associated with a particular chromosome, thereby increasing the number of detectable targets. Digital imaging microscopy was essential in the development of comparative genomic hybridization, in which a quantitative digital image processing system calculates ratios of fluorescence intensities generated by differentially labeled, competing DNA probes *(1)*. Regardless of the specific technique used, digital imaging is an ideal way to manipulate, enhance, analyze, and store microscopic images obtained by FISH.

4. APPLICATIONS OF FISH

4.1. FISH Applications in Tumor Pathology

The clinical applications of FISH include the diagnosis, prognosis, and monitoring of human malignancies *(4–7)*. Cytogenetic alterations associated with neoplastic disease have been identified in solid tumors and leukemias, and offer targets for FISH analysis. The relationship between genetic aberrations and tumor progression is understood best in human leukemias. FISH has been used to detect chromosome translocations associated with chronic and acute leukemias *(7)*. FISH was used to detect a common deletion in chromosome 5 in acute myeloid leukemia *(16)* and to identify deletions in the tumor suppressor gene p53 associated with poor prognosis in chronic B-cell leukemias *(17)*. Aneuploidy, including monosomy 7 and trisomy involving chromosomes 8, 12, and 17, are associated with leukemia and are readily detected by FISH using chromosome-specific satellite probes *(18–20)*. These studies demonstrate that FISH is an effective method for the analysis of chromosomal aberrations in hematologic malignancies. Several reports describe the detection of minimal residual disease and relapse in leukemia using FISH in cases in which patients appeared to be in complete remission *(7,21,22)*, whereas patients who did not exhibit chromosomal abnormalities by FISH remained in remission *(7,19)*. FISH probes specific for the X and Y chromosomes have been used to determine the origin of bone marrow cells following sex-mismatched transplantation *(6)*, in which the detection of hematopoietic cells of host origin often indicates relapse of leukemia.

The genetic abnormalities associated with solid tumors are less understood than those for the leukemias, because solid tumors are difficult to study by traditional cytogenetic techniques using metaphase chromosomes. The use of interphase FISH has contributed to important advances in the understanding of solid tumor cytogenetics, and was used to detect monosomy 9 in neoplasms of the bladder *(23)*, trisomy 7 in thyroid tumors *(24)*, aneuploidy in breast cancer *(25)*, and the deletion of loci in chromosome 17p in breast cancer *(18)*. A retrospective study using interphase FISH on paraffin-embedded tissues from patients with carcinoma of the prostate demonstrates that there is a strong correlation between the presence of trisomy 7 and poor prognosis in this cancer *(26)*. FISH has been used to detect gene amplification in solid tumors, including amplification of N-*myc* in neuroblastoma (Fig. 5; ref. *13*), and of *erb*B-2 (HER-2/*neu*) in cancers of the breast *(27)* and bladder *(28)*. Translocations have been identified in solid tumors using FISH, which is particularly useful in the diagnosis of Ewing's sarcoma and other "small round cell" tumors *(29)*. These reports demonstrate the utility of FISH for interphase cytogenetic analysis of chromosomal aberrations in solid tumors, which are often difficult or impossible to culture in vitro for standard karyotyping.

The ability to identify gene amplifications and deletions in solid tumors has been enhanced dramatically by comparative genomic hybridization *(1,30)*. This technique allows the detection of amplified or deleted sequences anywhere in the genome of human tumors, without prior knowledge of the aberration involved or possession of specific probes. Comparative genomic hybridization involves the competitive hybridization of differentially labeled tumor DNA and normal DNA to normal metaphase spreads. A quantitative digital image processing system calculates ratios of fluorescence intensities generated by the competing DNA along the medial axis of each chromosome. Amplification of a locus in the tumor genome results in an increase in signal from tumor DNA relative to normal DNA at that locus, whereas a deletion in the tumor genome results in a decrease in the ratio. Comparative genomic hybridization should help to expand knowledge rapidly of gene amplifications and deletions associated with various neoplasms. However, large clinical studies are required to correlate genetic abnormalities with disease progression, response to therapy, and overall clinical outcome in order to understand the significance of chromosome aberrations detected by FISH.

4.2. FISH Applications in the Prenatal and Postnatal Diagnosis of Genetic Disease

Traditional cytogenetic karyotyping of banded metaphase chromosomes provides a highly accurate method for detecting aneuploidies and gross structural rearrangements of chromosomes in amniocytes and chorionic villi. However, turnaround time is usually 1–2 wk, since cells must be cultured to generate metaphase chromosomes. FISH eliminates the need for cell culture in cases where interphase nuclei are suitable. Trisomies involving chromosomes 13 and 18 (multiple severe congenital malformations and rapid death in liveborn infants; *in utero* demise), trisomy 21 (Down's syndrome), and sex chromosome aneuploidies, such as XO (Turner's syndrome), XXY (Klinefelter's syndrome), XYY, and trisomy X, are readily detected in interphase nuclei by FISH using satellite probes *(8)*. Unbalanced translocations, complex rearrangements, duplications, and defects that fail to provide a distinct banding pattern are often difficult to ascertain by traditional karyotyping. These aberrations are detectable in prenatal studies by FISH, using chromosome-specific DNA libraries (paints), alone or in combination with karyotype analysis. (Fig. 3; ref. *8*). Unique sequence probes are available (Oncor) for the identification of deletions associated with several disorders with cytogenetic etiology, including Prader-Willi and Angelman syndromes, Cri-du Chat syndrome, X-linked ichthyosis, X-linked ocular albinism, Smith-Magenis syndrome, Elastin Williams syndrome, and DiGeorge syndrome (Fig. 6). These probes are prepared premixed with chromosome-specific control probes to assist in target chromosome verification.

5. LIMITATIONS OF FISH

There are several limitations associated with FISH technology. The use of FISH in monitoring minimal residual disease is limited, despite the success of some studies. For example, the false-positive rate can be as high as 5–10% when determining chromosome loss, making the analysis of minimal residual disease very difficult in leukemia characterized by a monosomy. Furthermore, because of technical artifacts, and the fact that some nonleukemic cells may be aneuploid, the overall sensitivity of FISH for the analysis of minimal residual disease is only about 1% *(31)*. FISH is far less sensitive than quantitative PCR methods, which can detect one residual disease cell in 10^6 normal cells *(32)*. Analysis of single-copy sequences requires specific probes, which may not be available for the locus of interest. This problem will become less relevant as the Human Genome Project progresses and makes available increasing numbers of newly cloned sequences. Cytogenetic analysis using FISH is limited to detecting aberrations that involve the target chromosomes. For example, unique sequence probes used to detect a translocation may not detect an accompanying aneuploidy, and chromosome-specific satellite probes will not detect aneuploidies involving other chromosomes. In contrast, traditional karyotyping displays all chromosomes for cytogenetic analysis. Comparative genomic hybridization and other multicolor techniques have increased the number of abnormalities that can be detected by FISH in a single assay. FISH is well suited to compliment standard cytogenetics in many situations, and may replace traditional techniques in specific circumstances, such as the detection of common aneuploidies.

6. ISH IN THE HISTOLOGICAL LOCALIZATION OF NUCLEIC ACIDS

ISH is used in combination with histochemical staining techniques to detect DNA or RNA targets in tissue sections or intact cells. Specific nucleic acid sequences can be analyzed in the context of morphologic information available from the analysis of specimens obtained by surgical biopsy. Tissue that has been properly fixed and embedded can be sectioned and analyzed immediately or can be archived for future analysis, including retrospective studies. The detection of mRNA by ISH is feasible in some cases in which immunohistochemical staining fails to detect protein. ISH has become an important method in molecular pathology *(33,34)*, with applications that include the cellular localization of viral nucleic acids *(5,35–38)* and the detection of tumor-specific gene expression in neoplasia *(5,37,39)*. The basic steps involved in ISH for the histological localization of nucleic acids in tissue sections are:

1. Fix tissue to preserve morphology and retain target nucleic acids;
2. Cytospin suspended cells onto slides or embed tissues in paraffin, cut sections, attach to slides, and deparaffinize;

3. Digest tissue with protease to render target sequences accessible to probe;
4. Denature double-stranded targets and probes;
5. Hybridize hapten-labeled probes to target DNA;
6. Wash to remove probe bound to nontarget sequences; and
7. Detect hybrids microscopically by immunohistochemical staining.

Morphology is best preserved by immersing fresh tissue in a chemical fixative. Tissue fixatives can be broadly classified as either crosslinking or precipitating. Crosslinking fixatives include buffered formalin, paraformaldehyde, and glutaraldehyde. Ethanol and acetic acid in a 3:1 mixture is a common precipitating fixative. In general, crosslinking fixatives are superior for ISH because they are more effective than precipitating fixatives for the preservation of tissue morphology. In addition, ethanol/acetic acid may be ineffective at retaining RNA in some tissues *(40)*. Crosslinking fixatives preserve RNA by limiting diffusion and by providing some protection from degradation by RNases. Buffered formalin is an excellent fixative for obtaining strong, reproducible ISH signals and maintaining morphology *(41)*, and is widely used in surgical pathology laboratories. Tissues can be fixed for several hours to several days. However, over-fixation can result in decreased adherence of tissue to slides and reduced accessibility of probes to nucleic acid targets, and should be avoided.

To ensure the best possible morphology, tissues are fixed in buffered formalin and embedded in paraffin prior to cutting sections. Surgical biopsy specimens are routinely prepared in this manner in most pathology laboratories, making formalin-fixed, paraffin-embedded tissues readily available for ISH. Paraffin blocks are cut with a microtome into sections 3-10 μm in thickness, which are attached to coated glass slides that promote adherence of tissue. Silane-coated slides can be prepared in the lab, but it is probably more time- and cost-effective to purchase pretreated slides. Vectabond (Vector Labs) and Superfrost/Plus slides (Fisher Scientific) performed well in tests of tissue adhesion *(42)*. Slides containing adhered tissue are deparaffinized in xylene and dehydrated in graded ethanols prior to protease digestion and ISH. Successful ISH is possible using fixed frozen tissue, without paraffin embedding, in some tissues *(42)*. In this case, tissues are immersed in a buffered solution of 15% sucrose, after fixation, to reduce freeze artifacts. Certain tissues, such as lung, are not appropriate for frozen sections and must be embedded in paraffin to maintain morphology.

Most tissues that are fixed in formalin or other crosslinking fixatives must be digested with a protease prior to ISH. Crosslinks between cellular macromolecules impede the penetration of probes and reduce accessibility to target nucleic acids. Optimal protease digestion will result in the degradation of enough crosslinks to allow penetration of probe while retaining acceptable morphology. Commonly used proteases for ISH include proteinase K and pepsin, which have different specific activities and pH optima. Pepsin is active at pH 2.0 and can be inactivated efficiently by washing in a neutral or slightly basic buffer. Proteinase K can be difficult to wash out of some tissues and can be heat-inactivated in formalin-fixed tissues if washing is insufficient. Different tissues exhibit distinct sensitivities to digestion with proteases. Therefore, protease concentration and time of treatment must be determined empirically for each tissue and protease used. Different lots of the same protease may also exhibit activity different from a previous lot and should be tested prior to use. In general, longer fixation times will require greater digestion with protease to obtain an optimal hybridiza-

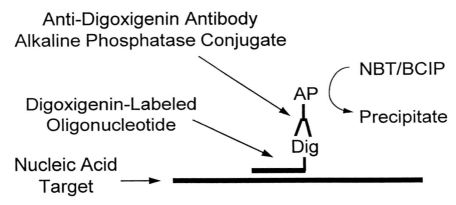

Fig. 8. Schematic representation of the detection of hapten-labeled ISH probes by immuno-histochemistry. In this example, an oligonucleotide probe is end-labeled with digoxigenin (designated Dig) and detected with an antidigoxigenin antibody conjugated with alkaline phosphatase (designated AP). A chromogenic mixture of nitroblue tetrazolium salt (designated NBT) and 5-bromo-4-chloro-3-indolyl phosphate (designated BCIP) is converted to a dark precipitate by alkaline phosphatase.

tion signal. Tissues can be viewed microscopically during protease treatment so that morphology can be monitored during digestion. The best indication of optimal protease treatment is a strong hybridization signal along with good tissue morphology.

Probes for ISH include:

1. Double-stranded genomic DNA cloned in a plasmid vector or amplified by PCR;
2. Single-stranded oligonucleotide DNA produced using a DNA synthesizer;
3. Single-stranded DNA cloned in a M13 bacteriophage vector or amplified by asymmetrical PCR; and
4. Single-stranded antisense RNA transcribed from DNA cloned in an expression vector (riboprobe).

Genomic probes can be labeled to a greater extent than oligonucleotide probes but do not necessarily increase sensitivity owing to reduced penetration compared to small oligonucleotide probes. The sensitivity of oligonucleotide probes can be increased by using multiple oligonucleotides specific for different regions of the same target. Oligonucleotide probes specific for short, unique sequences are useful for distinguishing targets with a high degree of homology. Detection of RNA targets is very sensitive using riboprobes because of the high thermal stability of RNA–RNA hybrids. Single stranded probes have advantages over double-stranded probes in that denaturing prior to use is unnecessary, and because the potential problem of reannealing to the complementary strand is eliminated.

Probes for ISH were originally labeled radioisotopically with ^{35}S, ^{32}P, or ^{125}I. However, probes labeled with the nonisotopic hapten digoxigenin are equally as sensitive, exhibit lower background, and provide greater resolution than radiolabeled probes *(43)*. Moreover, the use of nonisotopic labels eliminates the health hazards and disposal problems associated with radioactive probes. Digoxigenin-labeled probes are detected enzymatically with antidigoxigenin antibodies conjugated with alkaline phosphatase or horseradish peroxidase (Fig. 8). These enzymes convert soluble substrates into

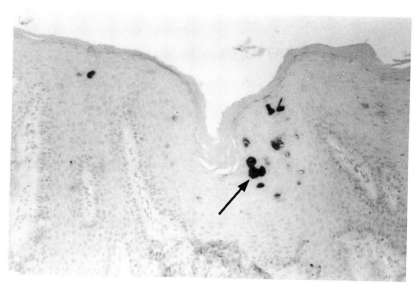

Fig. 9. Detection of HPV type 6 in a low-grade squamous intraepithelial lesion by *in situ* hybridization. A biotin labeled probe was used with an avidin/alkaline phosphatase conjugate to detect HPV 6 in a genital wart biopsy. Darkly stained cells containing HPV 6 are present near the surface of the lesion (photomicrograph contributed by Gerard Nuovo, State University of New York at Stony Brook).

insoluble precipitates, which appear as dark, localized cellular or subcellular staining when viewed microscopically (Fig. 9). Biotin is another popular nonisotopic label that can be detected with enzyme conjugates of avidin, streptavidin, or antibiotin antibodies. Endogenous biotin can cause high background staining in some tissues, particularly liver, kidney, and lymphoid tissues. Background signal is less likely with antidigoxigenin antibodies, because digoxigenin is not synthesized in mammalian tissue. Antibodies to digoxigenin and biotin can be labeled with gold particles and used for immunogold-silver staining, which has proven to be a very sensitive and reliable means to detect hapten-labeled probes in formalin-fixed, paraffin-embedded tissues *(44)*.

Labeled nucleotides, such as digoxigenin-11-dUTP or biotin-16-dUTP, are incorporated into double-stranded genomic probes by DNA polymerases using nick translation, random primed labeling, or PCR. Oligonucleotide probes are 3'-end-labeled using terminal deoxynucleotidyl transferase and a labeled dideoxynucleotide (digoxigenin-11-ddUTP), which prevents tailing of the probe with multiple labels. 3'-tailing enhances sensitivity by increasing the number of labels per probe molecule and can be accomplished by using terminal deoxynucleotidyl transferase with labeled dUTP. However, tailing may also increase background. Riboprobes are labeled during in vitro transcription by RNA polymerase. Nonisotopic labeling and detection kits are commercially available (Genius™ System, Boehringer Mannheim; BioProbe® and DETEK®, Enzo Diagnostics, Farmingdale, NY).

Hybridization is performed by transferring a small aliquot of a solution containing labeled probe (denatured in the case of double-stranded probes) to protease-digested tissue sections. A coverslip is then placed over the specimen to prevent evaporation. Double stranded targets must be denatured prior to hybridization, and denaturation enhances hybridization in mRNA by eliminating secondary structures. As with other forms of nucleic acid hybridization, the stability of the hydrogen bonds between probe and target molecules is dependent on temperature, salt, and formamide concentration, and the length and GC content of the hybrid. The hybridization reaction must be done at an optimal temperature relative to the target hybrid, yet higher than the melting temperature of potential nonspecific hybrids. The melting temperature of a given hybrid can be determined mathematically (*see* Chapter 6), however, the optimal hybridization temperature should be determined in the laboratory to maximize hybridization to target sequences and reduce nonspecific hybridization. Posthybridization washes of appropriate stringency (determined by temperature and concentrations of salt and formamide) further reduce nonspecific hybridization. Optimal stringency is particularly important for short probes, such as oligonucleotides. Following hybridization and washes, samples are incubated with ligand–enzyme conjugates, washed to reduce nonspecific ligand binding, and incubated with the appropriate enzyme substrates. The development of localized precipitate is monitored microscopically. When color development is sufficient, tissues are washed and counterstained to provide contrast for the visualization of morphology, or may be left without counterstain if morphology is visible. Detailed procedures and optimization protocols for ISH are available in the literature *(33,42,45,46)* and from companies that market ISH probes.

Controls are essential for the accurate interpretation of ISH data. Nonspecific signals from the hybridization of probe to nontarget sequences, or from the nonspecific binding of enzyme–antibody conjugates, produce false-positive signals which must be identified. Tissue specimens that are known to be positive or negative for the target nucleic acid are important controls that should be probed along with unknown samples. Probes should be used in Southern or Northern blot hybridization assays to demonstrate that the probes bind specifically to the target of interest. Probes that are noncomplementary to target sequences can be used as negative controls for ISH. For example, sense RNA probes are homologous to mRNA in tissue and should yield negative results, whereas antisense probes are complementary to mRNA and should be positive. Omission of probe will reveal nonspecific binding of the ligand–enzyme conjugate and exposes the presence of endogenous biotin when using avidin–enzyme conjugates. Omission of the ligand–enzyme conjugate exposes the presence of endogenous alkaline phosphatase or peroxidase, depending on the detection system. The preservation of RNA in paraffin-embedded tissue sections can be demonstrated by hybridization of a poly(dT) oligonucleotide probe *(33)* or by hybridization of a probe complementary to conserved sequences within 28S ribosomal RNA *(47)*. Moreover, these techniques are useful for optimizing ISH parameters, such as fixation and protease digestion, prior to the use of specific probes for mRNA. Treatment of specimens with RNase or DNase abolishes signal from RNA and DNA, respectively, and demonstrates the nature of the target sequence. Running the appropriate controls with each hybridization will ensure that the signals detected are a result of the specific hybridization of probe to the target sequence.

7. APPLICATIONS OF ISH
IN THE HISTOLOGIC LOCALIZATION OF NUCLEIC ACIDS

7.1. Detection and Localization of Viral Nucleic Acids

ISH is an important technique for identifying and localizing viral nucleic acids associated with infectious disease and cancer *(5,35–39,48)*. ISH has been used to determine the intracelluar localization of the hepatitis viruses, human papillomaviruses (HPV), and herpes simplex viruses (HSV) *(38)*, and to detect these viruses, as well as adenovirus, cytomegalovirus, and JC virus, in clinical specimens *(48)*. ISH was used to detect HSV in a duodenal biopsy in a patient described as having "nonspecific" inflammation, and to diagnose cytomegalovirus (CMV) infection in a patient originally suspected of being infected with HSV *(48)*. These cases demonstrate the ability of ISH to provide an unequivocal diagnosis in difficult clinical situations. Epstein-Barr virus (EBV)-encoded RNAs are expressed abundantly in latent EBV infections and are ideal ISH targets for detection and localization of EBV in a variety of malignancies *(37)*. ISH is particularly useful for the diagnosis of nasopharyngeal carcinoma in patients with neck metastases of unknown origin *(49)*. ISH can also provide important diagnostic information in equivocal cases of HPV, where it can be difficult to distinguish HPV-induced low-grade squamous intraepithelial lesions (condyloma) from non-HPV conditions in the lower genital tract (Fig. 9; ref. *48)*. Complete ISH assay systems for HPV, EBV, hepatitis B virus, HSV, adenovirus, and CMV are available from Enzo Diagnostics.

7.2. Detection and Localization of Gene Expression in Human Tumors

Carcinogenesis is a complex, multistep process in which the normal control of gene expression is altered, resulting in uncontrolled cell growth and metastatic neoplasia. ISH has been used to detect oncogene expression in neoplastic tissue *(5,39)*, including aberrant expression of c-*myc* in multiple myeloma and chronic lymphocytic leukemia *(50)*. Non-Hodgkin's lymphoma was typed based on oncogene expression as determined by ISH, which revealed a correlation between high-grade T-cell phenotype and Ki-*ras* expression *(51)*. c-*erb*B-2 mRNA was detected by ISH in paraffin-embedded sections of biopsies from patients with carcinoma of the breast in cases where cytosolic and immunohistochemical analyses of c-*erb*B-2 oncoprotein were negative *(33)*. ISH was used to analyze expression of insulin-like growth factor type II in hepatocellular carcinoma *(52)*, platelet-derived growth factor and platelet-derived growth factor receptor expression associated with primary human astrocytomas *(53)*, and epidermal growth factor receptors in colon carcinoma *(54)*. ISH has also been used to demonstrate a reduction in tumor suppressor gene expression. For example, ISH analysis of retinoic acid receptor mRNA revealed a significant reduction in retinoic acid receptor β expression in paraffin-embedded sections of human head and neck squamous cell carcinoma *(55)*.

Tumor-specific mRNAs are important markers in endocrine neoplasms, which have been studied extensively using ISH. Lactotrophic adenomas were shown to express prolactin mRNA, whereas somatotrophic adenomas expressed plurihormonal genes, including adrenocorticotropic hormone, follicle-stimulating hormone, and luteinizing hormone mRNAs *(56)*. These pituitary hormones were undetectable by immunohis-

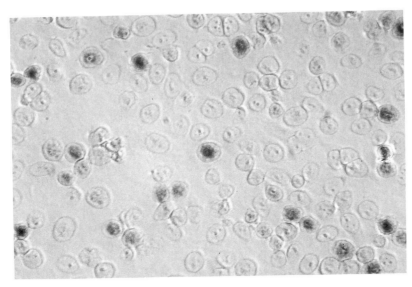

Fig. 10. Detection of an adenovirus DNA gene therapy vector by *in situ* hybridization. HeLa cells were grown in culture on glass microscope slides and exposed to replication-defective adenovirus. Cells were washed, fixed in 10% buffered formalin, permeabilized with pepsin, and probed with a digoxigenin-labeled oligonucleotide specific for adenovirus DNA. Dark staining nuclei indicate the subcellular localization of adenovirus DNA in transduced cells.

tochemical staining for protein in some cases in which mRNA was detected by ISH. mRNA for parathyroid hormone-related protein produced a strong hybridization signal in squamous cell carcinoma, but was not detected in basal cell carcinomas, demonstrating the tumor-specific expression of this peptide *(57)*. Chromogranin A has been used extensively as a marker for the diagnosis of neuroendocrine tumors, but is difficult to detect immunohistochemically in tumors with few secretory granules, such as neuroblastomas and small cell carcinoma of the lung. However, the chromogranin A gene is transcribed in these tumors, and chromogranin A mRNA is readily detectable by ISH *(58)*.

7.3. Cellular Localization of Expression Vectors for Gene Therapy

Diseases that result from mutations within the human genome are potentially curable by transducing effected cells with expression vectors containing a normal copy of the altered gene. Similarly, cancers might be cured by expressing, in tumor cells, foreign genes with therapeutic activity, such as tumor suppressor genes or genes that encode cytokines. The cellular location of transgenes and transgene expression must be ascertained for successful development of gene therapy vectors and protocols. ISH is an excellent method for localization of gene therapy vectors (Fig. 10) and has been used to detect transgene mRNA from a variety of expression vectors in transduced tissue. ISH detected neuron-specific expression of the *lacZ* reporter gene in a study that demonstrated the advantage of ISH over traditional X-gal staining for localization of gene therapy expression vectors *(59)*. Transgene expression has been detected by ISH in other systems, including vectors designed to express genes specifically in the hypoxic, glucose-deprived environment of solid tumors *(60)*, to treat cystic fibrosis

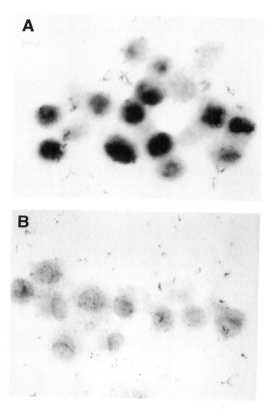

Fig. 11. Detection of HIV DNA in macrophages by PCR *in situ* hybridization. HIV DNA was readily detectable (dark staining) by PCR *in situ* hybridization using primers and a digoxigenin-labeled probe specific for the *gag* region of the HIV genome **(A)**. HIV DNA was undetectable in macrophages by standard ISH without prior amplification by PCR **(B)** (photomicrograph contributed by Gerard Nuovo, State University of New York at Stony Brook).

(61), and to inhibit the replication of human immunodeficiency virus (HIV) type I *(62)*. These investigations demonstrate the utility of ISH for sensitive detection of foreign gene expression in the development of gene therapy regimens for the treatment of human disease.

8. LIMITATIONS OF ISH IN THE HISTOLOGICAL LOCALIZATION OF NUCLEIC ACIDS

Although ISH is a sensitive technique for detecting nucleic acids in tissues, there is a lower limit to the copy number of mRNA or viral nucleic acid molecules detectable by this technique. It is generally accepted that approx 10 copies of RNA or foreign DNA/cell are required for successful detection by standard ISH methods *(48)*. Latent viral infections and low-level gene expression can be difficult, if not impossible, to detect if target copy number is below the detection threshold for ISH. This is evident in the difficulty encountered when one attempts to detect latent or occult viral infections by ISH (Fig. 11B). SiHa cells, a cervical carcinoma cell line latently infected with one integrated copy of HPV type 16/cell, typically do not exhibit a hybridization signal with standard ISH *(48,63)*. The HPV copy number is often below the detection threshold for ISH in invasive cancers and cannot be detected by ISH in occult HPV infections *(48)*. The general failure of ISH to detect DNA from HSV *(64)* and HIV *(65,66)* in latent infections has been a major impediment to understanding the pathogenesis of these diseases. However, studies of latent viral infections also demonstrate that low-level nucleic acid targets can be visualized by ISH following amplification of target sequences *in situ* by PCR. Low-level targets also may be detectable using recently developed signal amplification technology (Renaissance TSA Kit, Dupont NEN).

9. ISA

ISA was first reported in 1990 for the amplification and detection of viral DNA within intact cells *(67)*. Amplification of the target sequence *in situ* by PCR *(48,68)* or by other amplification techniques, such as 3SR *(69)*, can increase the target copy number to detectable levels in tissues with starting copy number below the detection threshold for ISH (Fig. 11A). ISA has been used to detect viral DNA in cells with only one copy per cell *(70,71)*, and was indispensable in studies describing the cell-specific distribution of proviral DNA in latent HIV infections *(65,66,72)*. ISA is, however, a technically demanding procedure that is difficult to standardize because of the large number of variables that can affect the final result. Numerous protocols for ISA have been published and the importance of certain steps have been debated, reflecting the lack of standardized procedures. However, ISA has great potential, which is becoming more apparent as the technical requirements for successful ISA are defined and new protocols are developed *(48,68)*. Applications of ISA include the elucidation of the histopathology of viral infections *(48,64–68,70–72)*, the diagnosis and prognosis of human malignancies *(73,74)*, and the localization of transgenes in the development of gene therapy protocols *(75)*.

The basic principles of ISA are similar to ISH, with the addition of the amplification step. Tissues must be fixed in a crosslinking fixative and digested with a protease prior to amplification. Crosslinking fixatives are required for successful ISA, because they promote the retention of amplification products within the tissue, whereas precipitating fixatives allow products to diffuse into the reaction mixture during amplification *(48)*. As with ISH, 10% buffered formalin is an excellent fixative for ISA. Some protocols include an additional fixation step following amplification (postfixation) to help localize the product *(76)*. Protease digestion is a critical step for successful ISA. Target sequences remain sequestered and unavailable for amplification in underdigested tissue, whereas overdigestion results in loss of tissue morphology and ISA signal. Pepsin and proteinase K are suitable proteases for tissue digestion. The extent of tissue digestion required for optimal signal is a function of the extent of tissue fixation, with longer fixation times requiring longer protease treatment *(48)*. Protease concentration and time of treatment must be optimized for each type of tissue owing to the individual sensitivity of different tissues to protease digestion.

The amplification step of PCR-based ISA is identical in principle to solution-based PCR in that one needs forward and reverse primers that are specific for the target sequence, an equimolar mixture of dNTPs, a thermostable DNA polymerase (for example *Taq*), and amplification buffer containing magnesium, which is required for

Taq polymerase activity. The reaction mixture is subjected to thermal cycling, during which double-stranded DNA denatures, primers anneal, and primer extension occurs by DNA synthesis. It is important to realize that amplification of nucleic acids *in situ* is much less efficient than solution-based PCR. The degree of amplification during ISA has been estimated to be from 50–200 copies after 30 cycles, compared with 1,000,000 after only 20 cycles in solution. Therefore, optimizing ISA reactions is critical for success. Optimal Mg^{2+} concentration for ISA is reported to be 4.5 mM for a wide range of tissues and targets *(48)*. This concentration of magnesium ion is higher than that required for most solution-based assays. Second, the concentration of *Taq* polymerase required for ISA is higher than that necessary for solution PCR, unless bovine serum albumin (BSA) (1 mg/mL) is added to the reaction. Maximum ISA signal was shown to require 2.0 U of *Taq* polymerase/μL of reaction volume, which is about 10 times the concentration required for solution-based amplification. However, the addition of 2 mg/mL BSA to the reaction mixture reduced the *Taq* requirement to 0.2 U/μL *(48)*. This effect is apparently the result of the ability of BSA to block the binding of *Taq* polymerase to the glass slide. The optimal magnesium ion and *Taq* polymerase concentration should be confirmed empirically to ensure that maximum amplification is obtained.

One of the main differences between solution-based PCR and ISA is in the method of thermal cycling and containment of the amplifying solution to prevent evaporation. Original methods of thermal cycling include the use of an aluminum foil boat to hold slides *(48)*. The amplification reaction mixture is transferred onto specimens and a coverslip is anchored over the tissue with nail polish to the corners. This allows bubbles to escape from under the coverslip during thermal cycling. A layer of mineral oil is added to the boat to prevent evaporation of the reaction solution, and the boats are placed on the heating block of a conventional thermal cycler. Another method, called localized ISA, employs tissue-culture cloning rings and a mineral oil overlay to contain reactants over the desired area of tissue, leaving areas outside the ring to serve as an unamplified control *(77)*. Several companies now manufacture thermal cyclers and containment vessels for ISA, including Perkin Elmer/Applied Biosystems (Foster City, CA).

Mispriming and DNA repair are two nonspecific pathways for DNA synthesis that may occur during PCR, and that can interfere with the specific amplification of the target sequence during ISA. Mispriming results from nonspecific annealing of primers to nontarget nucleic acid sequences and provides a starting point for nonspecific amplification. DNA synthesis resulting from mispriming competes with target-specific amplification and, thereby, reduces the sensitivity of the reaction. Mispriming can be decreased by optimizing the primer annealing temperature of the reaction. However, nonspecific primer annealing can occur during the setup of the reaction, and extension can occur as the reaction temperature increases during the first cycle. Mispriming can be eliminated by using the "hot-start" technique, in which DNA synthesis is blocked until the temperature of the reaction mixture reaches a level at which nonspecific primer annealing is eliminated. Hot starts are accomplished by withholding *Taq* polymerase until the reaction reaches 80°C, by using an anti-*Taq* antibody (Clonetech) that inhibits polymerase activity until the antibody is heat-denatured during the first cycle of the reaction, or by using a thermostable polymerase that remains inactive until the reaction obtains high temperature (AmpliTaq Gold, Perkin Elmer/Applied Biosystems). The hot start maneuver greatly increases the specificity and sensitivity of ISA, and is required for amplification of DNA targets. One copy of HPV DNA was detectable using a single primer pair in SiHa cells only when the hot-start technique was used *(48)*. The second nonspecific pathway for DNA synthesis during ISA is the result of primer-independent filling of nicks and large gaps in fragmented DNA by *Taq* polymerase. This is not a problem when amplification products are detected indirectly using labeled ISH probes, but is the primary obstacle to the use of direct labeling for *in situ* PCR of DNA targets in paraffin-embedded tissue.

Two basic methods have been described for the detection of ISA products. The first is direct incorporation of labeled nucleotides, such as digoxigenin-11-dUTP, into PCR products during the amplification reaction. Labeled amplification products are detected by antibody–enzyme conjugates as described for ISH. This method was originally described as a rapid, sensitive method for detection of DNA amplified *in situ*. However, numerous studies have shown that the direct detection method commonly results in false positive signals in cell nuclei caused by nonspecific incorporation of labeled nucleotides into genomic DNA *(63,78)*. Primer-independent labeling is especially problematic in paraffin-embedded tissues and results from the heat-induced damage of DNA during the embedding process *(78)*. Therefore, direct labeling of amplification products is not appropriate for the detection of DNA targets by ISA in paraffin-embedded tissues. The second method of detection is indirect, using ISH with labeled probes, and is the detection method of choice for DNA targets. This technique, called PCR ISH, combines the sensitivity of PCR with the specificity of ISH. Oligonucleotides or larger genomic probes are labeled with digoxigenin or biotin and detected immunohistochemically as described above in detail for ISH. Probes that are internal to the primer sequences will provide the most specific signal, since they are less likely to anneal to any misprimed sequences.

Reverse transcriptase *in situ* PCR can be used to detect mRNA in tissues in which low-level gene expression results in a target copy number below the detection threshold for ISH. Prior to the amplification reaction, cDNA is synthesized by reverse transcriptase using mRNA as template. The reverse transcription reaction and amplification of the resulting cDNA can be accomplished with separate enzymes (RT and *Taq* polymerase), or by using one enzyme with both activities, such as the polymerase from *Thermus thermopolis* (rTth, Perkin Elmer/Applied Biosystems). In paraffin-embedded tissue, products from RT *in situ* PCR can be detected by direct incorporation of labeled nucleotides, provided that specimens are treated with DNase prior to reverse transcription and amplification *(48)*. DNase treatment results in the digestion of genomic DNA and thereby eliminates nonspecific incorporation of labeled nucleotides and the false positive signals associated with direct detection of DNA targets in paraffin embedded tissue. However, DNase treatment may not be required for direct labeling with cytospins or tissue samples that have not been paraffin-embedded (Fig. 12).

The following positive and negative control reactions should be run on each slide to establish the specificity of direct labeling during RT *in situ* PCR in paraffin-embedded tissue *(48)*. The RT step is excluded in both controls to eliminate primer-specific signal. In the positive control, the DNase step is omitted, which should result in a strong nonspecific signal when the sample is subjected to thermal cycling. This reaction will demonstrate that the *Taq* polymerase and the detection system are functioning properly

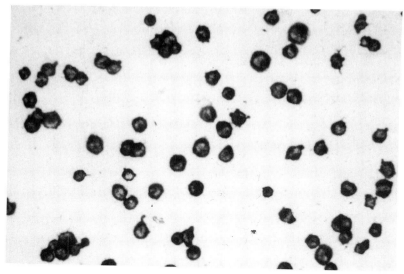

Fig. 12. Detection of bcr-abl mRNA in chronic myelogenous leukemia by reverse transcriptase *in situ* PCR and direct labeling. K562 cells containing the Philadelphia chromosome were fixed in 4% paraformaldehyde, centrifuged onto microscope slides, and permeabilized by proteinase K treatment. RT *in situ* PCR was performed using bcr-abl-specific primers, and digoxigenin was included in the PCR reaction. Intense cytoplasmic staining indicates the detection of bcr-abl mRNA. Genomic bcr-abl does not amplify in nuclei, because the PCR primers flank a large intron in the DNA. Specificity of the amplification reaction for mRNA target sequences could be verified by omitting the RT enzyme prior to the PCR reaction (not shown).

and have access to genomic DNA. In the negative control, the specimen is treated with DNase and thermal cycled. No signal should be associated with this sample owing to the effects of DNase treatment, if the protease treatment was optimal. However, if the protease treatment was suboptimal, then a nonspecific signal will be evident owing to gap filling in undigested genomic DNA. DNase apparently has limited accessibility to DNA under conditions of suboptimal protease digestion. Therefore, protease treatment must be optimized until the DNase treatment is capable of eliminating nonspecific signals in the negative control. Then, a specific primer-dependent signal is detectable when RT *in situ* PCR is performed. The hot start technique, which is required for PCR ISH to eliminate mispriming, is not required for RT *in situ* PCR providing that genomic DNA is adequately degraded by the DNase treatment.

Proper controls are essential for accurate interpretation of ISA because of the prevalence of false-positive and false-negative results. False positives occur owing to mispriming and gap filling during direct labeling as well as nonspecific binding of labeled probes or antibody–enzyme conjugates when detecting amplification products by ISH. False negatives can occur as the result of failure of any basic step in the procedure, from tissue fixation to product detection. Diffusion of amplification products can cause false negative results in cells that contain the target sequence, and can result in false positive signals in cells that did not originally contain the target. Therefore, the following controls should be run during the development of ISA protocols. Solution-based PCR or RT-PCR coupled with blot hybridization of nucleic acids extracted from the tissue of interest demonstrates the specificity of the reaction. Solution-based PCR is also useful to expose false negative results from ISA. Additional controls include tissue known to be positive and negative for the target nucleic acid, which provide information regarding the sensitivity and specificity of ISA reactions. The absence of a signal in the negative control tissue demonstrates the absence of mispriming, nonspecific annealing of probe, and nonspecific antibody binding in PCR ISH. Omission of *Taq* polymerase or magnesium exposes nonspecific hybridization of probes and nonspecific antibody binding. The latter is also revealed by omission of probes. Omission of antibody/enzyme conjugates reveals the presence of endogenous enzyme, which can cause false-positive staining in some tissues. Coamplification of known positive and negative control tissues in the same reaction exposes the presence of diffusional artifacts, which can cause staining in the negative control tissue. Amplification of endogenous control sequences serves as a positive control in negative tissue. Most tissues have internal negative controls, because in general, not all cells within the tissue will express the mRNA or contain the foreign DNA target of interest. Therefore, a generalized signal in most or all cells may indicate a nonspecific reaction. The failure to run appropriate controls will undoubtedly result in misinterpretation of ISA results.

10. APPLICATIONS OF ISA

10.1. Detection and Localization of Latent and Occult Viral Infections

ISA has been invaluable in elucidating latent HIV infections in helper T-lymphocytes and macrophages during the incubation period of AIDS. Early investigations using solution-based PCR greatly underestimated the number of cells containing proviral DNA in patients with latent HIV infections, because the destruction of cells during DNA extraction made direct association of viral DNA with individual cells impossible. Later, studies using PCR ISH demonstrated that the percentage of mononuclear cells and T-lymphocytes harboring HIV proviral DNA is much higher than was initially suspected *(65,66,72,79)*. HIV DNA was detected in activated macrophages in cervical biopsy specimens, suggesting that these cells may be a primary route of infection in women *(48)*. Muscle biopsies exhibited the presence of HIV DNA in patients with myopathy, as did CNS tissue from patients with AIDS dementia, only when specimens were subjected to ISA prior to hybridization *(48)*. HIV was also discovered in placental cells, which were not previously known to harbor HIV, suggesting a potential mode of mother–fetus transmission *(80)*. The combination of ISA and flow cytometry has been used to quantitate the number of peripheral blood mononuclear cells (PBMC) and CD4$^+$ T-cells harboring latent and active virus in patients infected with HIV *(71,81)*. These studies collectively demonstrate the utility of ISA to elucidate the histopathogenic progression of HIV infection.

ISA has also been used to detect HPV infection in genital tract lesions that are difficult to analyze by ISH without amplification *(48)*. HPV DNA is readily detectable by standard ISH in low grade squamous intraepithelial lesions, which typically have about 1000 copies of viral genome/cell (Fig. 9). However, ISA is more sensitive than ISH for the detection of HPV in invasive cancers, and is required for *in situ* detection of occult HPV infections, which are associated with from 1–<10 copies of HPV DNA/cell. PCR ISH was capable of detecting JC virus DNA in archival specimens from patients with leukoencephalopathy associated with chronic lymphocytic leukemia and AIDS, including an index case over 30 yr old *(82)*. RT ISA was used to demonstrate hepatitis C infection in hepatectomy specimens, which rarely show a positive signal with ISH *(83)*, and to detect RNA from polio, measles, influenza, and HTLV-1 in paraffin-embedded archival brain tissue, some of which were over 25 yr old *(84)*. RT ISA was used in lung autopsy specimens to ascertain parvovirus infection in a deceased child and to establish measles pneumonitis as the probable cause of death in a woman originally suspected to have died from CMV pneumonia *(48)*. The investigations described above demonstrate that ISA is capable of cell-specific localization of viral nucleic acids in retrospective studies, and in cases where insufficient sensitivity or destruction of cell morphology limits the ability of other techniques to detect low numbers of viral nucleic acids in a cell-specific manner.

10.2. Detection and Localization of Low-Level Gene Expression in Human Tumors

Several studies demonstrate the great potential value of ISA for the diagnosis and prognosis of human malignancies, based on the inherent sensitivity of ISA for the detection of tumor-specific transcripts. A case report describes a 63-yr-old female with a history of breast carcinoma who presented with symptoms of lung disease *(73)*. Adenocarcinoma of unknown origin was identified in pleural fluid from a thoracentesis. Estrogen and progesterone receptors were analyzed based on the patient's history of breast cancer, but the results were equivocal. RT ISA was performed using primers specific for surfactant protein A, based on the suspicion that the tumor might be a primary adenocarcinoma of the lung rather than metastic breast cancer. The results from RT ISA indicated the presence of mRNA for surfactant protein A, supporting the diagnosis of primary lung cancer.

ISA has also proven useful in elucidating the mechanisms of neoplastic progression. Gelatinases are potent metalloproteinases involved in the degradation of extracellular matrix proteins and endothelial cell basement membranes during the process of tumor metastasis. The relative level of expression between gelatinases and metalloproteinase inhibitors is thought to be either permissive or inhibitory to the development of metastatic tumors, depending on the balance between the two in the microenvironment of the tumor. The prognostic value of analyzing the relative expression of gelatinases and their inhibitors, by RT ISA, was examined in a retrospective study of surgical biopsy specimens from 23 women with cervical carcinoma *(74)*. In highly invasive tumors with poor prognosis, the gelatinase:inhibitor ratio was markedly greater than in well-differentiated, minimally invasive cancers with good prognosis. The two studies described above demonstrate the usefulness of ISA in the diagnosis and prognosis of human tumors.

10.3. Detection and Localization of Transgenes in Gene Therapy

Monitoring the cellular location and expression of transgenes is critical for the development of procedures for gene therapy. ISA offers a sensitive technique for the detection of vector nucleic acid sequences and reporter gene expression in transduced tissue. Primers specific for the bacterial *lacZ* gene have been used to detect viral transgene DNA by ISA in rat brain *(75)*. ISA has also been used to monitor transplanted cells in the development of *ex vivo* gene therapy protocols *(85)*, and a clinical protocol describes the use of ISA to monitor the fate of donor cells for autologous bone marrow transplantation *(86)*. RT ISA provides a sensitive method to detect mRNA from reporter gene expression in transduced tissues that do not exhibit a positive signal by less sensitive methods, such as colorimetric β-galactosidase assays and ISH. Thus, ISA has the potential to become an important method for the cell-specific localization of transgene DNA, and of mRNA from transgene expression in target tissues during the development of new gene therapy protocols.

11. LIMITATIONS OF ISA

The routine use of ISA for clinical diagnostic purposes is severely limited by the lack of established laboratory standards with respect to this technique and by the large number of variables that affect the final outcome, and is not recommended at this time. Leading investigators in the field use markedly different protocols, and debate persists regarding the significance and necessity of various steps of the procedure *(87)*. However, some limitations are clear. The use of direct incorporation of labeled nucleotides for the detection of ISA products is strictly limited to situations in which DNA repair mechanisms are inoperative, as described above. Amplification products can diffuse out of cells during thermal cycling, which leads to false-positive staining in cells that were previously target-negative *(88)*. Because of the relative difficulty in performing ISA, this technique should be avoided in circumstances where standard ISH, solution-phase PCR, or other techniques will suffice. However, the publication of detailed protocols greatly enhances the ability to perform ISA successfully *(48,68)*, and demonstrates the enormous potential of ISA for detecting nucleic acids present in low copy numbers in situations where cell-specific association of the target sequence is required.

ABBREVIATIONS

DAPI, 4,6-diamidino-2-phenylindole; FISH, fluorescence *in situ* hybridization; ISA, *in situ* amplification; ISH, *in situ* hybridization; PCR, polymerase chain reaction; RT, reverse transcriptase.

ACKNOWLEDGMENTS

The author thanks Georgette Dent, Peter Ferlisi, Kathleen Kaiser-Rogers, Gerard Nuovo, and Kathleen Rao for contributing excellent microscopic images.

REFERENCES

1. Kallioniemi, A., Kallioniemi, O.-P., Sudar, D., Rutovitz, D., Gray, J. W., Waldman, F., and Pinkel, D. Comparative genomic hybridization for molecular cytogenetic analysis of solid tumors. *Science* **258**:818–821, 1992.
2. Ried, T., Baldini, A., Rand, T. C., and Ward, D. C. Simultaneous visualization of seven different DNA probes by *in situ* hybridization using combinatorial flourescence and digital imaging microscopy. *Proc. Natl. Acad. Sci. USA* **89**:1388–1392, 1992.
3. Dekken, H. V., Arkesteijn, G. J. A., Visser, J. W. M., and Bauman, J. G. J. Flow cytometric quantification of human chromosome-specific repetitive DNA sequences by single and bicolor fluorescent *in situ* hybridization to lymphocyte nuclei. *Cytometry* **11**:153–164, 1990.
4. Fox, J. L., Hsu, P.-H., Legator, M. S., Morrison, L. E., and Seelig, S. A. Fluorescence *in situ* hybridization: powerful molecular tool for cancer research. *Clin. Chem.* **41**:1554–1559, 1995.

5. Uner, A. H., Hutchison, R. E., and Davey, F. R. Applications of *in situ* hybridization in the study of hematological malignancies. *Hematol. Oncol. Clin. North Am.* **8:**771–785, 1994.

6. Le Beau, M. M. Fluorescence *in situ* hybridization in cancer diagnosis, in *Important Advances in Oncology*, DeVita, V. T., Hellman, S., and Rosenbuerg, S. A., eds., Lippencott, Philadelphia, pp. 29–45, 1993.

7. Zhao, L., Chang, K.-S., Estey, E. H., Hayes, K., Deisseroth, A. B., and Liang, J. C. Detection of residual leukemic cells in patients with acute promyelocytic leukemia by the fluorescence *in situ* hybridization method: potential for predicting relapse. *Blood* **85:**495–499, 1995.

8. Kearns, W. G. and Pearson, P. L. Detection of chromosomal aberrations in interphase and metaphase cells in prenatal and postnatal studies, in In Situ *Hybridization Protocols. Methods in Molecular Biology*, vol. 33, Choo, K. H., ed., Humana, Totowa, NJ, pp. 459–476, 1994.

9. Lebo, R. V. and Su, Y. Positional cloning and multicolor *in situ* hybridization. Principles and protocols, in In Situ *Hybridization Protocols. Methods in Molecular Biology*, vol. 33, Choo, K. H., ed., Humana, Totowa, NJ, pp. 409–438, 1994.

10. Sandberg, A. A. and Bridge, J. A. Techniques in cancer cytogenetics. *Cancer Invest.* **10:**163–172, 1992.

11. Bentz, M., Schroder, M., Herz, M., Stilgenbaur, S., Lichter, P., and Dohner, H. Detection of trisomy 8 on blood smears using fluorescence *in situ* hybridization. *Leukemia* **7:**752–757, 1993.

12. Bentz, M., Cabot, G., Moos, M., Speicher, M. R., Ganser, A., Lichter, P., and Dohner, H. Detection of chimeric BCR-ABL genes on bone marrow samples and blood smears in chronic myeloid and acute lymphocytic leukemia by *in situ* hybridization. *Blood* **83:**1922–1928, 1994.

13. Misra, D. N., Dickman, P. S., and Yunis, E. J. Fluorescence *in situ* hybridization (FISH) detection of MYCN oncogene amplification in neuroblastoma using paraffin-embedded tissues. *Diagn. Mol. Pathol.* **4:**128–135, 1995.

14. Nederlof, P. M., Robinson, D., Abuknesha, R., Wiegant, J., Hopman, A. H. N., Tanke, H. J., and Raap, A. K. Three color fluorescence detection of multiple nucleic acid sequences. *Cytometry* **10:**20–27, 1989.

15. Morrison, L. E. Chromosome analysis by multicolor fluorescence *in situ* hybridization using direct-labeled fluorescent probes. *Clin. Chem.* **39:**733–734, 1993.

16. Le Beau, M. M., Espinosa, R., Neuman, W. L., Stock, W., Roulston, D., Larson, R. A., Keinanen, M., and Westbrook, C. A. Cytogenetic and molecular delineation of the smallest commonly deleted region of chromosome 5 in malignant myeloid diseases. *Proc. Natl. Acad. Sci. USA* **90:**5484–5488, 1993.

17. Dohner, H., Fischer, K., Bentz, M., Hansen. K., Benner, A., Cabot, G., Diehl, D., Schlenk, R., Coy, J., Stilgenbauer, S., Volkman, M., Galle, P. R., Poustka, A., Hunstein, W., and Lichter, P. p53 gene deletion predicts for poor survival and non-response to therapy with purine analogs in chronic B-cell leukemias. *Blood* **85:**1580–1589, 1995.

18. Matsumura, K., Kallioniemi, O., Kallioniemi, A., Chen, H. S., Smith, D., Pinkel, D, Gray, J. W., and Waldman, F. Deletion of chromosome 17p loci in breast cancer cells detected by fluorescence *in situ* hybridization. *Cancer Res.* **52:**3474–3477, 1992.

19. Anastasi, J., Vardiman, J. W., Rudinsky, R., Patel, M., Nachman, J., Rubin, C. M., and Le Beau, M. M. Direct correlation of cytogenetic findings with cell morphology using *in situ* hybridization: analysis of suspicious cells in bone marrow specimens of two patients completing therapy for acute lymphoblastic leukemia. *Blood* **77:**2456–2462, 1991.

20. Escudier, S. M., Pereira-Leahy, J., Drach, J. W., Weir, H. U., Goodare, A. M., Cork, A., Trujillo, J. M., Keating, M. J., and Andreeff, M. Fluorescence *in situ* hybridization and cytogenetic studies of trisomy 12 in chronic lymphocytic leukemia. *Blood* **81:**2702–2707, 1993.

21. Heerema, N. A., Argyropoulos, G., Weetman, R., Tricot, G., and Secker-Walker, L. M. Interphase *in situ* hybridization reveals minimal residual disease in early remission and return of the diagnostic clone in karyotypically normal relapse of acute lymphoblastic leukemia. *Leukemia* **7**:537–543, 1993.

22. Zhao, L., Kantarjian, H. M., Van, O. J., Cork, A., Trujillo, J. M., and Liang, J. C. Detection of residual proliferating leukemia cells by fluorescence *in situ* hybridization in CML patients in complete remission after interferon therapy. *Leukemia* **7**:168–171, 1993.

23. Sandberg, A. A. Chromosome changes in early bladder neoplasms. *J. Cell. Biochem.* **161(Suppl.)**:76–79, 1992.

24. Herrmann, M. E., and Lalley, P. A. Significance of trisomy 7 in thyroid tumors. *Cancer Genet. Cytogenet.* **62**:144–149, 1992.

25. Devilee, P. Detection of chromosome aneuploidy in interphase nuclei from human breast tumors using chromosome-specific repetitive DNA probes. *Cancer Res.* **48**:5825–5830, 1988.

26. Alcaraz, A., Takahshi, S., Brown, J. A., Herath, J. F., Bergstralh, E. J., Larson-Keller, J. J., Lieber, M. M., and Jenkins, R. B. Aneuploidy and aneusomy of chromosome 7 detected by fluorescence *in situ* hybridization are markers for poor prognosis in prostate cancer. *Cancer Res.* **54**:3998–4002, 1994.

27. Kallioniemi, O.-P., Kallioniemi, A., Kurisu, W., Thor, A., Chen, L.-C., Smith, H. S., Waldman, F. M., Pinkel, D., and Gray, J. W. ErbB-2 amplification in breast cancer analyzed by fluorescence *in situ* hybridization. *Proc. Natl. Acad. Sci. USA* **89**:5321–5325, 1992.

28. Sauter, G., Moch, H., Moore, D., Carroll, P., Kerschman, R., Chew, K., Mihatsch, M. J., Gudat, F., and Waldman, F. Heterogeneity of erbB-2 gene amplification in bladder cancer. *Cancer Res.* **53**:2199–2203, 1993.

29. Desmaze, C., Zuchman, J., Delattre, O., Melot,T., Thomas, G., and Aurias, A. Interphase molecular cytogenetics of Ewing's sarcoma and peripheral neuroepithelioma t(11;22) with flanking and overlapping cosmid probes. *Cancer Genet. Cytogen.* **74**:13–18, 1994.

30. du Manoir, S., Speicher, M. R., Joos, S., Schrock, E., Popp, S., Dohner, H., Kovacs, G., Robert-Nicould, M., Lichter, P., and Cremer, T. Detection of complete or partial chromosome gains and losses by comparative genomic *in situ* hybridization. *Hum. Genet.* **90**:590–610, 1993.

31. Campana, D. and Pui, C.-H. Detection of minimal residual disease in acute leukemia: methodologic advances and clinical significance. *Blood* **85**:1416–1435, 1995.

32. Lion, T. Clinical implications of qualitative and quantitative polymerase chain reaction analysis in the monitoring of patients with chronic myelogenous leukemia. *Bone Marrow Transplant.* **14**:505–509, 1994.

33. Szakacs, J. G. and Livingston, S. K. mRNA *in situ* hybridization using biotinylated oligonucleotide probes: implications for the diagnostic laboratory. *Ann. Clin. Lab. Sci.* **24**:324–338, 1994.

34. Lloyd, R. V., Jin, L., and Bonnerup, M. K. *In situ* hybridization in diagnostic pathology. *Mayo Clin. Proc.* **69**:597–598, 1994.

35. Negro, F., Pacchioni, D., Mondardini, A., Bussolati, G., and Bonino, F. *In situ* hybridization in viral hepatitis. *Liver* **12**:217–226, 1992.

36. Morey, A. L. and Fleming, K. A. The use of *in situ* hybridization in studies of viral disease, in In Situ *Hybridization: Medical Applications.* Coulton, G. R. and de Belleroche, J., eds., Kluwer, Boston, pp. 66–96, 1992.

37. Ambinder, F. and Mann, R. B. Epstein-Barr-encoded RNA *in situ* hybridization: diagnostic applications. *Hum. Pathol.* **25**:602–605, 1994.

38. Gowans, E. J., Arthur, J., Blight, K., and Higgins, G. D. Application of *in situ* hybridization for the detection of virus nucleic acids, in In Situ *Hybridization Protocols. Methods in Molecular Biology*, vol. 33, Choo, K. H., ed., Humana, Totowa, NJ, pp. 395–408, 1994.

39. DeLellis, R. A. In situ hybridization techniques for the analysis of gene expression: applications in tumor pathology. *Hum. Pathol.* **25**:580–585, 1994.

40. Biffo, S. *In situ* hybridization: optimization of the techniques for collecting and fixing the specimens. *Liver* **12**:227–229, 1992.

41. Nuovo, G. J. Buffered formalin is the superior fixative for the detection of human papillomavirus DNA by *in situ* hybridization analysis. *Am. J. Pathol.* **134**:837–842, 1989.

42. Wilcox, J. N. Fundamental principles of *in situ* hybridization. *J. Histochem. Cytochem.* **41**:1725–1733, 1993.

43. Komminoth, P. Digoxigenin as an alternative probe labeling for *in situ* hybridization. *Diagn. Mol. Pathol.* **1**:142–150, 1992.

44. Hacker, G. W., Zehbe, I., Hauser-Kronberger, C., Gu, J., Graf, A., Grimelius, L., and Dietz, O. Sensitive detection of DNA and mRNA sequences by *in situ* hybridization and immunogold-silver staining, in In Situ *Polymerase Chain Reaction and Related Technology*, Gu, J., ed., Eaton, Natick, MA, pp. 113–130, 1995.

45. Choo, K. H. (ed.) *In Situ* Hybridization Protocols. *Methods in Molecular Biology*, vol. 33, Humana, Totowa, NJ, 1994.

46. Guiot, Y. and Rahier, J. The effects of varying key steps in the non-radioactive *in situ* hybridization protocol: a quantitative study. *Histochem. J.* **27**:60–68, 1995.

47. Yoshii, A., Koji, T., Ohsawa, N., and Nakane, P. K. In situ localization of ribosomal RNAs is a reliable reference for hybridizable RNA in tissue sections. *J. Histochem. Cytochem.* **43**:321–327, 1995.

48. Nuovo, G. J. *PCR* In Situ *Hybridization. Protocols and Applications*, 2nd ed. Raven, New York, 1994.

49. Dictor, M., Siven, M., Tennvall, J., and Rambech, E. Determination of nonendemic nasopharyngeal carcinoma by *in situ* hybridization for Epstein-Barr virus EBER1 RNA: sensitivity and specificity in cervical node metastases. *Laryngoscope* **105**:407–412, 1995.

50. Greil, R., Fasching, B., Loidl, P., and Huber, H. Expression of c-myc proto-oncogene in multiple myeloma and chronic lymphocytic leukemia: an *in situ* analysis. *Blood* **78**:180–191, 1991.

51. Hamatani, K., Yoshida, K., Kondo, H., Toki, H., Okabe, K., Motoi, M., Ikeda, S., Mori, S., Shimaoka, K., Akiyama, M., Nakayama, E., and Shiku, H. Histologic typing of non-Hodgkin's lymphomas by *in situ* hybridization with DNA probes of oncogenes. *Blood* **74**:423–429, 1989.

52. Fiorentino, M., Grigioni, W. F., Baccarini, P., Errico, A. D., De Mitri, M. S., Pisi, E. and Mancini, A. M. Different *in situ* expression of insulin-like growth factor type II in hepatocellular carcinoma. An *in situ* hybridization and immunohistochemical study. *Diagn. Mol. Pathol.* **3**:59–65, 1994.

53. Maxwell, M., Naber, S. P., Wolfe, S. P., Galanopoulos, T., Hedley-Whyte, E. T., Black, P. M., and Antoniades, H. N. Platelet-derived growth factor (PDGF) and PDGF receptor genes in primary human astrocytomas may contribute to their development and maintenance. *J. Clin. Invest.* **86**:131–140, 1990.

54. Radinski, R., Bucana, C. D., Ellis, L. M., Sanchez, R., Cleary, K. R., Brigati, D. J., and Fidler, I. J. A rapid colorimetric *in situ* messenger RNA hybridization for analysis of epidermal growth factor receptor in paraffin-embedded surgical specimens of human colon carcinoma. *Cancer Res.* **53**:937–943, 1993.

55. Xu, X.-C., Clifford, J. L., Hong, W. K., and Lotan, R. Detection of nuclear retinoic acid receptor mRNA in histological tissue sections using nonradioactive *in situ* hybridization histochemistry. *Diagn. Mol. Pathol.* **3**:122–131, 1994.

56. Matsuno, A., Teramoto, A., Takekoshi, S., Sanno, N., Osamura, R. Y., and Kirino, T. Expression of plurihormonal mRNAs in somatotrophic adenomas detected using a nonisotopic *in situ* hybridization method: comparison with lactotrophic adenomas. *Human Pathol.* **26**:272–279, 1995.

57. Dank, J. A., McHale, J. C., Clark, S. P., Chou, S. T., Scurry, J. P., Ingleton, P. M., and Martin, T. J. *In situ* hybridization of parathyroid hormone-related protein in normal skin, skin tumors, and gynecological cancers using digoxigenin-labeled probes and antibody enhancement. *J. Histochem. Cytochem.* **43:**5–10, 1995.

58. Lloyd, R. V. and Long, J. *In situ* hybridization analysis of chromogranin A and B mRNAs in neuroendocrine tumors with digoxigenin-labeled oligonucleotide probe cocktails. *Diagn. Mol. Pathol.* **4:**143–151, 1995.

59. Anderson, J. K., Frim, D. M., Isacson, O., and Breakefield, X. O. Herpesvirus-mediated gene delivery into the rat brain: specificity and efficiency of the neuron-specific promotor. *Cell. Mol. Neurobiol.* **13:**503–515, 1993.

60. Gazit, G., Kane, S. E., Nichols, P., and Lee, A. S. Use of the stress-inducible grp78/BiP promoter in targeting high level gene expression in fibrosarcoma *in vivo. Cancer Res.* **55:**1660–1663, 1995.

61. Hyde, S. C., Gill, D. R., Higgins, C. F., Trezise, A. E. O., MacVanish, L. J., Cuthbert, A. W., Ratcliff, R., Evans, M. J., and Colledge, W. H. Correction of the ion transport defect in cystic fibrosis transgenic mice by gene therapy. *Nature* **362:**250–255, 1993.

62. Lisziewicz, J., Sun, D., Smythe, J., Lusso, P., Louie, A., Markham, P., Rossi, J., Reitz, M., and Gallo, R. C. Inhibition of human immunodeficiency virus type I replication by regulated expression of a polymeric Tat activation response RNA decoy as a strategy for gene therapy in AIDS. *Proc. Natl. Acad. Sci. USA* **90:**8000–8004, 1993.

63. Zehbe, I., Sallstrom, J. F., Hacker, G. W., Hauser-Kronberger, C., Rylander, E., and Wilander, E. Indirect and direct *in situ* PCR for the detection of human papillomavirus. An evaluation of two methods and a double staining technique. *Cell Vision* **1:**163–167, 1994.

64. Mehta, A., Maggioncalda, J., Bagasra, O., Thikkavarapu, S., Saikumari, P., Valyi-Nagy, T., Fraser, N. W., and Block, T. M. *In situ* DNA PCR and RNA hybridization detection of herpes simplex virus sequences in trigeminal ganglia of latently infected mice. *Virology* **206:**633–640, 1995.

65. Bagasra, O., Hauptman, S. P., Lischner, H. W., Sachs, M., and Pomerantz, R. J. Detection of human immunodeficiency virus type 1 provirus in mononuclear cells by *in situ* polymerase chain reaction. *New Engl. J. Med.* **326:**1385–1391, 1992.

66. Embretson, J., Zupancic, M., Ribas, J. L., Burke, A., Racz, P., Tenner-Racz, K., and Haase, A. T. Massive covert infection of helper T lymphocytes and macrophages by HIV during the incubation period of AIDS. *Nature* **362:**359–362, 1993.

67. Haase, A. T., Retzel, E. F., and Staskus, K. A. Amplification and detection of lentiviral DNA inside cells. *Proc. Natl. Acad. Sci. USA* **87:**4971–4975, 1990.

68. Gu, J. (ed.) In situ *Polymerase Chain Reaction and Related Technology.* Eaton. Natick, MA 1995.

69. Zehbe, I., Hacker, G. W., Sallstrom, J. F., Rylander, E., and Wilander, E. Self-sustained sequence replication-based amplification (3SR) for the *in situ* detection of mRNA in cultured cells. *Cell Vision* **1:**20–24, 1994.

70. Zehbe, I. E., Hacker, G. W., Sallstrom, J., Rylander, E., and Wilander, E. Detection of single HPV copies in SiHa cells by *in situ* polymerase chain reaction combined with immunoperoxidase and immunogold-silver staining techniques. *Anticancer Res.* **12:**2165–2168, 1992.

71. Patterson, B. K., Till, M., Otto, P., Gollsby, C., Furtado, M. R., McBride, L. J., and Wolinsky, S. M. Detection of HIV-1 DNA and mRNA in individual cells by PCR-driven *in situ* hybridization and flow cytometry. *Science* **260:**976–979, 1993.

72. Embretson, J., Zupancic, M., Beneke, J., Till, M., Wolinsky, S., Riba, J. L., Burke, A., and Hasse, A. T. Analysis of human immunodeficiency virus-infected tissues by amplification and in situ hybridization reveals latent and permissive infections at single-cell resolution. *Proc. Natl. Acad. Sci. USA* **90:**357–361, 1993.

73. Bibbo, M., Pestaner, J. P., Scavo, L. M., Bobroski, L., Seshamma, T., and Bagasra, O. Surfactant protein A mRNA expression utilizing the reverse transcription *in situ* PCR for metastatic adenocarcinoma. *Cell Vision* **1**:290–293, 1994.

74. Nuovo, G. J., MacConnell, P. B., Simsir, A., Valea, F., and French, D. Correlation of the *in situ* detection of polymerase chain reaction-amplified metalloproteinase complementary DNAs and their inhibitors with prognosis in cervical carcinoma. *Cancer Res.* **55**:267–275, 1995.

75. Yin, J., Kaplitt, M. G., and Pfaff, D. W. *In situ* PCR and in vivo detection of foreign gene expression in rat brain. *Cell Vision* **1**:58–59, 1994.

76. O'Leary, J. J., Browne, G., Landers, R. J., Crowley, M., Healy, I. B., Street, J. T., Pollock, A. M., Murphy, J., Johnson, M. I., Lewis, F. A., Mohamdee, O., Cullinane, C., and Doyle, C. T. The importance of fixation procedures on DNA template and its suitability for solution-phase polymerase chain reaction and PCR *in situ* hybridization. *Histochem. J.* **26**:337–346, 1994.

77. Tsongalis, G. J., McPhail, A. H., Lodge-Rigal, R. D., Chapman, J. F., and Silverman, L. M. Localized *in situ* amplification (LISA): A novel approach to *in situ* PCR. *Clin. Chem.* **40**:381–384, 1994.

78. Nuovo, G. J., MacConnell, P., and Gallery, F. Analysis of nonspecific DNA synthesis during *in situ* PCR and solution-phase PCR. *PCR Methods Appl.* **4**:89–96, 1994.

79. Bagasra, O., Seshamma, T., Oakes, J. W., and Pomerantz, R. J. High percentages of CD4-positive lymphocytes harbor the HIV-1 provirus in the blood of certain infected individuals. *AIDS* **7**:1419–1425, 1993.

80. Zevallos, E., Bard, E., Anderson, V., Carson, N, and Gu, J. Detection of HIV sequences in placentas of HIV-infected mothers by *in situ* PCR. *Cell Vision* **1**:116–121, 1994.

81. Re, M. C., Furlini, G., Gibellini, D., Vignoli, M., Rammazotti, E., Lolli, S., Ranieri, D., and La Placa, M. Quantification of human immunodeficiency virus type 1-infected mononuclear cells in peripheral blood of seropositive subjects by newly developed flow cytometry analysis of the product of an *in situ* PCR assay. *J. Clin. Microbiol.* **32**:2152–2157, 1994.

82. Ueki, K., Richardson, E. P., Henson, J. W., and Louis, D. N. In situ polymerase chain reaction demonstration of JC virus in progressive multifocal leukoencephalopathy, including an index case. *Ann. Neurol.* **36**:670–673, 1994.

83. Lidonnici, K., Lane, B., and Nuovo, G. J. Comparison of serologic analysis and *in situ* localization of PCR-amplified cDNA for the diagnosis of hepatitis C infection. *Diagn. Mol. Pathol.* **4**:98–107, 1995.

84. Isaacson, S. H., Asher, D. M., Gajdusek, D. C., and Gibbs, C. J. Detection of viruses in archival brain tissue by *in situ* RT-PCR amplification and labeled-probe hybridization. *Cell Vision* **1**:25–28, 1994.

85. Pereira, R. F., Halford, K. W., O'Hara, M. D., Leeper, D. B., Sokolov, B. P., Pollard, M. D., Bagasra, O., and Prockop, D. J. Cultured adherent cells from marrow can serve as long-lasting precursor cells for bone, cartilage, and lung in irradiated mice. *Proc. Natl. Acad. Sci. USA* **92**:4857–4861, 1995.

86. Deisseroth, A. B., Kavanagh, J., and Champlin, R. Use of safety-modified retroviruses to introduce chemotherapy resistant sequences into normal hematopoietic cells for chemoprotection during the therapy of ovarian cancer: a pilot trial. *Hum. Gene Ther.* **5**:1507–1522, 1994.

87. Teo, I. A. and Shaunak, S. Polymerase chain reaction *in situ*: an appraisal of an emerging technique. *Histochem. J.* **27**:647–659, 1995.

88. Teo, I. A. and Shaunak, S. PCR *in situ*: aspects which reduce amplification and generate false-positive results. *Histochem. J.* **27**:660–669, 1995.

9

Gene Therapy

Jeffrey S. Bartlett

1. INTRODUCTION

Genetic disorders account for a significant amount of human disease. About 4% of all infants born in the United States and Canada are affected by a birth defect. Approximately 1 in 200 births is affected by a chromosomal abnormality, whereas between 1 and 2 in 100 births are affected by a single gene disorder, most often recessive in character. The remainder of the disorders are presumed to be multifactorial in etiology, that is, involve more than one gene or are influenced by external factors. Although most genetic disorders are quite rare, there are several thousand of these disorders that are known, or suspected, to result from single gene defects. Many of these disorders are well known, such as sickle-cell anemia, CF*, muscular dystrophy, β-thalassemia, and PKU. Others are less common, but no less devastating to their victims; for example, the SCID syndromes, Lesh-Nyhan syndrome, and the various lipid and carbohydrate storage diseases.

Current therapy for genetic disease is terribly inadequate. This is largely because most current therapies only attempt to correct the symptoms or secondary biochemical effects of the primary disorder. In fact, such diseases as CF and sickle cell anemia can only be treated symptomatically. CF patients suffer from pancreatic exocrine insufficiency and develop frequent pulmonary infections because of thick mucus secretions in their lungs. This results from an impaired ability to regulate water balance across the airway epithelium. Pulmonary arrest is the major cause of death among these patients. During the last two decades, improved treatment has extended the average life expectancy of CF patients to 28 yr of age. However, a "cure" remains a challenge to be accomplished. Sickle cell anemia patients suffer from painful crises essentially owing to poor circulation. These individuals produce malformed red blood cells that are unable to oxygenate their tissue adequately. Such patients can benefit from antibiotics, hydration, and analgesia. However, this symptomatic therapy is not curative, and patients usually succumb to this disorder at a young age as well. These two examples serve to illustrate the need for new genetic disease therapy.

Gene therapy encompasses a broad range of technologies that are being applied to the clinical treatment of genetic diseases. Gene replacement therapy is the most com-

*See page 211 for list of abbreviations used in this chapter.

From: Molecular Diagnostics: For the Clinical Laboratorian
Edited by: W. B. Coleman and G. J. Tsongalis Humana Press Inc., Totowa, NJ

mon type of gene therapy. This form of therapy involves the transfer of genetic material to correct a patient's genetic defect. Essentially, this therapy involves the delivery to target cells of an expression cassette made up of one or more genes and the sequences that control their expression. This can be carried out ex vivo in a procedure in which the cassette is transferred to cells in the laboratory and the modified cells are then administered to the patient. Alternatively, human gene therapy can be done in vivo, in a procedure in which the expression cassette is transferred directly to cells within an individual. In both strategies, the transfer process is usually aided by a vector that helps deliver the therapeutic gene cassette to the desired target cells. Gene replacement therapy has theoretical appeal, since it is directed at the mutant gene itself rather than the symptoms or secondary events in the pathogenesis of the disease. It is anticipated that the diseases most amenable to gene therapy will be those in which a single gene product is missing (recessive inheritance) and where normal expression is constitutive. The majority of gene therapies fall into this classification

Any tissue is potentially amenable to genetic manipulation, although technical considerations suggest that those tissues with a high capacity for growth or self-renewal will have the best chance of permanently incorporating and expressing the exogenous genetic material. The targets of the gene therapies are the defective genes, which, of course, are present in every cell of the patient's body. However, gene transfer techniques for most disorders do not need to be 100% efficient to have a significant benefit. The diseases and tissues that will prove treatable by gene therapy can only be determined by an in depth study of the specific diseases and the techniques available for carrying out the genetic manipulations that are needed to treat these diseases, as discussed in more detail in the remainder of this chapter.

2. GENE TRANSFER AND EXPRESSION

In order to understand the methodology of human gene therapy, it is important to have an understanding of the components involved—genes, chromosomes, and cells—and the ways each is related to the other. Also important is an understanding of differentiation and development, and the way cells interact with each other to form tissues, organs, and entire organisms. Although a detailed discussion of these concepts is outside to scope of this chapter, several very good reviews on these subjects have appeared. Since gene therapy entails the molecular manipulation of cells at the DNA level, a short discussion of the basic fundamentals of molecular biology and gene expression, as they relate to human gene therapy, is presented here.

2.1. Eukaryotic Control Elements

As one attempts to express genes transferred into cells or into a patient, one must take into consideration the vast amount of information dealing with the various *cis*-acting DNA elements that either directly or indirectly affect gene expression. Each gene has not only a promoter, but often a matched enhancer, as well as splice signals, polyadenylation signals, and sequences that determine the stability of the messenger RNA. These elements exert their influence in a cooperative and tissue-specific manner, and serve to determine where in an organism the gene is expressed. These elements can be experimentally mixed and matched, leading to novel recombinant constructs with new patterns of gene expression that aid the development of gene-based therapeutics. It is important to recognize that promoters, enhancers, splice signals, and other *cis*-acting elements do not act as fully independent elements. It appears that there are preferred and nonfunctional combinations. In several cases, the appropriate tissue-specific expression is dependent on the assembly of a matched set of individual elements. Therefore, the selection and assembly of the correct elements in a recombinant gene cassette are critical in achieving the desired expression phenotype on transfer into the patient. The information that follows is provided to illustrate the range and behavior of *cis*-acting elements available to the gene therapist and the practical considerations involved in the construction of an appropriate transgene cassette for gene transfer experiments.

2.2. Promoters and Enhancers

Promoters are DNA sequence elements that control the initiation of transcription. Promoters for protein-encoding genes commonly contain two types of DNA sequence elements. These are core elements, which alone can support gene expression, and regulatory elements, which are recognized by gene-specific regulatory proteins and function to modulate the level of transcription initiated at the core element. Two types of core elements have been identified; the TATA box, which is found 25–30 bp upstream of the start site of transcription, and the initiator *(1)*, which fits a loose consensus sequence that overlaps the transcription start site *(2)*. Enhancers represent a second class of *cis*-acting sequences that modulate gene expression. Enhancers can not initiate transcription. Rather, they activate transcription from a linked promoter element. Enhancers are characterized by their ability to activate transcription in any orientation and at variable distances upstream or downstream of the promoter.

With few exceptions, the most critical variable in the design of a recombinant expression cassette is the selection of an enhancer and promoter element. Enhancers have been identified in association with both viral and cellular genes, and both are routinely included in gene transfer vectors. Viral enhancers, as a group, are the most active transcriptional enhancing elements. For this reason, they have been used in majority of human gene therapy vectors. However, recent evidence suggests that these viral elements may not be very good at driving transgene expression in vivo. Presumably the host cells have a mechanism by which they are able to recognize the viral sequences as foreign and downregulate their expression *(3,4)*. In studies using a viral LTR driving transgene expression in mouse liver, the mouse cells were able to shut off gene expression from this element completely, although the DNA remained intact *(5)*. Observations of this type have led to the use of eukaryotic enhancers or recombinant eukaryotic/viral enhancers as the elements of choice for modulating gene expression for gene therapy.

2.3. Inducible and Tissue-Specific Promoters and Enhancers

Genes that are not constitutively expressed in all cell types must possess a mechanism for regulating induction or repression of gene expression in response to physiological signals. The *cis*-acting sequences that control these effects reside in either the enhancer, promoter, or both elements. Tissue-specific control elements are attractive from a gene therapy point of view, because they can provide targeted expression of the therapeutic gene product. In addition, tissue-specific regulatory elements allow a greater latitude in the delivery of the vector, since only those vectors that are delivered to the appropriate cell type will become transcriptionally active. Similarly, inclusion of an inducible regulatory element in a transgene cassette may allow the transgene to respond to external stimuli.

2.4. Factors Influencing Transgene Expression

One of the peculiarities of the recombinant gene cassettes used for gene therapy is the observation that certain promoters function better if provided with a functional intron. Although this effect is promoter- and tissue-dependent, it can be tremendously important to include an intron in some vector constructions.

The stability of mRNAs in cells appears to vary widely, and it now appears that the rates of mRNA decay are important control points in the regulation of gene expression. The factors governing mRNA stability are structural in nature and are often contained within discrete sequence elements linked to the RNA transcript. An example of such a sequence is the 3'-noncoding region of β-globin mRNA, which is highly stable. These elements are often linked to protein coding sequences within the RNA component of gene expression cassettes to provide greater message stability. The role of poly-adenylation in mRNA stability is not quite as clear. However, it never appears that polyadenylation has a negative effect on gene expression, and in some instances, polyadenylation may be absolutely required for efficient transport and processing of the transcripts. Therefore, recombinant gene cassettes should carry polyadenylation signals to facilitate gene expression.

Several types of *cis*-acting elements that affect the efficiency of translation of mRNAs are used in expression constructs for gene therapy. These are of two main types: sequences based on the Kozak translation initiation signal sequence spanning the ATG start codon *(6)*, and sequences that function as IRES that facilitate the trans-lation of two or more coding sequences within a multicistronic mRNA *(7)*. Deviation from the Kozak consensus translation initiation sequence can have a profound effect on the quantity of therapeutic gene product produced. This effect is especially appar-ent when genes from lower eukaryotic, or prokaryotic, organisms are expressed in mammalian cells. Often the translation start codons within these genes are poorly recognized by the translational machinery of the mammalian cells and must be replaced by sequences more closely resembling the consensus Kozak sequences in order to be sufficiently expressed in human cells. IRES are based on adaptations from viral sequences. The insertion of an IRES into a recombinant DNA molecule at the appropriate location will allow the efficient translation of two or more genes from a single mRNA. Since only one enhancer and/or promoter is used to drive the expression of the multicistronic mRNA, this approach can be used when more than one gene is desired, but size constraints preclude the inclusion of a second set of transcriptional elements.

2.5. Assays for Gene Transfer and Expression

There are several methods that may be employed to monitor and quantitate success-ful gene transfer and determine the efficacy of gene therapy. Each disease will, of course, have its own clinically determinable therapeutic efficacy. However, short of an easily discernible clinical effect, it is often difficult to determine the true efficiency of gene transfer. One can assay for the presence of transferred DNA by Southern hybridization or PCR using genomic DNA obtained from a patient biopsy or blood sample. Additionally, it is possible to monitor successful gene transfer by examining mRNA expression from the exogenous transgene through northern analysis of cellular RNA or by RT-PCR. Similarly, protein production can be monitored through the application of either immunoprecipitation or Western blotting techniques, as well as immunofluorescence analysis or bioassay where appropriate.

3. METHODS OF GENE TRANSFER

Before describing the collection of gene transfer vectors available, it is important to discuss the two fundamentally different approaches to gene therapy and the desired expression characteristics of the transferred gene. When cells are removed from a patient and genetic material is transferred into these cells in the laboratory prior to their introduction back into the patient, this is referred to as ex vivo gene therapy. When gene transfer is accomplished directly within the patient, it is referred to as in vivo gene therapy, or gene transfer having taken place *in situ*. These are two fundamentally different approaches to gene therapy, and the methods used for each differ significantly. For example, the ex vivo approach allows for selection of a particular cell type prior to gene transfer as well as selection of transduced cells prior to introduction back into the patient. In vivo gene therapy, on the other hand, has a whole host of other obstacles associated with its success. These include immune response against the gene transfer vector, targeted delivery of the vectors to the appropriate cell/tissue type, and high enough frequency of gene delivery to be of therapeutic value.

In the laboratory, the experimental introduction of DNA into cells is accomplished by methods that:

1. Form DNA precipitates that can be internalized by the target cell, such as the calcium phosphate transfection method *(8,9)*;
2. Create DNA-containing complexes whose charge characteristics are compatible with DNA uptake by the target cell, like the DEAE dextran transfection method; or
3. Result in the transient formation of pores in the plasma membrane of a cell exposed to an electric pulse which allow DNA to enter the target cell.

However, the introduction of DNA into the cells of a patient for therapeutic purposes is accomplished by different methods that must speak to the inherent difficulties and requirements of this type of gene transfer. There are two major classes of techniques for introducing DNA into cells: those utilizing physical or chemical methods to transfect DNA and those utilizing biological-viral vectors to introduce foreign DNA. In addition, some methods have been optimized for transient expression, whereas others are preferred for the stable expression required for gene therapy in vivo.

3.1. Physical Methods of Gene Transfer

3.1.1. Direct Injection of DNA

One of the most straightforward ways of introducing DNA into cells is to inject the sequences of interest directly into a target tissue. Direct gene transfer has been achieved in vivo by appropriately engineered circular plasmid DNA in skin, striated muscle, and myocardium, as well as in several other less well-studied tissues. Different tissues have different abilities to take up naked DNA. However, in some instances, only a small number of cells are needed to take up and express the transferred gene. This technique is currently being used for the purposes of vaccination and cancer immunotherapy. Direct intramuscular or intradermal injection of naked DNA-encoding microorganism-derived antigens can result in a specific, potent, and lasting immunity of both humoral and cell-mediated type. Particle bombardment with DNA bound to microparticles represents an analogous method for directly introducing genes into cells. Particle bombardment involves precipitating DNA onto microparticles that are projected into cells using explosive or gas-driven ballistic devices. When DNA-coated particles land within the cell, the DNA is gradually released from the particle leading to gene expression.

3.1.2. Liposome-Mediated Gene Transfer

Cationic lipids have become important reagents for gene transfer. The prototype cationic lipid for gene transfer is DOTMA *(10,11)*. Formulations of DNA with cationic lipids, such as DOTMA, and a neutral phospholipid, commonly DOPE, produce lipid–DNA complexes that are capable of introducing DNA into cells at high efficiency. These methods provide transfection efficiencies of >90% in some cell lines and primary cells in vitro. Commercially available cationic lipid mixtures, such as Lipofectin and Lipofectamine (Gibco-BRL, Gaithersburg, MD), are used routinely in basic research. The lipid–DNA complex in these formulations is not a true liposome in which compounds are encapsulated within a lamellar lipid structure. Rather, the cationic lipid forms a particle by condensing DNA through the ionic interactions between the cationic lipid and DNA, and form a particulate complex that may contain several plasmids through the hydrophobic interactions among the bound lipids. The size and charge of the lipid–DNA complex and the efficiency of gene delivery can be optimized by altering the composition of lipids and DNA within the complex. A variety of cationic lipids have been synthesized and used for gene transfer. These include cationic lipids with structures analogous to DOTMA, such as DMRIE *(12)* and DOTAP *(13)*, as well as cationic lipids containing polylysine *(14,15)*, cholesterol *(16)*, lipopolyamides *(17,18)*, and quaternary ammonium detergents *(19)*. Although various cationic lipids and lipid combinations exhibit quantitatively different gene delivery efficiencies in different cells, no clear patterns have emerged concerning features of the lipid carriers that are necessary for optimal gene delivery.

Plasmid–liposome complexes have several advantages as gene transfer vectors, in that they can be used to transfer expression cassettes of varying size, do not replicate or recombine to form infectious agents, and generally provoke less immune response than viral vectors because of the lack of protein components (Fig. 1). The disadvantage of these vectors is that they are very inefficient in vivo and often require thousands of plasmid molecules per target cell to achieve successful gene transfer. Nonetheless, cationic lipids have been used to deliver genes to several tissues in vivo. Successful expression of α1-antitrypsin and CFTR transgenes in animal lungs has led to clinical trials of gene therapy for genetic deficiencies of these proteins in humans. Several other studies have employed cationic lipid–DNA complexes administered directly into tumor masses for anticancer gene therapy. Initial studies were aimed at expressing a foreign antigen within tumor cells to enhance the immunogenicity of tumor or presentation of tumor-specific antigens.

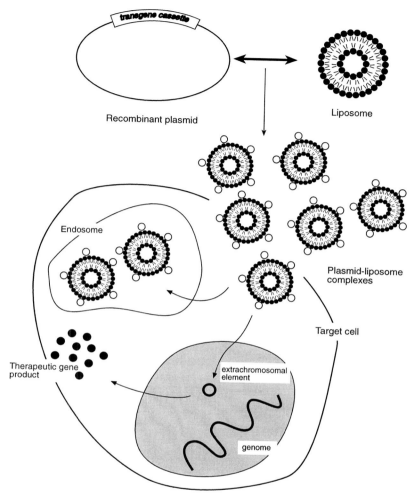

Fig. 1. Gene transfer with plasmid–liposome complexes. Although the lipid components of these complexes can have different compositions, the general scheme is consistent. The positively charged lipid is complexed to the negatively charged plasmid DNA containing the desired transgene cassette, and the complexes enter the cell by an unknown mechanism. Genetic material that is able to avoid degradation in cytoplasmic vesicles reaches the nucleus and is expressed.

3.1.3. Molecular Conjugates

Another method for introducing genes into cells is to complex DNA with ligands able to bind to the surface of a target cell. Such complexes are commonly prepared by covalently coupling the ligand to polylysine and then condensing the polylysine to DNA by the ionic interaction between the positively charged polylysine and the negatively charged DNA *(20–23)*. The resulting complexes retain their ability to interact specifically with the receptors on the target cell leading to receptor-mediated internalization of the complex into the cell. One of the factors that limits the efficiency of receptor-mediated gene delivery, as well as lipid-mediated gene delivery, is the rapid degradation of DNA within the endosome. Several methods have been described for enhancing the release of DNA from endosomes. One approach has been to include adenoviral particles in the transfection mixture. This is based on the observation that adenoviral particles are capable of inducing endosomal lysis during the process of adeno-viral infection *(24)*. Adenovirus-enhanced gene delivery is most effective when the DNA is complexed to the adenoviral particles. This is accomplished by covalently binding polylysine to the surface of adenovirus, which allows binding of the DNA, and the ligand-polylysine components of the molecular conjugates by ionic attraction. Despite the importance of enhancing endosomal release to improve the efficiency of gene transfer in vitro, methods for enhancing endosomal release have not been effec-tively employed in vivo. This may be because of the large size of the adenoviral–DNA–ligand complexes or because of the concentration of these conjugates in vivo cannot approach that commonly used in vitro.

3.2. Gene Transfer Using Biological Vectors

Biological vectors are constructed from naturally occurring DNA molecules, for example, animal viruses. The ideal vector will carry a therapeutic gene of interest into a high percentage of target cells and facilitate integration and expression of the gene. The development of biological vectors is a field that has received a great deal of atten-tion lately, and future vectors may be able to deposit the gene of interest in a tissue-specific manner and impart either the normal physiologic or regulatable expression of the transferred gene.

3.2.1. Retrovirus-Mediated Gene Transfer

Retroviruses contain single-stranded RNA genomes and replicate in animal cells via DNA intermediates called proviruses. Because of their unique lifestyles, retroviruses can be used to shuttle genetic material into cells. After infecting a susceptible cell, the retrovirus begins to replicate in the cytoplasm where a viral encoded enzyme, reverse transcriptase, synthesizes a DNA copy of the single-stranded RNA genome. Subse-quently, the viral DNA is transferred to the nucleus, where it becomes integrated ran-domly into the host genome as a provirus. LTR sequences contained in the genome of a retrovirus are important for virus replication and expression of viral genes. The inte-grated provirus utilizes regulatory elements contained within the LTR sequence to direct host enzymes to make new retroviral particles. These regulatory elements include a strong promoter, an enhancer, and sequences for the addition of a 5'-CAP and 3'-polyadenosine tail to viral RNAs. In addition there is a packaging sequence that is required for the incorporation of viral RNA genomes into new virion particles. An infectious retrovirus has three translation units:

1. *gag*, encoding the group-specific antigen internal structural proteins;
2. *pol*, encoding reverse transcriptase and viral integrase, which facilitates proviral insertion into the host cell genome; and
3. *env*, encoding the envelope glycoproteins essential for the entry of virus particles into cells.

Mature retroviral particles bud from the cell surface without killing the cell in which they were produced.

The DNA form of the retroviral genome does not appear to have any preference regarding where it integrates in the cellular genome. This random entry into the host cell chromatin can have serious consequences for the cell. It is well known that some types of neoplasia are caused by integration of proviral DNA adjacent to cellular proto-oncogenes. The proximal integration of proviral DNA adjacent to a proto-oncogene can result in enhanced proto-oncogene expression owing to the presence of retroviral control elements. This insertional oncogenesis is a potential stumbling block for the safe use of retroviral vectors in human gene therapy.

A number of features make retroviruses attractive candidates to carry DNA into cells for gene therapy. Retroviruses converted into vectors offer the potential for effective introduction, integration, and expression of new genes. In addition, tissue specificity may be determined at several levels. First, viruses gain entry into only those cells bearing specific receptors, and second, viral RNA is transcribed in a tissue-specific manner, since transcription is regulated by specific enhancer and promoter elements in the LTR. Potentially these characteristics offer a way of targeting genes to affected tissues for gene therapy. To exploit retroviruses as vectors for therapeutic purposes, it has been necessary to delete essential viral structural genes to make room for exogenous genetic material. This also renders these viral vectors replication-defective. Defective replication means that these viruses are not infectious in the absence of a helper virus that can supply the missing viral genes required to complete the viral life cycle. However, the viral RNA must be "packaged" within an infectious virion to capitalize on the capacity of the virus to transfer and express a gene of interest efficiently. There are two solutions to the problem of propagating replication-defective retroviruses bearing foreign genes. In nature, similar viruses propagate by means of helper viruses. For gene therapy, viral structural genes are best supplied by means of helper cell lines. Helper cell lines contain integrated provirus sequences that supply viral structural proteins (Fig. 2). Such lines do not produce progeny virus independently, because the RNA they produce is defective for packaging because of the deletion of necessary sequence elements. When a helper cell line is infected with a replication-defective retroviral vector carrying a foreign gene, the vector RNA is copied into DNA by the host cell reverse transcriptase, and the host cell integrase facilitates integration at a random site. The vector RNA is transcribed from its own LTR. Since the vector RNA contains the necessary packaging sequences, it is able to form viable infectious virions utilizing the structural proteins provided in trans by the helper cell line. When such particles infect a normal cell, they are able to reverse transcribe their RNA into DNA because of the reverse transcriptase supplied by the packaging cell line and carried along in the viral particle, and efficiently integrate into the genomic DNA of recipient cells using the supplied integrase. Integrated provirus DNA presumably will express mRNA because it has functional LTR or alternative promoter sequences (Fig. 2). Transmissible viral particles will not be produced, however, because the target cells lack the structural genes for *gag*, *env*, and *pol*, and so forth. Theoretically, the target cells for gene therapy receive a cloned replacement gene regulated by its own promoter carried to recipient cells by a defective retrovirus vector packaged in a helper cell line. To increase the efficiency of retroviral-mediated gene transfer, a major aim of recent work has been to increase the viral titer of the producer cell lines. Typical helper cell lines produce 10^4–10^6 CFU/mL. In practice, it has proven difficult to concentrate virus-containing cell supernatants to increase their titers additionally. High-titer vectors are important for efficient infection of most cell types. The highest titers have been obtained with small retroviral constructs, whereas retrovirus vectors that contain larger exog-

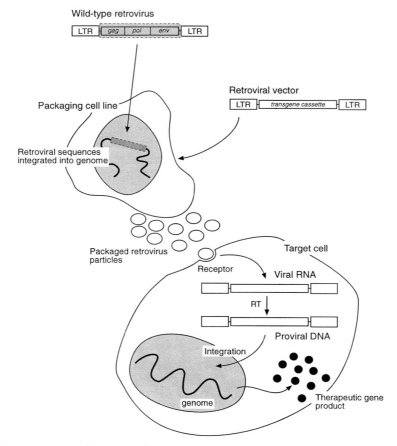

Fig. 2. Gene transfer with recombinant retrovirus vectors. The *gag*, *pol*, and *env* sequences are removed from the virus, rendering it replication-defective. These functions are supplied in *trans* by a packaging cell line. A recombinant transgene cassette is inserted in place of these sequences in the virus. When the recombinant virus is transfected into the packaging cell line, replication-defective retroviral vectors are produced. The vectors, with their transgene cassettes, enter target cells via a specific receptor. In the target cells, the viral RNA is converted to DNA and integrated into the target cell genome, where the transgene cassette makes its product.

enous gene cassettes are not packaged as efficiently by helper cell lines. Vectors that contain long *gag* sequences also are produced at higher titer, perhaps because they contain more of the natural packaging signal.

The majority of retroviral vectors currently in use are derived from murine retroviruses, most commonly the Mo-muLV. The types of cells a retrovirus can infect (called its tropism) are determined by the envelope glycoprotein that facilitates attachment of the virus to cell-surface receptors and the viral LTR, in particular, the enhancer sequences that determine in which tissues viral genomes can be expressed. The envelope protein can be manipulated by introducing the appropriate *env* sequences into helper cell "packaging" cell lines. Three categories of viruses can be distinguished: Ecotropic viruses infect murine and some other rodent cells, xenotropic viruses infect nonrodent cells, and amphotropic viruses infect both rodent and nonrodent cells, including human cells. A prototypic retroviral vector, N2, developed by Gilboa and coworkers at Sloan Kettering Memorial Cancer Center in New York, NY, contains the bacterial neomycin resistance gene derived from the TN5 transposon cloned into a skeleton Mo-MuLV virus consisting of the 5'- and 3'-LTR sequences, the packaging signal, and a small portion of the viral *gag* sequences. N2 has been used as a basis for the construction of many vectors expressing a variety of human and other vertebrate genes.

Vectors with internal promoters can utilize the viral LTR to express one gene, whereas a second promoter can be linked to a second gene in *cis* directs its expression. The second promoter unit may be in either orientation with respect to the LTR if the second gene is a cDNA. Genomic DNA (containing introns) placed in the 5' to 3' orientation will lose its introns via splicing during propagation in the helper cell lines and therefore must be inserted in the 3' to 5' orientation. Examples of internal promoters include certain viral derivatives (e.g., the SV40 early promoter), the HSV-tk promoter, the early promoter of cytomegalovirus, and promoters derived from human or other vertebrate genes (e.g., histone H4 or, β-actin promoters). An advantage of internal promoter vectors over the LTR expression vectors is that control over exogenous gene expression may be obtained by varying the nature of the second promoter. Additional modifications of retroviral vectors include:

1. Exchange of enhancer sequences; for example, exchange of the Mo-MuLV-enhancer or Friend LV enhancer sequences for those from a murine myeloproliferative sarcoma virus can increase expression of exogenous genes in murine hematopoietic cells;
2. Use of a polyoma early region to amplify transient expression after transfection;
3. Employment of alternative eukaryotic promoters, i.e., those from avian β-actin, human histone H4, or phosphoglycerate kinase genes to attempt to increase expression of introduced genes in murine bone marrow cells in vivo.

Retroviral vectors have been used successfully to introduce and express diverse genes in a wide variety of cells in vitro and in many in vivo systems. General problems that have arisen include:

1. Far better expression of introduced genes in vitro than in vivo;
2. No single retroviral vector is universally useful for introducing genes into a variety of cell types; and
3. In some cases, when two genes are expressed from the same vector, there is interference with expression of the LTR-driven gene by the second promoter (and vice versa).

It appears that each application of gene therapy will require a distinct retroviral vector that can optimally introduce and express the therapeutic gene in the particular cells to be repaired.

3.3. Adenovirus-Mediated Gene Transfer

Adenoviruses are widespread in nature. Clinical illness associated with adenovirus infection depends on the serotype of virus, but is usually mild and is rarely life-threatening. For this reason, adenovirus-based vectors are good candidates for human gene therapy. Adenovirus contains a double-stranded linear DNA genome of about 36 kb packaged into a rigid protein capsid with a diameter of about 60–90 nm (the size of the capsid depends on the serotype of adenovirus). The capsid is icosahedral in shape and

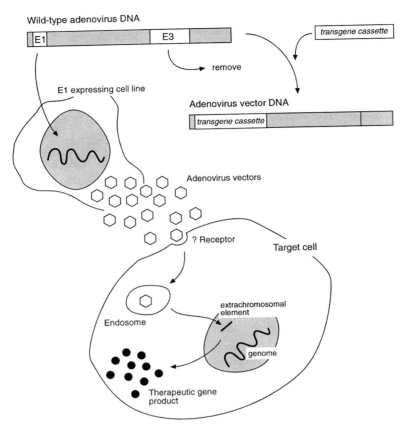

Fig. 3. Gene transfer with adenovirus vectors. The E1 region (and E3 region if space is needed) of the adenovirus genome is removed to accommodate the transgene cassette. Deletion of the E1 regions makes the vector replication-defective, and it must be grown on a E1-expressing cell line. When the virus genome containing the transgene cassette is transfected into the complementing cell line, adenovirus vectors containing the foreign gene are produced. The vectors probably enter cells through a specific receptor and deposit their DNA into the nucleus, where it functions in an epichromosomal fashion to direct the synthesis of the therapeutic gene product.

has protein fibers protruding from each vertex that are responsible for attachment of the virus to cells. Each viral chromosome has a 100–140 bp long-terminal redundancy, the ITR, which is necessary for viral replication. Adjacent to the ITR are several specific sequences that direct the packaging of the viral DNA into the protein capsids. The requirement for these encapsidation signals makes adenovirus virion assembly specific and precludes entry of cellular DNA into adenovirus capsids.

Our understanding of the molecular genetics of adenovirus has allowed us to use adenovirus as a cloning vector for the transfer of genes in cell culture and in vivo. In order to block the genetic program of the virus so that the targeted cells do not die, the E1A region of the virus is removed (Fig. 3). This deletion renders the vectors replication-defective. The adenovirus E1A gene is located in the left-most end of the adenovirus genome adjacent to the packaging signals and left ITR. This region is transcribed by cellular factors immediately after infection (also called the immediate early gene

[IEG] region), and codes for two related, multifunctional proteins. These proteins are responsible for the transcriptional activation of several other adenovirus genes. Therefore, without E1A, the adenovirus is unable to go through a productive infection. In this case, the propagation of recombinant adenovirus vectors requires the use of an E1-complementing cell line, such as the 293 cell line, which is a human embryonic kidney cell line expressing the E1 gene functions. High-titer stocks of E1A-deleted viruses can be obtained by propagation in 293 cells and purification by centrifugation through CsCl buoyant density gradients (Fig. 3). Replication-defective adenovirus vectors typically have additional deletions to provide room for cloning foreign DNA. At a minimum, the E1, E3, and part of the E4 regions of the adenoviral genome can be replaced by a foreign gene cassette. Adenovirus vectors in current use accommodate expression cassettes up to about 7.5 kb.

Adenovirus vectors are well suited for in vivo applications, because they efficiently transfer genes to nonreplicating and replicating cells. The transferred genetic material remains extrachromosomal, thus avoiding the risk of insertional mutagenesis common to the retrovirus vectors. However, the recombinant adenovirus genomes are, by the same mechanism, unstable and eventually lost from the target cell population. Therefore, adenoviral vectors have to be repeatedly administered to patients, which is problematic because of antivector immunity and nonspecific vector-mediated inflammatory responses. Nonetheless, adenovirus vectors have been used extensively for in vivo human gene therapy trials *(25–29)*.

3.3.1. AAV-Mediated Gene Transfer

The development of gene transfer vectors from the human parvovirus, AAV, has provided yet another way of delivering genes into mammalian cells. The AAV genome is encapsidated as a single-stranded DNA molecule of plus or minus polarity. Strands of both polarities are packaged, but in separate virus particles, and both strands are infectious. The genome of AAV is 4675 bp in length and is flanked by ITR sequences of 145 bp each similar to the adenovirus ITR. However, the AAV ITR sequences fold back on themselves to form "T"-shaped hairpin structures that are used to initiate DNA replication. The terminal repeats also contain the sequences necessary to package the viral DNA into virions. Early characterization of AAV replication, latent viral chromosomes, and defective interfering particles all point to the viral terminal repeats as key *cis*-acting elements required for the AAV life cycle.

AAV is a defective member of the parvovirus family. AAV can be propagated as a lytic virus or maintained as a provirus that is integrated into the host cell genome. In a lytic infection, replication requires coinfection with either adenovirus or herpes simplex virus, hence the classification of AAV as a "defective" virus. The requirement of a helper virus for a productive infection has made understanding the AAV life cycle more difficult. However, from a vector point of view, it has added a level of control when generating nonreplicative vectors, in that they can be propagated under controlled conditions, thereby reducing unwanted spread, and providing a margin of safety. One of the most interesting aspects of the AAV life cycle is the virus' ability to integrate into the host genome in the absence of helper virus. When AAV infects cells in the absence of helper virus, it establishes latency by persisting in the host cell genome as an integrated provirus. It is this aspect of the AAV life cycle that is exploited to provide long-term stable transfer of exogenous genes for gene therapy.

The first use of AAV as a vector for the transduction of a foreign gene into the host chromosome was demonstrated by Hermonat and Muzyczka in 1984 *(30)*. An rAAV viral stock was produced using an infectious plasmid vector containing a double-stranded version of the virus cloned into a plasmid backbone in which the neomycin resistance gene was substituted for the AAV capsid genes. The ability to generate large quantities of plasmid DNA, which is basically inert until introduced into adenovirus-infected human cells, provides a safe and efficient way of manipulating this system. This rAAV was able to transduce neomycin resistance to both murine and human cell lines *(30)*. Since these first studies, AAV has been used as a viral vector system to express a variety of genes in a number of different eukaryotic cells *(31–33)*. All of these experiments have used plasmid vectors in which portions of the AAV genome were replaced by a foreign gene of interest. However, the size of the inserted foreign DNA is limited by the ability of the rAAV vector to be packaged into infectious virions (4.7 kb), which depends on the size of the retained AAV sequences.

The present method for producing stocks of recombinant AAV utilizes a two-component plasmid system: AAV plasmid vector, which contains little more than the AAV ITR flanking the desired transgene cassette, and AAV helper plasmid, which provides the necessary AAV capsid and replication proteins in *trans* (Fig. 4). An important consideration is that the vector and helper plasmid DNAs should be sufficiently non-homologous to preclude homologous recombination events between the two that could generate wild-type AAV. By cotransfecting the helper plasmid and the recombinant vector plasmid in the presence of adenovirus, rescue, replication and packaging of the foreign gene into AAV particles occur. The result of such a packaging scheme is an adenovirus helper and AAV particle carrying the recombinant expression cassette. The adenovirus helper can be removed by a number of physical and genetic techniques.

rAAV is among the newest of the gene therapy vectors. This once obscure virus possesses several properties that distinguish it from other vectors. Its advantages include the ability to integrate into the host cell genome and the lack of any known pathogenicity. In addition, its ability to carry regulatory elements (i.e., tissue-specific enhancers/promoters, splice sites, and so on) without interference from the viral genome allows for greater control of transferred gene expression *(34,35)*. In vitro experiments demonstrate that rAAV vectors can transduce a number of different primary cell types and support the development of this vector system for gene therapy *(36,37)*. However, no human gene therapy protocols using AAV are currently being conducted. One reason for this has been the inferior packaging systems, which yield low numbers of recombinant virions that are often contaminated with wild-type adenovirus. Fortunately, this difficulty does not seem to be an insurmountable technical problem, and AAV may be in routine clinical use as a gene therapy vector in the near future.

3.3.2. Other Viral Vectors for Gene Delivery

Other viruses being studied for use as gene transfer vectors include herpes virus, HDV, and poxvirus. Although the development of these viruses for use in gene therapy has not progressed as far as that of the viruses discussed above, there may be distinct advantages to the development of these viruses for human gene therapy. For example, the recombinant viral genomes of HDV vectors are self-replicating and could facilitate the delivery of very high copy numbers of biologically active sequences. Additionally,

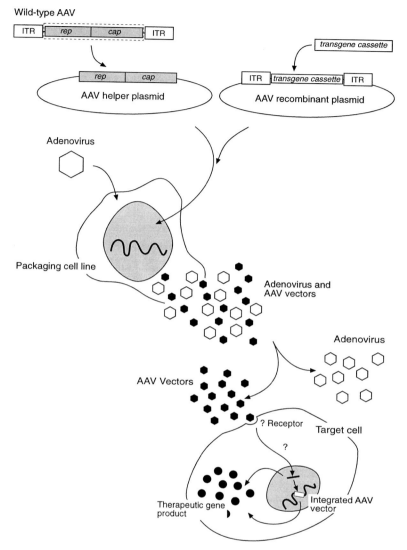

Fig. 4. Gene transfer with AAV vectors. The AAV genome is divided into two components. The *trans*-acting AAV function is supplied by a "helper" plasmid, whereas the *cis*-acting AAV ITRs flank the transgene cassette in a second AAV plasmid. When these two plasmids are transfected into cells, in conjunction with adenovirus infection, progeny adenovirus and rAAV vectors are produced. The adenovirus must be physically removed from the preparation. The AAV vectors containing the transgene cassette are internalized by the target cells, and the foreign DNA is inserted into the genome where the therapeutic gene product can be expressed.

human herpes viruses are very large viruses, and offer the potential of transferring very large genes or entire chromosomal regions into a patient. Of course, the complex biology of these viruses and the poorly understood pathology of HDV and herpes viral infection necessitate additional research in order to construct safe and efficient virus vectors for gene therapy.

4. GENE TRANSFER IN THE TREATMENT OF HUMAN GENETIC DISEASE

The components necessary for successful gene therapy include choice of an appropriate disease and knowledge of the molecular defect involved, as well the cloning of the normal gene needed to correct the disorder, development of an appropriate vector system, and adequate expression of the transferred gene. It is also useful if the pathogenesis of the disease is well understood and an appropriate animal model is available. Human diseases that are amenable to gene therapy can be grouped into two main categories. The first grouping includes the inherited genetic diseases characterized by single gene defects, and the second category is made up of acquired and infectious diseases. Although these diseases may not be considered truly genetic in origin, their genetic components allow them to be treated by gene therapy.

4.1. Inherited Genetic Diseases Involving Single-Gene Defects

Inherited genetic diseases caused by single-gene defects were among the first to be considered for gene therapy. Of these, the SCID syndromes characterized by an autosomal-recessive deficiency of the purine catabolic enzyme ADA were the first inherited human genetic diseases treated by gene transfer. About 25% of SCID cases are caused by a defect in the gene for ADA, and another small percentage are the result of another purine metabolic disorder caused by PNP deficiency. These deficiencies were the perfect candidates for the initial trials of human gene therapy for a number of reasons. First, ADA and PNP deficiencies are fatal in all untreated cases, and alternative therapies are inadequate. Bone marrow transplantation can be curative for these defects. However, few patients are treated in this manner because of either clinical deterioration or lack of suitable sibling or histocompatible donors. Second, it has been shown that enzyme replacement therapy could correct the clinical manifestations of disease during the time that the enzyme is present. Therefore, a case could be made that transfer of the genes encoding these enzymes should also be able to correct the disorder. Additionally, it had been shown that individuals could tolerate a wide range of ADA or PNP activity, such that even modest gene transfer that provided only 5–10% of the normal enzyme activity should be curative. Finally, gene transfer vectors carrying the ADA or PNP gene could be constructed and tested for their ability to transfer these genes in tissue-culture systems that were defective in these enzyme activities. The original gene therapy experiments for the treatment of ADA deficiency were carried out ex vivo using autologous bone marrow cells that had been removed from individual patients. These cells were separated and incubated with recombinant retrovirus carrying the normal ADA gene. Following infection and removal of excess virus, cells were infused intravenously back into the patient. The ex vivo approach allowed for the selection of the appropriate target cell, controlled administration of the gene transfer vectors, and selection and expansion in vitro of the transduced cells prior to reintroduction into the patient. Diseases of hematopoietic cell lineages are particularly amenable to this type of gene therapy, since the technology for removing, cultivating, and reinfusing these cells back into patients is already part of routine medical practice. Other single-gene disorders that can be treated by ex vivo gene therapy include the hemoglobinopathies, sickle cell anemia, and β-thalassemia, as well as some plasma protein deficiencies, such as the hemophilia and α1-antitrypsin deficiency. Some of the storage diseases that are recessively inherited single-gene defects resulting in the inability to degrade complex carbohydrates and lipids have also been treated by ex vivo gene transfer into blood cell lineages. These include the glycogen storage diseases, mucopolysaccharidoses, and Gaucher's disease.

Other inherited single-gene defects cannot be treated ex vivo. Of these, CF is a good example. CF is an autosomal-recessive disorder and one of the most common genetic ailments among Caucasians. Mutations in the CFTR gene result in the clinical manifestation of CF. The major cause of morbidity and mortality in CF patients is respiratory disease. Thus, the lung is the principal target for gene therapy in CF patients. It is the lung airway epithelium that must be transduced with the CFTR gene to provide an effective therapy. Since this tissue is not amenable to transplantation, gene transfer must be carried out *in situ* within the patient's lung. The natural tropism of adenovirus vectors for respiratory epithelia and the ability of adenovirus to enter quiescent cells make them attractive candidates for gene therapy of CF. Currently, several clinical gene transfer studies in CF patients utilizing recombinant adenovirus vectors are being conducted. In the present human studies, preparations of the viral vector are administered directly to small areas of the airway epithelium. However, in the future it may be possible to aerosolize the vector and have the patient inhale the vector preparation. This should result in a substantially larger surface area being treated and better chance of achieving a therapeutic level of gene transfer.

4.2. Cancer

Several gene therapy strategies dealing with the study or treatment of cancer are currently being developed and have already entered into clinical trials. In general, these clinical trials can be divided into two types: gene-marking and gene therapy protocols. All of the gene-marking studies to date have been accomplished using replication-defective retroviruses. Gene-marking protocols are intended to determine the in vivo fate of the genetically marked cells, whereas other protocols have genetically modified cells with a therapeutic intent.

The number of gene therapy protocols for the treatment of human cancer has grown rapidly since gene therapy was first applied to the treatment of brain tumors *(38,39)*. A survey of the treatments currently being pursued reveals five general approaches. The first approach involves the insertion of a cytokine gene into tumor cells ex vivo. This is basically a tumor vaccination in which the transduced gene increases the immunogenicity of the tumor cells on autologous transplantation back into the affected patient. At least five cytokine genes are presently under active clinical study: interleukin-2, interleukin-4, tumor necrosis factor, granulocyte-macrophage colony-stimulating factor, and interferon-γ *(40–43)*. A variation on this approach as proposed by Rosenberg and colleagues *(44,45)* has been to insert a cytokine gene into tumor-infiltrating lymphocytes in order to make these cells more effective in destroying tumors. Of the approved cancer gene therapy protocols, approximately half fall into this first category.

The second approach has been the insertion of a "suicide" gene into tumor cells *in situ*, with subsequent activation by prodrug therapy. The strategy here is that the transferred gene will confer susceptibility to a drug that will then kill the tumor cells. The therapeutic gene that is most widely used is the HSV-tk gene *(39,46,47)*, although several other genes, including the bacterial genes encoding cytosine deaminase, PNP, and xanthine/guanine phosphoribosyltransferase, have been proposed *(48–51)*. Each of these genes provides activities not present in mammalian cells that are capable of converting relatively nontoxic prodrugs to toxic substances. A important phenomenon here is the "bystander effect." It has been observed by several investigators studying different kinds of tumors that not all of the tumor cells need to be transduced with the suicide gene for the tumor cells to be killed. In some cases, tumors can be completely eliminated if only 10–20% of the tumor cells carry the transduced gene. In the case of the HSV-tk gene, it has been suggested that the toxic metabolites might cross gap junctions to kill neighboring cells that are not transduced.

The third approach has been the *in situ* insertion of an HLA gene into a tumor that is negative for the inserted HLA gene *(38,52,53)*. The objective here has been to induce an immune response to the foreign HLA antigen with hope that tumor-surface antigens will also be recognized and illicit a simultaneous immune response.

The fourth approach has relied on the use of tumor suppresser genes, antioncogenes, or oncogene-directed ribozymes *(54–56)*. Although it seems like an attractive strategy to inactivate expression of an oncogene in tumor cells, or replace a functioning tumor suppresser gene, the effectiveness of this approach depends on the transduction of all or most of the cells of a tumor, a goal not readily achievable using current vector delivery systems. However, a similar form of bystander effect may be active in this strategy also.

The final category has involved the use of a drug resistance or multidrug resistance gene to protect bone marrow cells, facilitating the use of higher doses of chemotherapy in the treatment of the primary tumor *(57,58)*. One concern with this approach has been that metastatic tumor cells present in the bone marrow could acquire the transferred gene and become drug-resistant. This will be especially relevant to vectors that require cell division, since they would be expected to transduce the actively dividing tumor cells at a much higher efficiency than nondividing bone marrow cells.

4.3. Infectious Disease

A number of infectious diseases have recently been proposed to be candidates for treatment by gene therapy. Of these, the diseases caused by HIV and hepatitis viral infection are examples. In these cases, gene therapy will not be curative. However, the transfer of genetic material can still be used to combat infection. In some instances, the transferred genes can provide immunizing antigen, so that the patient is protected from subsequent exposure. Other approaches attempt to overexpress gene products that will interfere with the biological processes of the infectious agent. Such as overexpression of the HIV transdominant rev protein or antisense TAR elements.

4.4. Other Acquired Diseases

Still other acquired diseases have been proposed to be treatable by gene transfer. Although several ethical questions remain to be addressed concerning the use of gene transfer for the treatment of nonlife-threatening afflictions, a number of such uses are the subject of recent clinical trials. These include arterial gene transfer for therapeutic angiogenesis in patients with peripheral artery disease, and transfer of a potentially antiarthritic cytokine gene to human joints for the treatment of rheumatoid arthritis.

5. VACCINATION

One of the more promising applications of gene therapy is vaccination. The in vivo delivery of antigen-encoding expression vectors can result in *de novo* antigen production in the target tissue and development of specific antibody responses. The target tissues for this type of gene therapy are usually the skin or muscle. However, the highest levels of both protein expression and antibody production have been correlated with delivery to the epidermis, whereas deliveries extending into the dermis, or underlying muscle, typically result in decreased protein and antibody production. Optimal immune responses have been shown to be dependent on the delivery of a sufficient number of DNA molecules, indicating that a dose–response relationship exists between the number of genes delivered and the resultant levels of protein expression and antibody production. Further, maximal protein expression and associated antibody titers have been elicited with surprisingly small amounts of gene transfer. The practicality of targeting skin demonstrates the potential utility of this emerging technology for development of a new class of human clinical vaccines based on direct DNA delivery.

ABBREVIATIONS

AAV, adeno-associated virus; ADA, adenosine deaminase; CF, cystic fibrosis; CFTR, CF transmembrane conductance regulator; HDV, hepatitis delta virus; HSV-tk, herpes simplex virus thymidine kinase; IRES, internal ribosome entry site; ITR, inverted terminal repeat; LTR, long-terminal repeat; Mo-MuLV, Moloney murine leukemia virus; PGK, phosphoglycerate kinase; PKU, phenylkentonuria; PNP, purine nucleoside phosphorylase; rAAV, recombinant AAV; SCID, severe combined immunodeficiency.

REFERENCES

1. Smale, S. T. and Baltimore, D. The "initiator" as a transcriptional control element. *Cell* **57**:103–113, 1989.
2. Javahery, R., Khachi, A., Lo, K., Zenzie-Gregory, B., and Smale, S. T. DNA sequence requirements for transcriptional initiator activity in mammalian cells. *Mol. Cell. Biol.* **14**:116–127, 1994.
3. Palmer, T. D., Rosman, G. J., Osborne, W. R. A., and Miller, A. D. Genetically modified skin fibroblasts persist long after transplantation but gradually inactivate introduced genes. *Proc. Natl. Acad. Sci. USA* **88**:4626–4630, 1991.
4. Scharfmann, R., Axelrod, J. H., and Verma, I. M. Long-term *in vivo* expression of retrovirus-mediated gene transfer in mouse fibroblast implants. *Proc. Natl. Acad. Sci. USA* **88**:1330–1334, 1991.
5. Challita, P.-M. and Kohn, D. B. Lack of expression from a retroviral vector after transduction of murine hematopoietic stem cells is associated with methylation *in vivo*. *Proc. Natl. Acad. Sci. USA* **91**:2567–2571, 1994.
6. Kozak, M. An analysis of 5'-noncoding sequences from 699 vertebrate messenger RNAs. *Nucleic Acids Res.* **15**:8125–8148, 1987.
7. Jang, S. K., Krausslich, H., Nicklin, M. J. H., Duke, G. M., Palmenberg, A. C., and Wimmer, E. A segment of the 5' nontranslated region of encephalomyocarditis virus RNA directs internal entry of ribosomes during *in vitro* translation. *J. Virol.* **62**:2636, 1988.
8. Graham, F. L. and van der Eb, A. A new technique for the assay of infectivity of human adenovirus IV DNA. *Virology* **102**:420, 1973.
9. Wigler, M., Silverstein, S., Lee, L. S., Pellicer, A., Cheng, V. C., and Axel, R. Transfer of purified herpes virus thymidine kinase gene to cultured mouse cells. *Cell* **11**:223, 1977.

10. Felgner, P. L., Gadek, T. R., Holm, M., Roman, R., Chan, H. W., Wenz, M., Northrop, J. P., Ringold, G. M., and Danielson, M. Lipofectin: a highly efficient, lipid-mediated DNA-transfection procedure. *Proc. Natl. Acad. Sci. USA* **84:**7413–7417, 1987.

11. Felgner, P. L. and Ringold, G. M. Cationic liposome-mediated transfection. *Nature* **337:**387,388, 1989.

12. Felgner, J. H., Kumar, R. , Sridhar, C. N., Wheeler, C. J., Tsai, Y. J., Border, R., Ramsey, P., Martin, M., and Felgner, P. L. Enhanced gene delivery and mechanism studies with a novel series of cationic lipid formulations. *J. Biol. Chem.* **269:**2550–2561, 1994.

13. McLachlan, G., Davidson, H., Davidson, D., Dickenson, P., Dorin, J., and Porteous, D. DOTAP as a vehicle for efficient gene delivery *in vitro* and *in vivo*. *Biochemica* **11:**19–21, 1994.

14. Zhou, X. H., Klibanov, A. L., and Huang, L. Lipophilic polylysines mediate efficient DNA transfection in mammalian cells. *Biochim. Biophys. Acta* **1065:**8–14, 1991

15. Zhou, X. and Huang, L. DNA transfection mediated by cationic liposomes containing lipopolylysine: characterization and mechanism of action. *Biochim. Biophys. Acta* **1189:**195–203, 1994.

16. Gao, X. A. and Huang, L. A novel cationic liposome reagent for efficient transfection of mammalian cells. *Biochem. Biophys. Res. Commun.* **179:**280–285, 1991.

17. Behr, J. P., Demeneix, B., Leoffler, J. P., and Perez-Mutul, J. Efficient gene transfer into mammalian primary endocrine cells with lipopolyamine-coated DNA. *Proc. Natl. Acad. Sci. USA* **86:**6982–6986, 1989.

18. Barthel, F., Remy, J. S., Leoffler, J. P., and Behr, J. P. Gene transfer optimization with lipospermine-coated DNA. *DNA Cell Biol.* **12:**553–560, 1993.

19. Pinnaduwage, P., Schmitt, L., and Huang, L. Use of a quaternary ammonium detergent in liposome mediated DNA transfection of mouse L-cells. *Biochim. Biophys. Acta* **985:**33–37, 1989.

20. Wu, G. Y. and Wu, C. H. Receptor-mediated *in vitro* gene transformation by a soluble DNA carrier system. *J. Biol. Chem.* **262:**4429–4432, 1987.

21. Wu, G. Y. and Wu, C. H. Evidence for targeted gene delivery to HepG2 hepatoma cells *in vitro*. *Biochemistry* **27:**887–892, 1988.

22. Wagner, E., Zenke, M., Cotten, M., Beug, H., and Birnstiel, M. L. Transferrin-polycation conjugates as carriers for DNA uptake into cells. *Proc. Natl. Acad. Sci. USA* **87:**3410–3414, 1990.

23. Wagner, E., Cotten, M., Foisner, R., and Birnstiel, M. L. Transferrin-polycation-DNA complexes: the effect of polycations on the structure of the complex and DNA delivery to cells. *Proc. Natl. Acad. Sci. USA* **88:**4255–4259, 1991.

24. Blumenthal, R., Seth, P., Willingham, M. C., and Pastan, I. pH-Dependent lysis of liposomes by adenovirus. *Biochemistry* **25:**2231–2237, 1986.

25. Rosenfeld, M. A., Yoshimura, K., Trapnell, B. C., Yoneyama, K., Rosenthal, E. R., Dalemans, W., Fukayama, M., Bargon, J., Stier, L. E., Stratford-Perricaudet, L., Perricaudet, M., Guggino, W. B., Pavirani, A., Lecocq, J.-P., and Crystal, R. G. *In vivo* transfer of the human cystic fibrosis transmembrane conductance regulator gene to the airway epithelium. *Cell* **68:**143–55, 1992.

26. Engelhardt, J. F., Simon, R. H., Yang, Y., Zepeda, M., Weber-Pendleton, S., Doranz, B., Grossman, M., and Wilson, J. M. Adenovirus-mediated transfer of the CFTR gene to lung of nonhuman primates: biological efficacy study. *Hum. Gene Ther.* **4:**759–769, 1993.

27. Akli, S., Caillaud, C., Vigne, E., Stratford-Perricaudet, L. D., Poenaru, L., Perricaudet, M., Kahn, A., and Peschanski, M. R. Transfer of a foreign gene into the brain using adenovirus vectors. *Nature Genet.* **3:**224–228, 1993.

28. Brody, S. L. and Crystal, R. G. Adenovirus-mediated in vivo gene transfer. *Ann. NY Acad. Sci.* **31:**90–101, 1994.

29. Setoguchi, Y., Jaffe, H. A., Danel, C., and Crystal, R. G. Ex vivo and in vivo gene transfer to the skin using replication-deficient recombinant adenovirus vectors. *J. Invest. Dermatol.* **102:**415–421, 1994.

30. Hermonat, P. L. and Muzyczka, N. Use of adeno-associated virus as a mammalian DNA cloning vector: transduction of neomycin resistance into mammalian tissue culture cells. *Proc. Natl. Acad. Sci. USA* **81:**6466–6470, 1984.

31. LaFace, D., Hermonat, P. L., Wakeland, E., and Peck, A. Gene transfer into hematopoietic progenitor cells mediated by an adeno-associated virus vector. *Virology* **162:**483–486, 1988.

32. Muzyczka, M. Use of adeno-associated virus as a general transduction vector for mammalian cells. *Curr. Top. Microbiol. Immunol.* **158:**97–129, 1992.

33. Tratschin, J.-D, West, M. H. P., Sandbank, T., and Carter, B. J. A human parvovirus, adeno-associated virus, as a eukaryotic vector: transient expression and encapsidation of the prokaryotic gene for chloramphenicol acetyltransrerase. *Mol. Cell. Biol.* **4:**2072–2081, 1984.

34. Kumar, S. and Leffak, M. Conserved chromatin structure in c-myc 5' flanking DNA after viral transduction. *J. Mol. Biol.* **222:**45–57, 1991.

35. Walsh, C. E., Liu, J. M., Xiao, X., Young, N. S., Nienhuis, A. W., and Samulski, R. J. Regulated high level expression of a human γ-globin gene introduced into erythroid cells by an adeno-associated virus vector. *Proc. Natl. Acad. Sci. USA* **89:**7257–7261, 1992.

36. Goodman, S., Xiao, X., Donahue, R. E., Moulton, A., Miller, J., Walsh, C., Young, N. S., Samulski, R. J., and Nienhuis, A. W. Recombinant adeno-associated virus-mediated gene transfer into hematopoietic progenitor cells. *Blood* **84:**1492–1500, 1994.

37. Walsh, C. E., Nienhuis, A. W., Samulski, R. J., Brown, M. G., Miller, J. L., Young, N. S., and Liu, J. M. Phenotypic correction of Fanconi anemia in human hematopoietic cells with a recombinant adeno-associated virus vector. *J. Clin. Invest.* **94:**1440–1448, 1994.

38. Nabel, G. J., Chang, A., Nabel, E. G., and Plautz, G. Immunotherapy of malignancy by *in vivo* gene transfer into tumors. *Hum. Gene Ther.* **3:**399–410, 1992.

39. Oldfield, E. H., Culver, K. W., and Anderson, W. F. A clinical protocol: gene therapy for the treatment of brain tumors using intratumoral transduction with thymidine kinase gene and intravenous ganciclovir. *Hum. Gene Ther.* **4:**39–69, 1993.

40. Gansbacher, B., Houghton, A., and Livingston, P. A pilot study of immunization with HLA-A2 matched allogeneic melanoma cells that secrete interleukin-2 in patients with metastatic melanoma. *Hum. Gene Ther.* **3:**677–690, 1992.

41. Gansbacher, B., Motzer, R., Houghton, A., and Bander, N. A pilot study of immunization with interleukin-2-secreting allogeneic HLA-A2 matched renal cell carcinoma cells in patients with advanced renal cell carcinoma. *Hum. Gene Ther.* **3:**691–703, 1992.

42. Rosenberg, S. A. The immunotherapy and gene therapy of cancer. *J. Clin. Oncol.* **10:**180–199, 1992.

43. Rosenberg, S. A., Anderson, W. F., Asher, A. L., Blaese, M. R., Ettinghausen, S. S., Hwu, P., et al. Immunization of cancer patients using autologous cancer cells modified by insertion of the gene for tumor necrosis factor. *Hum. Gene Ther.* **3:**57–73, 1992.

44. Rosenberg, S. A., Anderson, W. F., Asher, A. L., Blaese, M. R., Ettinghausen, S. S., Hwu, P., et al. TNF/TIL human gene therapy clinical protocol. *Hum. Gene Ther.* **1:**443–462, 1990.

45. Rosenberg, S. A., Packard, B. S., Aebersold, P. M., Solomon, D., Topalian, S. L., Toy, S. T., Simon, P., Lotze, M. T., Yang, J. C., Seipp, C. A., Simpson, C., Carter, C., Bock, S., Schwartzentruber, D., Wei, J. P., and White, D. E. Use of tumor-infiltrating lymphocytes and interleukin-2 in the immunotherapy of patients with metastatic melanoma. *New Engl. J. Med.* **319:**1676–1680, 1988.

46. Culver, K. W., Ram, Z., and Walbridge, S. *In vivo* gene transfer with retroviral vector producer cells for treatment of experimental brain tumors. *Science* **256:**1550–1552, 1992.

47. Moolten, F. L. Tumor chemosensitivity conferred by inserted herpes thymidine kinase genes: paradigm for a prospective cancer control strategy. *Cancer Res.* **46:**5276–5281, 1986.

48. Austin, E. A. and Huber, B. E. A first step in the development of gene therapy for colorectal carcinoma: cloning, sequencing, and expression of *Escherichia coli* cytosine deaminase. *Mol. Pharmacol.* **43**:380–387, 1993.

49. Mroz, P. J. and Moolten, F. L. Retrovirally transduced *Escherichia coli gpt* genes combine selectability with chemosensitivity capable of mediating tumor eradication. *Hum. Gene Ther.* **4**:589–595, 1993.

50. Mullen, C. A., Coale, M. M., Lowe, R., and Blaese, R. M. Tumors expressing the cytosine deaminase suicide gene can be eliminated *in vivo* with 5-fluorocytosine and induce protective immunity to wild type tumor. *Cancer Res.* **54**:1503–1506, 1994.

51. Mullen, C. A., Kilstrup, M., and Blaese, R. M. Transfer of a bacterial gene for cytosine deaminase to mammalian cells confers lethal sensitivity to 5-fluorocytosine: a negative selection system. *Proc. Natl. Acad. Sci. USA* **89**:33–37, 1992.

52. Nabel, G. J., Nabel, E. G., Yang, Z., Fox, B. A., Plautz, G. E., Gao, X., Huang, L., Shu, S., Gordon, D., and Chang, A. E. Direct gene transfer with DNA-liposome complexes in melanoma: expression, biologic activity, and lack of toxicity in humans. *Proc. Natl. Acad. Sci. USA* **90**:11307–11311, 1993.

53. Ostrand-Rosenberg, S., Thakur, A., and Clements, V. Rejection of mouse sarcoma cells after transfection of MHC class II genes. *J. Immunol.* **144**:4068–4071, 1990.

54. Fujiwara, T., Grimm, E. A., Cai, D. W., Owen-Schaub, L. B., and Roth, J. A. A retroviral wild-type p53 expression vector penetrates human lung cancer spheroids and inhibits growth by inducing apoptosis. *Cancer Res.* **53**:4129–4133, 1993.

55. Kashani-Sabet, M., Funato, T., Florenes, V. A., Fodstad, O., and Scanlon, K. J. Suppression of the neoplastic phenotype *in vivo* by an anti-ras ribozyme. *Cancer Res.* **54**:900–902, 1994.

56. Zhang, Y., Mukhopadhyay, T., Donehower, Georges, R. N., and Roth, J. A. Retroviral vector-mediated transduction of K-ras antisense RNA into human lung cancer cells inhibits expression of the malignant phenotype. *Hum. Gene Ther.* **4**:451–460, 1993.

57. McLachlin, J. R., Eglitis, M. A., Ueda, K., Kantoff, P. W., Pastan, I. H., Anderson, W. F., and Gottesman, M. M. Expression of a human complementary DNA for the multidrug resistance gene in murine hematopoietic precursor cells with the use of retroviral gene transfer. *J. Natl. Cancer Inst.* **82**:1260–1263, 1990.

58. Sorrentino, B. P., Brandt, S. J., Bodine, D., Gottesman, M., Pastan, I., Cline, A., and Nienhuis, A. W. Selection of drug-resistant bone marrow cells *in vivo* after retroviral transfer of human MDR-I. *Science* **257**:99–103, 1992.

Part III
Applications to Molecular Pathology

An Overview of Molecular Genetics

Gregory J. Tsongalis

1. INTRODUCTION

Sir Archibald Garrod concluded in the early 1900s that predisposition to disease is dependent on each individual's chemical composition *(1)*. Beadle later described the one gene–one enzyme concept, which emphasized the genetic control of biochemical processes and theorized that mutations in any given gene would result in a defective biochemical reaction *(2)*. In 1953, Watson and Crick described for the first time the structure of the DNA molecule, which is now recognized as the "blueprint" of all living things *(3)*. As part of their report, they described in detail the nature of complementary base pairing as part of the stoichiometry necessary for this structure to maintain its integrity. The current concepts of molecular mechanisms of disease have evolved from these early observations. Our ability to detect various alterations, both intra- and extra-chromosomal, at the molecular level has led to a revolution in laboratory medicine giving way to our understanding of molecular mechanisms of disease processes or molecular pathology. The fact that these alterations play significant roles in disease inheritance and that many human diseases can now be associated with defects at the gene level has expanded our knowledge of the mechanism of inheritance based on the acquisition of half of our genetic makeup from each parent. Thus, molecular genetics provides an avenue for examining inheritance patterns at the level of nucleic acids and provides a vehicle for dissecting complex pathophysiological processes into gene defects.

2. THE HUMAN GENOME

Biological information exists as three fundamental forms: DNA, RNA, and protein. Each is accompanied by a wide degree of structural and functional complexity. In part because of the major strides made by researchers in the development of recombinant DNA technologies and the unprecedented successes of the Human Genome Project, we are now capable of providing direct and indirect molecular diagnostic assays for many human diseases at the level of the nucleic acid. It is estimated that the human genome is comprised of between 50,000 and 100,000 genes neatly packaged into a total of 46 chromosomes; 22 pairs of autosomes and one pair of sex chromosomes (X or Y). A haploid genome (23 chromosomes) containing only half of the total genetic material, as in sperm and egg cells (gametes), contains approx 3×10^9 bp. On average, each chromosome will then contain 2000–5000 genes dispersed within 1.3×10^8 bp.

From: Molecular Diagnostics: For the Clinical Laboratorian
Edited by: W. B. Coleman and G. J. Tsongalis Humana Press Inc., Totowa, NJ

Table 1
Types of Noncoding "Junk" DNA Sequences

Intron	DNA sequences that interupt the coding (exon) sequences of a gene
Satellite	Short repetitive DNA sequences that occur at the ends (telomeres) and centers (centromeres) of a chromosome
Minisatellite	Repetitive sequences that are shorter than satellites and found throughout the genome (VNTRs)
Microsatellite	Even shorter repetitive sequences; di-, tri-, and tetranucleotides (STRs)
3'-Untranslated regions	DNA that is transcribed into RNA at the end of a gene but is not translated into protein; function in regulation of gene expression
Short interspersed elements (SINEs)	These repetitive sequences are well represented by the 300-bp Alu repeat that occurs approx 500,000 times within the genome
Long interspersed elements (LINEs)	Up to 700 bp in length and scattered throughout the genome

The majority of human DNA exists within the nucleus of the cell. Through interactions with specific histone and other nuclear proteins, DNA is condensed into chromosomal structures. The packaging efficiency provided by these DNA:protein interactions is analogous to the packaging efficiency necessary to place approx several hundred miles of cable wire (DNA) into the center of a basketball (nucleus). Some of these specific protein–DNA interactions function in structural roles, whereas others regulate expression of genes. Of the 3×10^9 bp of genomic DNA, only 3–5% account for coding sequences (exons) that result in protein. The remaining 95–97% has been termed "junk" DNA and consists of intervening sequences (introns), of which 75% is unique and 25% is repetitive (Table 1) *(4)*. Another source of human DNA resides within the cell's mitochondria. The mitochondrial DNA consists of approx 16,500 bp that are unique to this organelle.

DNA is considered the "blueprint" of living organisms, because it contains the information needed to construct the vast array of proteins needed for cellular function and vitality. The ultimate result, therefore, of an alteration to DNA sequences (genotype) in many cases results in an alteration to the amino acid sequence of the protein, which renders it nonfunctional (phenotype). As the continuous discovery of new genes and proteins becomes a routine segment of the medical and scientific communities, so too will the application of nucleic acid technologies to diagnostic laboratory medicine.

3. CATEGORIES OF GENETIC DISORDERS

Currently there is an enormous amount of information with respect to numbers of and characteristics of various genetic diseases and syndromes. To this list are added the growing numbers of diseases for which genetic mechanisms of disease are being identified almost daily. Genetic diseases can be categorized into three major groups, which include chromosomal disorders, monogenic, or single-gene disorders, and polygenic or multifactorial disorders.

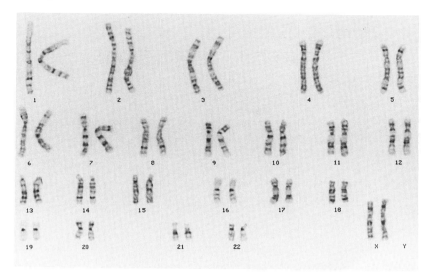

Fig. 1. A human female karyotype showing the 22 pairs of autosomes and the two sex chromosomes (X) (courtesy of Peter Benn, University of Connecticut Health Center).

Chromosomal disorders are the result of the loss, gain, or abnormal arrangement of one or more chromosomes, which results in the presence of excessive or deficient amounts of genetic material. Syndromes characterized by multiple birth defects and various forms of hematopoietic malignancy are examples of chromosomal disorders. An individual's karyotype (number and structure of chromosomes) contains 46 chromosomes, 44 of which are the autosomes and designated by number from 1–22 and two are sex chromosomes designated X or Y (Fig. 1). The individual chromosomes can be distinguished from one another by size, location of centromere, and unique banding patterns after special staining methods. These types of alterations usually involve large segments of DNA containing numerous genes and can be classified into four groups:

1. Aneuploidy refers to excess or loss of one or more chromosomes;
2. Deletion owing to breakage and/or loss of a portion of a chromosome;
3. Translocation refers to breakage of two chromosomes with transfer of broken parts to the opposite chromosome; and
4. Isochromosome formation results from the splitting at the centromere during mitosis so that one arm is lost and the other duplicated to form one chromosome with identical arms.

Monogenic disorders are the result of a single mutant gene and display traditional Mendelian inheritance patterns, including autosomal-dominant or -recessive and X-linked types. The overall population frequency of monogenic disorders is thought to be approx 10/1000 live births. The impact of modern molecular technologies and the Human Genome Project on molecular genetic testing for single gene disorders is well appreciated with the discovery of increasing numbers of disease-associated genes. Biochemical lesions characteristic of monogenic disorders result from defects in a wide array of proteins, many of which are not yet characterized.

Polygenic or multifactorial disorders consist of chronic diseases of adulthood, congenital malformations, and dysmorphic syndromes. These disorders result from multiple genetic and/or epigenetic factors that do not conform to traditional Mendelian

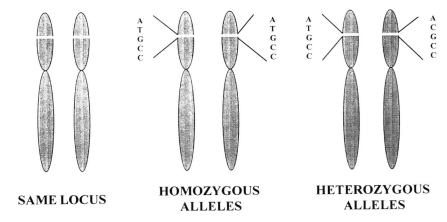

SAME LOCUS   **HOMOZYGOUS ALLELES**   **HETEROZYGOUS ALLELES**

Fig. 2. Schematic representation of chromosomes differentiating a genetic locus from homozygous and heterozygous genetic alleles.

inheritance patterns. Such diseases as hypertension, ischemic heart disease, Alzheimer's disease, diabetes mellitus, and cancer develop from the interaction of numerous altered genes and environmental factors. The molecular dissection of the genetic complexity of most polygenic disorders is only in its infancy.

4. DNA SEQUENCE VARIATIONS: MUTATION AND/OR POLYMORPHISM

It has been suggested that only 5% of the approx 3 billion base pairs that constitute the human genome codes for proteins. Only recently have scientists begun to understand the significance of the sequences that comprise the remaining 95%.

One interesting aspect of these noncoding repetitive sequences is the amount of interindividual variation that they exhibit. In some instances, these variants are the result of mutation, the permanent alteration of DNA sequences. However, when two or more variants are present in a given population with a frequency of >1%, then they are said to be polymorphic. At the molecular level, DNA polymorphism refers to differences in nucleotide sequences between two chromosomes at a similar locus. A genetic locus designates the position or location of a particular sequence on a chromosome, whereas different sequences that are present at the same locus are called alleles. Homozygosity, then, refers to having the same allele present on each of two chromosomes, and heterozygosity refers to different alleles at the same locus (Fig. 2).

Genetic polymorphism most often is a normal occurrence without grave consequences, except defining those traits that establish our individuality. Common mutations can be classified as polymorphisms. However, many mutations are not polymorphic, by virtue of the fact that they represent a rare genetic event. The first types of polymorphisms to be described were those that resulted in fragment length variations when DNA was digested with restriction endonucleases *(5,6)*. These enzymes cleave DNA at specific recognition sites so that smaller DNA fragments are produced. Restriction fragment length polymorphisms (RFLPs) occur when a restriction endonuclease recognition sequence varies between alleles at the same locus within the same

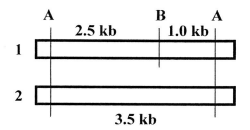

ALLELE	POLYMORPHIC RESTRICTION SITE	FRAGMENT SIZE
1	PRESENT (B)	2.5 kb, 1.0 kb
2	ABSENT	3.5 kb

Fig. 3. RFLP analysis for alleles 1 and 2 of a given genetic sequence. Allele 1 has restriction enzyme recognition sequences, which are invariant **(A)** and variant **(B)**. This variant site is the site of the sequence polymorphism. When digested with the enzyme, 2.5- and 1.0 kb-fragments are detected by gel electrophoresis. In contrast, allele 2 contains only the two invariant sites. Thus, after restriction enzyme digestion, only a 3.5-kb fragment is detected.

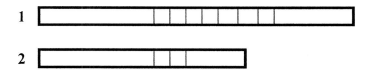

ALLELE	NUMBER OF VNTRs PRESENT	FRAGMENT SIZE
1	7	900 bp
2	2	400 bp

Fig. 4. Schematic diagram describing length polymorphisms of VNTR sequence. Alelel 1 contains 7 VNTR repeats (open boxes), whereas allele 2 only contains two repeats. These result in different size fragments, 900 or 400 bp, being detected by gel electrophoresis.

individual or between individuals at the same locus (Fig. 3). These are commonly referred to as sequence polymorphisms. A second type of polymorphism is based on sequence length and consists of hypervariable regions of DNA characterized by many copies of the same DNA sequence. Minisatellite sequences were the first of these types of polymorphisms to be identified and are referred to as variable numbers of tandem repeats (VNTRs) which can be from 10–100 bp in length (Fig. 4) *(7)*. Microsatellites or small tandem repeats (STRs) consist of di-, tri-, and tetranucleotide repetitive sequences, which are distributed throughout the genome with a frequency of approx 1 locus/10 kb of sequence *(8,9)*. Polymorphic DNA sequences can be used as markers for determining allelic inheritance of disease causing genes and for identity testing.

Mutations represent permanent alterations to a DNA sequence. The clinical significance of a mutation is determined by the type of mutation, its location within the gene, and the tissue involved, since not all tissues express all genes. Germline mutations are those that occur in germ cells, and are thus inheritable and present in every cell of the body. In contrast, an acquired mutation by a cell other than a germ cell is referred to as a somatic mutation. These mutations are only passed on to daughter cells and are not inheritable. Transition and transversion refer to the general category of point mutations that result in purine to purine or pyrimidline to pyrimidine substitutions and purine to pyrimidine substitution, respectively.

5. GENE INHERITANCE PATTERNS

Inheritance patterns of single-gene disorders are based on traditional Mendelian laws of segregation and independent assortment. The following assumptions are made as a result of these laws:

1. An offspring inherits one autosomal chromosome from each parent and thus one of any given allele from each parent;
2. Both alleles, regardless of inheritance are equally expressed and heterozygotes can transmit equally either allele to their offspring; and
3. The phenotypic pattern of inheritance is dependent on the type of chromosome, autosome or sex chromosome, the allele in question is located on.

The latter is also dependent on which category of expressivity the phenotype is attributed to, dominant or recessive.

Dominant phenotypes are those in which the mutated allele is expressed over the normal allele in heterozygotes. Both heterozygotes and homozygotes of an autosomal-dominant disorder express the disease phentoype. However, individuals homozygous for a dominant disorder are relatively rare. Recessive phenotypes, on the other hand, are those in which heterozygotes are indistinguishable from normal. It is important to note that in recessive disorders, heterozygotes may have subtle phenotypic differences at the biochemical level that often go unnoticed.

A mutant allele, dominant or recessive, results from the effect of the mutation on the role of a gene product associated with any given biological system. Disease phenotypes can be caused by the total loss or gain of protein function as a result of a single base mutation. In some cases a total or partial loss of protein function is observed, whereas in others, there is a retention of abnormal or gain in excessive normal function. Most mutant alleles whose phenotype is expressed because of a loss of protein function are recessive in origin. A dominant allele typically results in a gain of function, either abnormal or normal. In addition, dominant negative phenotypes have been described that refer to a mutant protein interfering with the normal function of the protein produced by the normal allele in heterozygotes.

The typical patterns of autosomal-dominant and recessive inheritance are depicted in the following pedigrees. Autosomal-dominant disorders are characterized by verti-

AUTOSOMAL DOMINANT DISORDERS

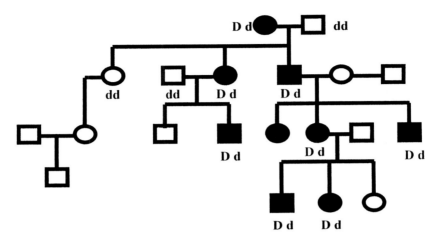

Fig. 5. Family pedigree showing autosomal dominant inheritance pattern of a genetic disease. Examples include Huntington's disease, neurofibromatosis, myotonic dystrophy, familial hypercholesterolemia, Marfan syndrome, adult polycystic kidney disease, and multiple endocrine neoplasia (MEN). Circle, female; square, male; open, unaffected; solid, affected; D, dominant mutant allele; d, normal allele.

cal transmission of the disease from generation to generation, equal expressivity in males and females, an affected individual having a 50% chance of offspring being affected or unaffected, lack of affected children from unaffected parents, and most affected individuals having an affected parent, except in the case of a new mutation (Fig. 5). In contrast, autosomal-recessive disorders are characterized by horizontal penetrance, affected homozygous individuals having unaffected heterozygous parents, and heterozygous parents having a 25% chance of offspring being affected (Fig. 6).

Several exceptions to these classic, Mendelian rules of inheritance have been recognized, and include recently described unstable mutations, uniparental disomy, and genetic imprinting *(9–11)*. Unstable mutations refer to the trinucleotide repeat expansions responsible for such disorders as Fragile X syndrome, myotonic dystrophy, and Huntington's disease. The identification of this type of mutation at the molecular level helped to define the phenomenon of anticipation, in which there is an increase in severity of a disease phentoype from one generation to the next. Premutations or a slight increase in trinucleotide repeat number exist without phenotypic expression. However, these premutations are prone to further expansion, which then results in a full mutation and the disease phenotype. Uniparental disomy and genetic imprinting contradict assumptions that each individual inherits one copy of a single chromosome from each parent. Uniparental disomy refers to the inheritance of two copies of a chromosome from one parent and none from the other parent. This can result from differential expression of genes in one or the other parent, in which only the expressed genes are inherited (imprinting). Parental dependency, however, can also result from the normal distribution of genetic material in male and female gametes (i.e., X vs Y chromosomes,

AUTOSOMAL RECESSIVE DISORDERS

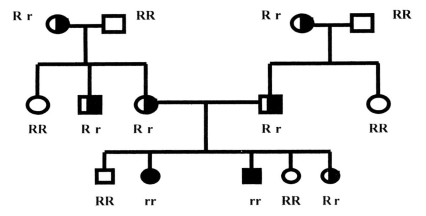

Fig. 6. Family pedigree showing autosomal recessive inheritance pattern of a genetic disease. Examples include cystic fibrosis, Tay-Sachs disease, phenylketonuria, α1-antitrypsin deficiency, and sickle-cell anemia. Circle, female; square, male; open, unaffected; solid, affected; half-shaded, carrier; R, normal allele; r, recessive mutant allele.

Table 2
Human Genes Exhibiting Differential Parental Expression *(10)*

Gene	Expressed allele
WT-1 (Wilms' tumor suppressor)	Maternal
INS (insulin)	Paternal
IGF2 (insulin-like growth factor)	Paternal
SNRPN (small nuclear riboprotein particle)	Paternal
IGF2R (insulin-like growth factor receptor)	Maternal

mitochondrial genes). More commonly, parental-dependent traits are the result of genetic imprinting in which male and female alleles are present, but not equally expressed. Several human genes exhibit parental-dependent expression or imprinting which is thought to be the result of methylation patterns of specific alleles (Table 2) *(10)*.

Other patterns of inheritance include those for X-linked disorders and mitochondrial disorders. Genes responsible for X-linked disorders are located on the X chromosome. Because females have two X chromosomes and males only one X chromosome, the severity and risk for developing these disorders are different for the two sexes. Females can be heterozygous or homozygous for a mutant X-linked gene, so that the associated trait can be either dominant or recessive. Males, on the other hand, express the mutant gene whenever they inherit it. As seen in the pedigree for X-linked disorders, there is absence of male-to-male transmission, and all daughters of an affected male inherit the mutant gene. If the disorder is X-linked recessive, then affected individuals are primarily male (Fig. 7). In X-linked dominant disorders, all daughters of affected males are

X-LINKED RECESSIVE DISORDERS

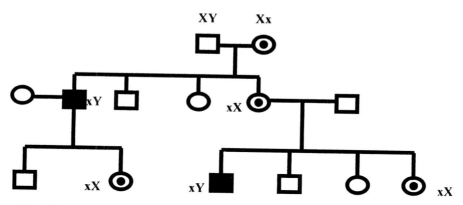

Fig. 7. Family pedigree showing X-linked recessive inheritance pattern of a genetic disease. Examples include muscular dystrophy and retinitis pigmentosa. Circle, female; square, male; open, unaffected; solid, affected; circle with dot, carrier female; X, normal allele; x, recessive mutant allele.

X-LINKED DOMINANT DISORDERS

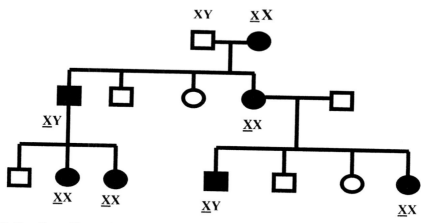

Fig. 8. Family pedigree showing X-linked dominant inheritance pattern of a genetic disease. Examples include several mental retardation syndromes. Circle, female; square, male; open, unaffected; solid, affected; X, dominant mutant allele.

affected, an affected female has a 50% chance of having an affected offspring, and affected individuals have an affected parent (Fig. 8). X-inactivation or Lyonization refers to the expression of X-linked genes in females. One X chromosome is irreversibly inactivated in females early in embryonic development, and thus genes on only one X chromosome are expressed. Thus, expression of a mutant allele is dependent on

MITOCHONDRIAL - ASSOCIATED DISORDERS

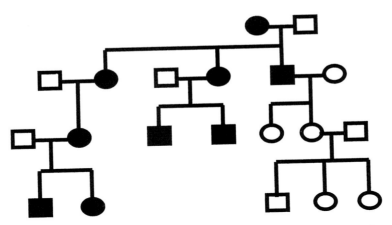

Fig. 9. Family pedigree showing mitochondrial DNA inheritance pattern of a genetic disease. Examples include Leber's hereditary optic neuropathy and Kearn-Sayre syndrome. Circle, female; square, male; open, unaffected; solid, affected.

its location on either an active or inactive X chromosome. Unlike X-linked disorders, inheritance of mitochondrial associated disorders is strictly maternal (Fig. 9). Thus, females transmit these traits to all of their offspring.

6. DIRECT VS INDIRECT MOLECULAR DIAGNOSTIC TESTS

Chapters 3–9 of this textbook describe the many molecular tools used in the analysis of nucleic acids. Many procedures can be used in either a direct or indirect mutation analysis. In so doing, it has become very common for analyses to rely on some form of in vitro amplification before proceeding with the actual analysis. Direct analysis refers to those procedures that detect the specific disease-causing mutations or foreign DNA sequence. These assays are dependent on the mutation and/or the gene sequence being known. In such cases, allele-specific oligonucleotide probes, DNA sequencing, and a wide array of PCR-mediated procedures can be employed.

Indirect detection methods, on the other hand, are utilized when the sequence of a disease-associated gene or disease-causing mutation is not known. Thus, polymorphic markers or gene sequences closely associated with the disease-causing gene are used to assess whether an individual has inherited the gene responsible for the disease phenotype. This is commonly referred to as linkage analysis. Linkage analysis is based on tracking the inheritance of polymorphic markers in a family with a genetic disease. If the marker and disease-associated gene are in close proximity, then the likelihood of a recombination event occurring between them is minimal. Thus, it is more likely that the marker and gene are inherited together. The advantage of linkage analysis is that the gene of interest needs only to be mapped to a chromosomal location, but not sequenced. Limitations to this technology include increased labor and turnaround times, the need to obtain samples from many family members, and the possibility of having to use numerous markers to obtain information.

7. CONCLUSION

This chapter was intended to provide the reader with some of the basic concepts of molecular genetics. One should keep in mind not only the applications of this technology, which will be discussed in the following chapters, but also the "nonscience" consequences that arise because of genetic disease testing. Nucleic acid-based laboratory testing can be performed as a diagnostic procedure, for carrier testing, as a prenatal diagnostic test, or for presymptomatic and susceptibility testing. As more of these diagnostic tests become available for genetic diseases, the laboratorian must also be aware of patterns of inheritance, risk assessment, family counseling issues, and the ethical issues associated with genetic testing. It is imperative, therefore, that the molecular genetics diagnostic laboratory function in close association with certified medical geneticists and genetics counselors. This will ensure the proper dissemination and interpretation of test results as well as maximize the benefits of such testing to family members.

As the identification of disease-associated mutations and genetic sequences continues to increase, so does the potential for clinical laboratorians to apply the discussed technologies to the diagnosis and monitoring of the resulting pathology in a traditional clinical laboratory fashion. Health care professionals must become familiar with the advantages, disadvantages, and limitations of molecular genetic technologies when applied to the diagnosis of disease. The following chapters discuss the current applications of molecular techniques to the diagnosis of human diseases. It would be impossible, even at this early stage of molecular diagnostics, to cover all of the possibilities for molecular diagnostic testing in an up-to-date fashion. As clinical laboratorians, we must not only be aware of these rapid advances, but embrace these new technologies as the "next generation" of assays we will be performing. Rapid advances in automation promise to make in vitro amplification, probe assays, and sequencing as routine in the clinical laboratory as the once not so popular immunoassay.

REFERENCES

1. Garrod, A. E. The incidence of alkaptonria: a study in chemical individuality. *Lancet* **2**:1616, 1902.
2. Beadle, G. N. Biochemical genetics. *Chem. Rev.* **37**:15, 1945.
3. Watson, J. D. and Crick, F. H. C. Molecular structure of nucleic acids. *Nature* **171**:737–738, 1953.
4. Nowak, R. Mining treasures from "junk' DNA. *Science* **263**:608–610, 1994.
5. Kan, Y. W. and Dozy, A. M. Polymorphism of EDNA sequence adjacent to the human Betaglobin structural gene: relationship to sickle mutation. *Proc. Natl. Acad. Sci. USA* **75**:5631–5635, 1978.
6. Butstein, D., White, R. L., Skolnick, M., and Davis, R. W. Construction of a genetic linkage map in man using restriction fragment length polymorphisms. *Am. J. Hum. Genet.* **32**:314–331, 1980.
7. Jeffreys, A. J., Wislon, V., and Thein, S. L. Hypervariable minisatellite regions in human DNA. *Nature* **314**:67–73, 1985.
8. Lareu, M. V., Phillips, C. P., Carracedo, A., Lincoln, P. J., Syndercombe, Court, D., and Thomson, A. Investigation of STR locus HUMTH01 using PCR and two electrophoresis formats: UK and Galacian caucasian population surveys and usefulness in paternity investigations. *Forensic Sci. Int.* **66**:41–52, 1994.

9. Sutherland, G. R. and Richards, R. I. DNA repeats: a treasury of human variation. *New Engl. J. Med.* **331:**191–193, 1994.
10. Barlow, D. P. Genetic imprinting in mammals. *Science* **270:**1610–1613, 1995.
11. Tsongalis, G. J. and Silverman, L. M. Molecular pathology of the fragile X syndrome. *Arch. Pathol. Lab. Med.* **117:**1121–1125, 1993.

SUGGESTED REFERENCE BOOKS

Bernstam, V. A., ed. *Handbook of Gene Level Diagnostics in Clinical Practice.* CRC, Boca Raton, 1992.

Heim, R. A. and Silverman, L. M., eds. *Molecuar Pathology.* Carolina Academic, Durham, NC, 1994.

Leder, P., Clayton, D. A., and Rubenstein, E., eds. *Introduction to Molecular Medicine.* Scientific American, New York, 1994.

Scriver, C. R., Beaudet, A. L., Sly, W. S., and Valle, D., eds. *The Metabolic and Molecular Bases of Inherited Disease.* McGraw-Hill, New York, 1995.

Thompson, M. W., McInnes, R. R., and Willard, H. F., eds. *Genetics in Medicine.* W. B. Saunders, Philadelphia, 1991.

11

Genetic Basis of Neurologic and Neuromuscular Diseases

Myra J. Wick, Pamela A. Crifasi, Zhenyuan Wang, and Stephen N. Thibodeau

1. INTRODUCTION

Traditionally, the diagnosis of neurological and neuromuscular disorders was based on patient history, clinical findings, and pedigree analysis. As the result of the Human Genome Project and advances in the fields of cytogenetics and molecular genetics, genes involved in both normal and pathologic processes have been mapped, cloned, and characterized. The types of DNA mutations that have been implicated in neurological diseases include trinucleotide repeat expansions, point mutations, insertions, deletions, and duplications. This chapter describes selected disorders that exemplify the types of mutations and molecular mechanisms involved in neurological and neuromuscular disorders that have been identified to date.

2. TRINUCLEOTIDE REPEAT DISORDERS

Trinucleotide repeat expansions, initially described in 1991 *(1,2)*, are responsible for a number of neurological diseases, including Fragile X syndrome (FRAXA), myotonic dystrophy (DM), spinal and bulbar muscular atrophy (SBMA), Huntington disease (HD), spinocerebellar ataxia type 1 (SCA1), Machado-Joseph disease (MJD)/ spinocerebellar ataxia type 3 (SCA3), and dentatorubral-pallidoluysian atrophy (DRPLA) *(3–5)*. Clinical and molecular features of these disorders are described in the following section and are summarized in Table 1.

2.1. Clinical Features

2.1.1. FRAXA

FRAXA is the most frequent form of inherited mental retardation, with an incidence of about 1 in 1500 males and 1 in 2500 females. It is associated with a fragile site on Xq27.3. FRAXA syndrome exhibits X-linked dominant inheritance with reduced penetrances of 80% in males and 30% in females. Dysmorphic features associated with FRAXA include large ears, a long and narrow face, and moderately increased head circumference. Macro-orchidism is a common finding in postpubescent affected males. Other common features include hyperactivity, attention deficit disorder, and autism.

From: Molecular Diagnostics: For the Clinical Laboratorian
Edited by: W. B. Coleman and G. J. Tsongalis Humana Press Inc., Totowa, NJ

Table 1
Genetic and Molecular Characteristics of Trinucleotide Repeat Diseases[a]

Disorders	FRAXA	DM	SBMA	HD	SCA1	MJD/SCA3	DRPLA
Inheritance	X-linked	AD	X-linked	AD	AD	AD	AD
Chromosome location	Xq27.3	19q13.3	Xq21.3	4p16.3	6p24	14q32	12p12ter
Repeat sequence	CGG	CTG	CAG	CAG	CAG	CAG	CAG
Repeat location	5'UTR	3'UTR	Coding region	Coding region	Coding region?	Coding region	Coding region?
Gene product	FMR-1	Myotonin protein kinase	Androgen receptor	Huntington	Ataxia-1	Unknown	Unknown
Normal allele	6–50	5–37	11–34	6–38	6–39	13–41	7–35
Premutation	50–200	—	—	—	—	—	—
Disease allele	>200	>200	36–62	27–121	40–81	61–84	49–75
Transmission sex bias	Maternal	Maternal	Paternal	Paternal	Paternal	Paternal	Paternal

[a]Size ranges of different alleles (normal, premutation, disease) are subject to change with additional data available.

2.1.2. DM

DM is the most common form of adult muscular dystrophy, with a prevalence of 1 in 8000. DM is characterized by progressive muscle weakness, myotonia, cataracts, cardiac arrhythmia, and diabetes. Phenotypic expression of DM is variable both within and between families. Individuals who have the congenital form of DM display myopathic facial appearance, hypotonia, feeding difficulties, delayed motor development, and mental retardation.

2.1.3. HD

HD is a progressive neurodegenerative disorder affecting 1/10,000 individuals, and is characterized by choreic movements, impaired cognition, and personality changes. This disorder is inherited as an autosomal-dominant trait with complete penetrance and variable age of onset, with a mean age of onset at approx 40 yr. Personality changes and dementia, followed by chorea, are the presenting symptoms of the disease. Minor motor abnormalities, including clumsiness, hyperreflexia, and eye movement disturbances, are also early manifestations of HD. As the disease progresses, features of bradykinesia, rigidity, dystonia, and epilepsy may become evident.

2.1.4. SCA1

The autosomal dominant spinocerebellar ataxias currently comprise a group of six separate neurodegenerative disorders. Two of the SCAs (SCA1 and SCA3) have been identified as trinucleotide repeat disorders. SCA1 is an autosomal-dominant, progressive neurodegenerative disease of the cerebellum, brainstem, and spinal cord. SCA1 typically begins in adulthood and progresses over 10–20 yr. Its clinical features include ataxia, ophthalmoparesis, and weakness. The clinically distinct MJD and SCA3 are both characterized by ataxia with ophthalmoparesis and variable pyramidal-extrapyramidal findings. However, dystonia and facial fasciculations, which are present in MJD patients, are rarely observed in SCA3 patients. The recent identification of a CAG repeat expansion within the same gene in both MJD and SCA3 patients suggests that these two disorders are allelic.

2.1.5. X-Linked SBMA

The X-linked recessive disorder SBMA (Kennedy disease) is a rare neuromuscular disorder affecting approx 1/50,000 males. The disease is characterized by the adult onset of proximal muscle weakness, atrophy, and fasciculations. Affected males often have signs of androgen insensitivity, such as gynecomastia, reduced fertility, and testicular atrophy; female carriers have few or no symptoms. The pathological findings in SBMA include degeneration of anterior horn cells and bulbar motor neurons. SBMA progresses slowly and is complicated by the involvement of the bulbar muscles.

2.1.6. DRPLA

DRPLA is a rare neurodegenerative disorder characterized by ataxia, choreoathetosis, myoclonus, epilepsy, and dementia. This disease demonstrates anticipation and has a variable age of onset that ranges from the first to the seventh decade.

2.2. Genetics

2.2.1. Repeat Instability

Each of the disorders described above is characterized by the presence of a trinucleotide repeat within the gene responsible for that disorder. For FRAXA, the trinucleotide repeat is localized to the 5'-untranslated region. For SBMA, HD, SCA1, SCA3/MJD, and DRPLA, on the other hand, the repeat is within the coding region, and for

DM, it is present in the 3'-untranslated region. Common to each of these is that the trinucleotide repeat is polymorphic within the normal population, with alleles stably inherited from one generation to another *(6)*. Also common to each of these is that expansion of the repeat beyond the normal range results in either abnormal gene function or abnormal levels of gene product, and ultimately disease.

In the disease state, the trinucleotide repeat for each of these disorders demonstrates instability when transmitted from parents to offspring. Expansion of unstable trinucleotide repeats during transmission is most often the case, although contractions have also been documented. In general, instability of trinucleotide repeats is directly related to their size, i.e., the longer the repeat, the more likely it is to undergo expansion *(1,6,7)*. This is particularly well documented for FRAXA and DM. Stability of repeats also appears to be related to the primary sequence. In FRAXA and SCA1, for example, the trinucleotide repeat sequences are not perfect sequences, but are interrupted: interspersed AGG (rather than CGG) for FRAXA and 1–3 CAT repeats within the CAG repeat for SCA1 *(8,9)*. Absence of these interruption sequences appears to render the resulting repeat to greater instability with minimal expansion. However, when a repeat reaches a critical size threshold, the repeat becomes very unstable. For example, a repeat size of 100 or greater in FRAXA almost always leads to a full mutation (>200 repeats) in subsequent generations *(10)*.

2.2.2. Genotype and Phenotype Correlation

For each of the trinucleotide repeat disorders, there is a correlation between increasing repeat size and disease severity *(1,11,12)*. Anticipation (worsening of disease severity and decreasing of age of onset over successive generations) is well documented and correlates with increasing expansion size *(1,6,11–13)*. For example, both congenital DM patients and the most severely retarded FRAXA patients nearly always have dramatic repeat expansions, whereas those with smaller expansions typically have milder disease *(1,6,14)*. In the five CAG repeat disorders, increasing repeat length correlates with earlier disease onset *(11–13,15,16)*. This correlation is strongest for SCA1, for which approx 70% of the variability in age of disease onset is accounted for by repeat length *(15)*. Although strong correlations exist in all triplet repeat diseases, other factors apparently also influence the severity and age onset of the diseases *(11,14,16)*. For example, in SBMA and HD, it has been reported that affected siblings with very similar repeat lengths have had onset of symptoms at very different ages *(11,16)*.

FRAXA and DM also have repeat sizes considered to be in a "premutation" range. The premutation, which is intermediate between normal repeat and "full mutation", usually causes minimal (if any) phenotypic abnormalities. However, the premutation is unstable and often leads to further expansion and full phenotypic expression in subsequent generations *(1)*. In addition, there is evidence for the existence of a "gray zone" in which normal and abnormal repeat sizes may overlap. The stability of repeats in this range differs between families, and thus for a particular family, repeat stability cannot be determined until other generations are evaluated. Stability of gray zone repeats can be affected by interruption of the trinucleotide repeat sequence.

2.2.3. Bias of Parental Transmission

Interestingly, parental bias has been observed with respect to expansion in subsequent generations. For several disorders (SBMA, HD, SCA1, SCA3/MJD, and

DRPLA), **paternal** transmission of an abnormal allele often produces expansions that are relatively large, whereas maternal transmission may result in expansions of only a few repeats *(11,13,17,18)*. Hence, affected males are more likely to transmit a greatly expanded repeat, which may cause juvenile-onset disease. On the other hand, the untranslated CTG and CGG repeats of DM and FRAXA tend to have **maternal** bias of transmission *(19,20)*. Almost all cases of congenital DM are maternally transmitted and, in FRAXA, the expansion from premutation to full mutation occurs through a female. The mechanism responsible for transmission bias of trinucleotide repeat diseases has not yet been elucidated.

2.2.4. Molecular Mechanisms

The five CAG repeat neurodegenerative disorders (SBMA, HD, SCA1, SCA3/MJD, and DRPLA) are caused by modest expansions of CAG repeats, which are subsequently translated into enlarged polyglutamine tracts *(21–23)*. It has been proposed that these mutations result in an abnormal protein that is directly responsible for the observed neuronal toxicity. This "gain of function" hypothesis is supported by the finding that mutations other than (CAG) repeat expansions within the androgen receptor gene result in phenotypes (i.e., testicular feminization and androgen insensitivity syndrome) distinct from the SBMA phenotype *(24)*. Additionally, the "gain of function" hypothesis is consistent with the dominant pattern of inheritance that is observed for these diseases.

Altered protein function is unlikely to be the underlying mechanism for those trinucleotide repeat diseases in which the repeat is not translated (FRAXA and DM). Rather, $(CGG)_n$ repeat expansion in the FMR-1 gene is associated with decreased mRNA and protein levels. These decreases are often accompanied by increased DNA methylation of an adjacent CpG island *(1,25)*. Increased methylation itself may cause decreased transcription of the FMR-1 gene. In DM, it is generally believed that repeat expansion results in a reduction of steady-state Mt-PK mRNA and protein *(26–28)*.

2.3. Molecular Diagnosis

The understanding of trinucleotide repeat diseases at the molecular level has had a major impact on the laboratory diagnosis of these diseases. Molecular testing has greatly improved the accuracy of the diagnosis, and has allowed for accurate presymptomatic testing of at-risk family members and for the differential diagnosis of those diseases with overlapping clinical features. Laboratory diagnosis of the trinucleotide repeat diseases generally involves two approaches, polymerase chain reaction (PCR) and Southern blot analysis.

Primers flanking the region of DNA that contains the trinucleotide repeat are used to amplify that region by PCR. The PCR product is analyzed by gel electrophoresis, and the size of the product is determined by comparison with a standardized sizing ladder. Utilizing this approach, one can accurately determine numbers of repeats up to 200 (Fig. 1). This includes both normal and abnormal alleles of CAG repeat disorders (SCA1, MJD/ SCA3, SBMA, HD, and DRPLA), and normal alleles and premutations in FRAXA and DM. Because the efficiency of PCR is inversely correlated with the number of repeats in each allele, alleles with more than 200 repeats (including full mutations in FRAXA and DM) are more difficult to amplify and may yield no PCR products. PCR analysis, however, is simple and inexpensive, and quickly provides accurate sizing of most alleles.

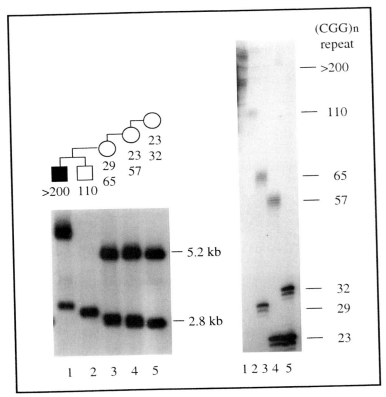

Fig. 1. Example of Southern blot and PCR analysis of DNA from individuals of a Fragile X family. Left: Southern blot of DNA digested with *Eco*RI and *Nru*I, and hybridized with the DNA probe StB12.3; right: PCR amplification of CGG repeat followed by denaturing gel electrophoresis. Lane numbers on the right panel correspond to those on the left. Numbers below the pedigree correspond to the CGG repeat number. The great grandmother in lane 5 has two normal alleles (CGG repeat sizes of 23 and 32). Her daughter (lane 4) has a normal allele of 23 and an expanded allele of 57. In subsequent transmissions, the abnormal allele of 57 expanded to 65 in one generation (lane 3) and then to 110 and >200 in the next generation (lanes 2 and 1, respectively).

Southern blot analysis, on the other hand, allows detection of full mutations in those diseases with large repeat expansion (FRAXA and DM) (Fig. 1). Additionally, for FRAXA, Southern blot analysis provides information concerning the methylation status of an abnormal allele. The methylation status may be of diagnostic importance when the number of repeats is near the upper end of the premutation range *(29,30)*. Southern blot analysis is more labor-intensive than PCR and requires larger quantities of genomic DNA. Southern blot can detect alleles in most size ranges, but does not allow for precise sizing of trinucleotide repeats in the normal and premutation range.

For diseases with small repeat expansions (SBMA, SCA1, HD, SCA3/MJD, and DRPLA), PCR analysis alone is generally adequate for diagnosis. However, for those disorders with larger repeat expansions (FRAXA and DM), combined Southern blot and PCR analysis are most often used. For some of the trinucleotide repeat disorders, additional studies may be recommended. For example, the stability of an SCA1 allele with CAG repeats at the upper end of the normal range can be assessed by *Snf*II restriction endonuclease digestion, which detects the presence of CAT interruptions. In SCA1, the normal-sized (CAG) alleles are nearly always interrupted by 1–3 CAT trinucleotide repeats, whereas the expanded or unstable gray zone SCA1 repeat is an uninterrupted sequence of CAG repeats *(9)*. Routine cytogenetic analysis is recommended as part of a comprehensive genetic evaluation of patients referred for FRAXA testing. This testing strategy enables detection of constitutional chromosome abnormalities that may have overlapping phenotypic features of FRAXA.

Finally, it should be realized that disease-causing mutations other than trinucleotide repeat expansion may occur within the aforementioned genes. Thus, the absence of trinucleotide repeat amplification does not necessarily rule out the diagnosis. This implies that for presymptomatic testing, it is important first to document the presence of a repeat amplification in an affected family member, which then verifies the underlying mechanism of disease.

3. SMA

SMA is an autosomal-recessive disorder that affects 1/6000–1/10,000 live-born children. Thus, SMA is the second most common autosomal-recessive lethal disease after cystic fibrosis. In this disorder, anterior horn cells degenerate, resulting in hypotonia, symmetrical muscle weakness, and wasting of voluntary muscles. The childhood spinal muscular atrophies, which will be discussed here, are divided into three types (I, II, III) according to age of onset, rate of progression, and age at death. Historically, the diagnosis and classification have been made on clinical and pathological findings. Recent advances in the understanding of the genes responsible for SMA may allow confirmation of the diagnosis of SMA in symptomatic individuals, and prenatal or presymptomatic diagnosis in family members.

SMA I or Werdnig-Hoffman disease represents 25% of all SMA cases *(31)*. Onset occurs prenatally or in early infancy, with the mean onset at 1.5–3 mo. Muscle weakness and hypotonia are severe and reflexes are absent. The disease progresses rapidly with death occurring between 9 mo and 3 yr.

SMA II is an intermediate form; infants usually develop normally for 6 mo before onset disease. These infants may learn to sit alone, but do not walk unassisted. Survival into adulthood has been reported.

SMA III, Kugelberg-Welander juvenile spinal muscular atrophy, has onset between the ages of 3 and 18 yr or later, and has a slower clinical course *(32)*. Atrophy and weakness of proximal muscles occur first, and may be followed by distal involvement.

3.1. Genetics

All three forms of SMA are linked to 5q12–13 and may be allelic *(33,34)*. Two genes, the survival motor neuron gene (SMN) *(35)* and the neuronal apoptosis inhibitory protein (NAIP) *(36)*, are mapped to this region. Both have been shown to be deleted in affected patients. Single-strand conformation polymorphism (SSCP) analysis of the SMN gene has shown that approx 96% of SMA type I, 94% of type II, and 82% of type III patients have homozygous deletions of exons 7 and/or 8 *(37)*. However, there have been reports of asymptomatic parents of affected children who have the same homozygous deletions in this region *(37)*. Additionally, there has been a report of one member of a sibpair having SMA type I and the other having SMA type III *(38)*. This implies that there may be other modifying genes involved in the expression of SMA. NAIP, which is located in the proximal portion of the SMA region, is reported to have deletions in 67% of type I SMA chromosomes, but only 2% of non-SMA chromosomes *(36)*. NAIP is more commonly deleted in SMA I than in types II or III *(39)*. The role of these two genes in the development of SMA is not yet clearly defined, although it has been postulated that a mutation in NAIP could lead to a failure of normally occurring inhibition of motor neuron apoptosis *(36)*.

3.2. Molecular Diagnosis

Historically, linkage analysis has been utilized for prenatal diagnosis of SMA in affected families *(40)*. Currently, a testing strategy using SSCP analysis to screen for abnormalities of exons 7 and 8 in the SMN gene followed by confirmatory sequencing studies is being developed *(41)*. These studies will detect homozygous deletions in the SMN gene and so can be used to confirm the diagnosis in affected individuals, but cannot be used for carrier testing. Use of this assay for prenatal detection of SMA is currently hampered by reports of asymptomatic individuals with homozygous deletions *(41)*. Improved molecular diagnosis of this disorder will require elucidation of the molecular mechanisms of SMA.

4. NEUROFIBROMATOSIS 1 (NF 1)

NF 1 is an autosomal-dominant disorder affecting approx 1/3500 individuals. It is characterized by tumors of neural crest origin. Predominant manifestations include cafe au lait spots and cutaneous or subcutaneous neurofibromas (benign tumors of peripheral nerves). Other findings include axillary freckling, Lisch nodules (iris hamartomas), scoliosis, plexiform neurofibromas, macrocephaly, short stature, seizures, and localized hypertrophy. Over half of individuals report learning problems. Patients are at increased risk for malignant tumors, including neurofibrosarcoma, astrocytoma, pheochromocytoma, embryonic rhabdomyosarcoma, and leukemia. Malignancy risk is currently estimated to range from 2–5% *(42)*. Affected individuals may have cafe au lait spots at birth, and 97% of these individuals are symptomatic by age 20. Cutaneous neurofibromas appear in the second decade.

Neurofibromatosis 2 (NF 2) or central NF is a separate disorder, which is mapped to 22q12. It is characterized by acoustic neuromas and meningiomas. Cafe au lait spots and neurofibromas are not prominent features of NF 2. This discussion will focus on NF 1.

4.1. Genetics

The gene for NF 1, which has been localized to 17q11.2 *(43)*, is extremely large, spanning 350 kb and containing at least 51 exons *(44)*. The introns range in size from 6 bp to more than 40 kb. Intron 27 contains genes for three other proteins whose role in NF 1, if any, has not been determined *(45)*. The mutation rate for the NF 1 gene is approx $1 \times 10^{-4}/$ generation (approx 50% of the affected individuals have a new mutation).

Neurofibromin, the 2818 amino acid protein encoded by NF 1, contains a domain that shares sequence homology with mammalian *Ras* p21 **G**TPase-**a**ctivating **p**rotein (GAP) *(45)*. This domain is denoted NF1GRD for **G**TPase-activity protein **r**elated

domain of the human *NF* type 1 protein. GAP functions to stimulate the conversion of the active GTP-bound form of *Ras* (p21 *ras*-GTP) to the inactive GDP bound form (p21 *ras*-GDP) *(46)*, *Ras* p21 proteins stimulate DNA synthesis and changes in cell morphology in response to mitogenic growth factors *(47)*. Thus, NF1GRD is believed to act as a tumor suppressor gene by stimulating the conversion of p21 *ras* to its inactive form.

4.2. Molecular Diagnosis

Screening the neurofibromin gene from affected patients has resulted in detection of a limited number of mutations. The mutations include translocations, deletions, insertions, and nonsense and missense mutations *(48)*. "Hot spots" for mutagenesis have not been identified. A consortium was formed in 1993 to consolidate NF 1 mutation data *(45)*. In 1994, the consortium reported only 45 mutations detected in screening over 500 NF 1 patients. This low detection rate may be the result of several factors, including mutations outside the exons or inability to pick up subtle mutations *(45)*. The size of the NF 1 gene has hindered development of direct mutation analysis for use in the clinical setting.

Recently, laboratories have focused on the protein truncation test (PTT) for the molecular diagnosis of NF1. The PTT assay involves generation of NF1 cDNA from cellular mRNA. This is accomplished through the use of overlapping primer sets. Coupled in vitro transcription/translation reactions generate a protein product that is then analyzed by electrophoresis. The location of the protein truncation can be estimated by comparing the migration patterns of the aberrantly migrating polypeptides with proteins of known molecular weight. Subsequent sequencing of the cDNA can be done through the use of primers designed for the region of the suspected mutation. Heim et al. *(49)* reported a 60% mutation detection rate with the NF1 PTT assay.

Linkage analysis is available for those individuals who are part of an NF 1 pedigree. However, for the 50% of affected individuals representing sporadic cases, linkage analysis cannot be utilized. New techniques and technologies will hopefully allow for the efficient and accurate detection of mutations in affected and at-risk individuals, as well as assist in the understanding of the function and regulation of the NF1 gene.

5. ATAXIA TELANGIECTASIA (AT)

AT is an autosomal recessive disorder that affects 1/40,000 to 1/100,000 individuals. It is characterized by cerebellar ataxia, oculocutaneous telangiectasias, immune defects, endocrine abnormalities, sensitivity to ionizing radiation, chromosome rearrangements, and a predisposition to malignancy. The thymus may be embryonic or hypoplastic in appearance. Defects in both humoral and cellular immunity are present and may be responsible for severe morbidity. Although prenatal growth retardation may occur, the usual onset of symptoms occurs in early childhood. Progressive ataxia is generally the first symptom, followed by choreiform movements (in approx 90% of patients) and conjunctival telangiectasias, which usually appear between 3 and 5 yr of age. AT results in a decreased life expectancy, with few patients reaching the age of 50 *(50)*.

The predisposition to malignancy, primarily B-cell lymphomas and chronic T-cell leukemias, is well described *(51)*. Approximately one-third of patients will develop a malignancy in their lifetime with 15% of these cases resulting in death *(52,53)*. AT patients are also more sensitive to radiotherapy used in treatment of cancer, and are at risk for early and late complications *(54,55)*. Interestingly, heterozygotes are also at increased risk for malignancy *(56)*; increased rates of breast cancer in mothers of affected individuals have been noted *(56,57)*.

Cytogenetic evaluation provides evidence for a high degree of chromosome breakage, translocations, and inversions involving regions other than the gene locus. The translocations often involve chromosomes 7 and 14 at the sites of T-cell receptor genes and immunoglobulin heavy-chain genes *(58)*. Defective DNA repair mechanisms, including abnormal progression through cell-cycle checkpoints, are thought to be responsible for the chromosome rearrangements *(59)*.

5.1. Genetics

In the late 1970s, complementation studies demonstrated the existence of at least four AT complementation groups, which suggested the possible involvement of four distinct genes *(60)*. Linkage analysis, which mapped AT to 11q22–23, indicated that all four complementation groups were linked to the same locus *(61)*. The gene responsible for AT, ataxia telangiectasia mutated (ATM), has recently been identified and ATM mutations have been found in all four complementation groups, suggesting a single AT gene *(62)*. ATM encodes a 12-kb transcript that has sequence homology to mammalian and yeast cell regulatory proteins *(62)*. Although these proteins appear to play a part in the cellular response to DNA damage, the specific function of the ATM gene product has not yet been elucidated.

5.2. Molecular Diagnosis

Historically, confirmation of a clinical diagnosis of AT has been done in the cytogenetics laboratory. Bleomycin or radiation stress tests have been utilized to demonstrate the abnormal response of AT chromosomes. Karyotypes are analyzed for increased numbers of chromosome rearrangements, with particular attention paid to the chromosome 7;14 translocations commonly seen in AT. Prenatal diagnosis in affected families has traditionally been done by linkage analysis using a fetal sample collected by amniocentesis or chorionic villi sampling *(54)*. The recent identification of the putative AT gene, however, will likely result in the development of direct molecular analyses in the future.

6. CMT1A AND HEREDITARY NEUROPATHY WITH LIABILITY (OR TENDENCY) TO PRESSURE PALSIES (HNPP)

In 1886, two reports published simultaneously by Charcot and Marie, and by Tooth described a hereditary disorder known as peroneal muscular atrophy *(63,64)*. Charcot-Marie-Tooth (CMT) disease, as it is now known, encompasses a group of adolescent to late-onset, slowly progressive peripheral neuropathies. Patients have peripheral nerve and spinal cord abnormalities, including axonal degeneration and gliosis. There are a number of forms of CMT; all share the basic features of distal limb muscle atrophy and pes cavus. Patients with CMT1 tend to present with gait abnormalities in adolescence or early adulthood, whereas CMT2 patients have later onset of symptoms. The disorders are distinguished by slow nerve conduction velocities in CMT1 and normal nerve conduction velocities in CMT2. This discussion includes only CMT1A, an autosomal dominant form of CMT that has been mapped to 17p11.2–12.

HNPP, a second type of peripheral neuropathy that also mapped to 17p11.2–12, is distinguished from CMT1A based on clinical features and electrophysiological and pathological findings. HNPP patients have episodes of prolonged weakness following minor pressure on peripheral nerve tracks. Recovery usually requires weeks to months, but patients do not manifest major neurologic deficit. HNPP patients also have normal to moderately decreased nerve conduction velocity, with areas of focal slowing. Pathologically, segmental nerve demyelination and focal thickening of the myelin sheath are common.

6.1. Genetics

Approximately 70% of CMT patients *(65)* have a 1.5-Mb duplication of the 17p11.2–12 region, whereas patients with HNPP have a deletion of this same 1.5-Mb region. Unequal meiotic crossing-over, mediated by two low-copy-number repeat elements, is the mechanism believed to be responsible for the duplication and deletion *(66)*. The crossover event results in a 500-kb *Sac*II junction fragment *(67)*, which, to date, has been detected in the DNA of all CMT1A duplication patients *(65)*. Experimental evidence suggests that duplication or deletion (i.e., dosage imbalance) of the peripheral myelin protein 22 gene (PMP22), which maps to 17p11.2, is responsible for CMT and HNPP, respectively *(68,69)*. Although the mechanism by which dosage imbalance of the PMP22 gene results in two distinct peripheral neuropathies has not yet been elucidated, it is believed that CMT1A mutations result in gain of protein function, whereas HNPP mutations result in loss of protein function.

6.2. Molecular Diagnosis

Currently, the most efficient method for the detection of duplication in CMT1A patients appears to be Southern blot analysis in which *Msp*I-digested DNA is hybridized with the probe VAW409R3a, which maps to 17p11.2 (D17S122) *(70)*. This probe/enzyme combination detects three polymorphic restriction fragments and has a heterozygosity of 70%. It is interesting to note that approx 8% of CMT1A duplication patients have all three fragments *(65)*. Duplication is detected as a dosage difference between restriction fragments. A second method which offers definitive detection of CMT1A duplications, is pulsed-field gel electrophoresis (PFGE) of *Sac*II-digested DNA followed by hybridization with the VAW409R3a probe. Although this method detects the previously described 500-kb fragment in all CMT1A duplication patients, it is much more time- and labor-intensive than routine Southern blot analysis. PCR analysis utilizing simple sequence repeats in the CMT1A region is a third method for the detection of duplications. This method is informative in 80% of duplication cases, and 46% of these patients are fully informative, having three detectable alleles *(65)*. However, because it is difficult to detect duplications by PCR analysis, PCR is not the preferred method for the molecular diagnosis of CMT1A. Another method for the detection of duplications of the CMT1A locus is by fluorescent *in situ* hybridization (FISH) analysis with the VAW409R3a probe in combination with a control probe. Currently, the most commonly used testing strategy for detection of CMT1A duplications is Southern blot analysis followed by PFGE in those cases in which the patient is uninformative for the *Msp*I polymorphism *(71)*. FISH analysis, on the other hand, is recommended for the molecular diagnosis of HNPP *(72,73)*. Molecular diagnosis of

CMT1A and HNPP patients with alterations other than duplication or deletion requires alternative testing strategies *(74)*.

7. DUCHENNE MUSCULAR DYSTROPHY (DMD)

DMD is a neuromuscular disorder that also involves gene deletion and duplication. DMD is a devastating, progressive, muscle-wasting disorder that is not usually diagnosed before 3 yr, but often results in wheelchair confinement by 12 yr, and death in the early 20s *(75)*. Manifestations of this disease include pseudohypertrophy of muscles, joint contractures, scoliosis, respiratory compromise, cardiomyopathy, and markedly increased serum creatine kinase (CK) levels owing to leakage of CK from diseased muscle into the bloodstream. The brain is also affected, and as a consequence, the IQ range of DMD patients is approx 20 points below average. Aggressive symptom management may extend the survival of DMD patients into their mid-20s. It was once believed that patients with a milder form of the disease were affected with a distinct disorder, Becker Muscular Dystrophy (BMD). However, molecular analysis has demonstrated that mutations in the same gene are responsible for both disorders. BMD patients may remain ambulatory through adulthood. Individuals with phenotypes intermediate to DMD and BMD have also been described *(76)*. The DMD gene has been mapped to Xq21, and although DMD is an X-linked recessive disorder, studies have demonstrated that 8% of DMD carrier females are mildly affected owing to skewed X-inactivation *(75)*.

7.1. Genetics

The DMD gene was one of the first genes to be cloned by positional cloning *(77)*. The gene is extremely large, spanning approx 2300 kb, and contains 79 exons. The gene encodes the protein dystrophin. The normal protein product is not expressed in DMD patients. In skeletal muscle, dystrophin is located in the sarcolemma membrane, where it is believed to play a crucial role in linking the contractile apparatus of myocytes to the sarcolemma membrane *(78)*. Isoforms of dystrophin, produced by the use of alternative splice sites and alternative promotors, are expressed in cardiac muscle and in the brain. The finding that dystrophin is expressed in the brain offers a possible explanation for the mental subnormality that is often present in DMD patients *(79)*. Approximately 60% of DMD patients have deletions and 6% have duplications within the DMD gene. Although the deletions are distributed throughout the DMD gene, two deletional "hot spots" have been identified. One of these regions extends over the first 20 exons and the second region includes exons 45–53 *(80)*. Although regions of clustered deletions suggest the presence of specific sites of breakage and recombination, such sites have not been identified. There is no correlation between the size of deletion and severity of disease. However, deletions resulting in frameshift mutations are generally associated with a severe phenotype, and most nonframeshift mutations are associated with a BMD phenotype *(81)*. Duplications are associated with severe phenotypes, since they often result in frameshift mutations or protein truncation. Point mutations that have been identified in DMD patients are distributed throughout exons 8–70 *(82)*.

7.2. Molecular Diagnosis

Prior to cloning of the DMD gene and identification of the protein product, diagnosis of DMD was based primarily on clinical features, muscle biopsy, and CK levels.

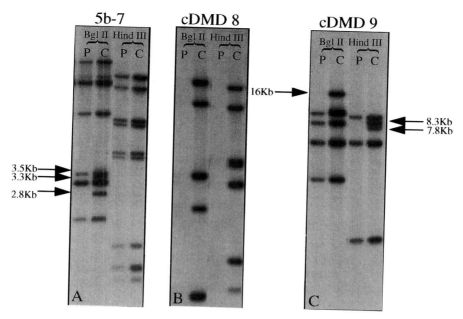

Fig. 2. Southern blot analysis of a DMD patient (P) and a normal control (C). The probe cDMD 5b-7 in combination with the *Bgl*II digest **(A)** shows absence of the 2.8-, 3.3-, and 3.5-kb bands, consistent with the deletion of exons 45–47. The probe cDMD 8 with either the *Bgl*II or the *Hind*III digest **(B)** shows the absence of all bands, consistent with the deletion of exons 48–52. The probe cDMD 9/*Bgl*II digest shows absence of the 16 kb band, and cDMD 9/*Hind*III digest shows the absence of the 7.8- and 8.3-kb bands **(C)**; both are consistent with the deletion of exons 53 and 54. These results indicate that the deletion spans exon 45–54.

Carrier testing involved examination of CK levels, which is often equivocal in carriers, and linkage analysis. Current diagnostic and carrier testing strategies include direct examination of the DMD gene and/or dystrophin analysis. Direct analysis of the DMD gene is accomplished by PCR or Southern blotting techniques. The Southern-based assay typically utilizes both *Hind*III and *Bgl*II restriction enzyme digestion and hybridization with the following cDNA probes: 1–2a (exons 1–9), 2b-3 (exons 10–20), 4–5a (exons 21–33), 5b–7 (exons 34–48), 8 (exons 47–52), and 9 (exons 53–59). Each exon is represented by a specific band on the autoradiogram (Fig. 2) *(76)*. The 3'-end of each exon has been characterized with regard to whether the exon ends with the first, second, or third nucleotide of a codon *(83)*. This information, along with Southern blot results for an individual patient, can be used to determine whether a particular deletion will cause a shift in the translational reading frame. Southern blot detection of carrier females and patients with duplications is based on dosage differences and usually requires quantitative analysis. In a small percentage of DMD patients, the junction of the deletion or duplication creates a novel restriction fragment. Carrier status determination is easily accomplished in these families.

PCR analysis typically involves multiplex reactions in which the promoter region and multiple exons are amplified (Fig. 3). The multiplexes described by Chamberlain et al. *(84)* and Beggs et al. *(85)* are commonly used in the clinical laboratory. PCR detects

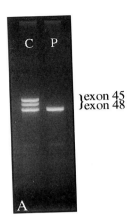

Fig. 3. PCR analysis of the DNA from a normal control (C) and the DMD patient (P) described in Fig. 2. The PCR results indicate deletion of exons 45 and 48.

approx 98% of the deletions detected by Southern blot analysis. However, PCR-based detection of duplications and of carrier females is difficult, and PCR analysis cannot be used to distinguish between frameshift and nonframeshift deletions. It should be noted that in the prenatal setting, the speed and smaller specimen requirements of PCR may render it the method of choice for the evaluation of at risk male fetuses. For males with a suspected diagnosis of DMD, many molecular genetics laboratories begin the analysis with the PCR-based assay. If PCR fails to detect a deletion, Southern analysis can be used for further investigation. If a deletion is detected by PCR, Southern analysis with the appropriate probes can be used to confirm the extent of the deletion, as well as to distinguish between frameshift and nonframeshift mutations. The information derived from the molecular analysis can subsequently be utilized by at-risk family members.

Approximately 35% of DMD patients have no detectable deletions or duplications. For families of these patients, linkage analysis can often be used for prenatal evaluation and to determine the carrier status of at-risk females. Linkage analysis can involve a number of approaches; the most informative are PCR-based assays in which extragenic $(CA)_n$ repeats on the 5'- and 3'-ends of the DMD gene, as well as intragenic (CA)n repeats are utilized *(86)*. Although linkage analysis is highly accurate, it requires the participation of key family members, which may eliminate its utility for certain families. At risk females who are in this situation will require alternative testing strategies for the evaluation of carrier status. This testing may include determination of CK values and dystrophin analysis. It should be noted that dystrophin analysis offers the advantage that it is not dependent on the type of mutation present in the DMD gene *(82)*. For additional information concerning DMD testing strategies, a reference by Beggs and Kunkel *(87)* is recommended.

8. SUMMARY

Representative neurologic and neuromuscular genetic disorders, the disease-causing mutations, and current molecular testing strategies were discussed. The ongoing progress and ultimate completion of the human genome project will undoubtedly identify additional genes involved in neurological function. Characterization of newly identified genes, further analysis of previously identified genes, and improved technologies will allow for the design of improved molecular diagnosis and the understanding of genotype/phenotype correlations.

REFERENCES

1. Fu, Y. H., Kuhl, D. P. A., Pizzuti, A., Pieretti, M., Sutcliffe, J. S., Richards, S., Verkerk, A. H. M. H., Holden, J. J. A., Fenwick, R. G., Jr., Warren, S. T., Oostra, B. A., Nelson, D. L., and Caskey, C. T. Variation of the CGG repeat at the fragile X site results in genetic instability: resolution of the Sherman paradox. *Cell* **67**:1047–1058, 1991.

2. La Spada, A. R., Wilson, E. M., Lubahn, D. B., Harding, A. E., and Fischbeck, K. H. Androgen receptor gene mutations in X-linked spinal and bulbar muscular atrophy. *Nature* **352**:77–79, 1991.

3. La Spada, A. R., Paulson, H. L., and Fischbeck, K. H. Trinucleotide repeat expansion in neurological disease. *Ann. Neurol.* **36**:814–822, 1994.

4. Bates, G. and Lehrach, H. Trinucleotide repeat expansions and human genetic disease. *BioEssays* **16**:277–284, 1994.

5. Plassart, E. and Fontaine, B. Genes with triplet repeats: a new class of mutations causing neurological diseases. *Biomed. Pharmacother.* **48**:191–197, 1994.

6. Caskey, C. T., Pizzuti, A., Fu, Y. H., Fenwick, R. J., Jr., and Nelson, D. L. Triplet repeat mutations in human disease. *Science* **256**:784–789, 1992.

7. Zuhlke, C., Riess, O., Bockel, B., Lange, H., and Thies, U. Mitotic stability and meiotic variability of the $(CAG)_n$ repeat in the Huntington disease gene. *Hum. Mol. Genet.* **2**:2063–2067, 1993.

8. Snow, K., Tester, D. J., Kruckeberg, K. E., Schaid, D. J., and Thibodeau, S. N. Sequence analysis of the fragile X trinucleotide repeat: implications for the origin of the fragile X mutation. *Hum. Mol. Genet.* **9**:1543–1551, 1994.

9. Zoghbi, H. Y. and Orr, H. T. Spinocerebellar ataxia type 1. *Semin. Cell Biol.* **6**:29–35, 1995.

10. Snow, K., Doud, L. K., Hagerman, R., Pergolizz, R. G., Erster, S. H., and Thibodeau, S. N. Analysis of a CGG sequence at the FMR-1 locus in fragile X families and in the general population. *Am. J. Hum. Genet.* **53**:1217–1228, 1993.

11. La Spada, A. R., Roling, D. B., Harding, A. E., Warner, C. L., Spiegel, R., Hausmanowa-Petrusewicz, I., Yee, W.-C., and Fischbeck, K. H. Meiotic stability and genotype-phenotype correlation of the trinucleotide repeat in X-linked spinal and bulbar muscular atrophy. *Nature Genet.* **2**:301–304, 1992.

12. Maciel, P., Gaspar, C., DeStefano, A. L., Silveira, I., Coutinho, P., Radvany, J., Dawson, D. M., Sudarsky, L., Guimaraes, J., Loureiro, J. E. L., Nezarati, M. M., Corwin, L. I., Lopes-Cendes, I., Rooke, K., Rosenberg, R., MacLeod, P., Farrer, L. A., Sequeiros, J., and Rouleau, G. A. Correlation between CAG repeat length and clinical features in Machado-Joseph disease. *Am. J. Hum. Genet.* **57**:54–61, 1995.

13. Nagafuchi, S., Yanagisawa, H., Sato, K., Shirayama, T., Ohsaki, E., Bundo, M., Takeda, T., Tadokoro, K., Kondo, I., Murayama, N., Tanaka, Y., Kikushima, H., Umino, K., Kurosawa, H., Furukawa, T., Nihei, K., Inoue, T., Sano, A., Komure, O., Takahashi, M., Yoshizawa, T., Kanazawa, I., and Yamada, M. Dentatorubral and pallidoluysian atrophy expansion of an unstable CAG trinucleotide on chromosome 12p. *Nature Genet.* **6**:14–18, 1994.

14. Tsilfidis, C., MaKenzie, A. E., Mettler, G., Barcelo, J., and Korneluk, R. G. Correlation between CTG trinucleotide repeat length and frequency of severe congenital myotonic dystrophy. *Nature Genet.* **1**:192–195, 1992.

15. Orr, H. T., Chung, M., Banfi, S., Kwiatkowski, T. J., Jr., Servadio, A., Beaudet, A. L., McCall, A. E., Duvick, L. A., Ranum, L. P. W., and Zoghbi, H. Y. Expansion of an unstable trinucteotide CAG repeat in spinocerebellar ataxia type 1. *Nature Genet.* **4**:221–226, 1993.

16. Andrew, S. E., Goldberg, Y. P., Kremer, B., Telenius, H., Theilmann, J., Adam, S., Starr, E., Squitieri, F., Lin, B., Kalchman, M. A., Graham, R. K., and Hayden, M. R. The relationship between trinucleotide (CAG) repeat length and clinical features of Huntington's disease. *Nature Genet.* **4**:398–403, 1993.

17. Chung, M., Ranum, L. P. W., Duvick, L. A., Servadio, A., Zoghbi, H. Y., and Orr, H. T. Evidence for a mechanism predisposing to intergenerational CAG repeat instability in spinocerebellar ataxia type 1. *Nature Genet.* **5**:254–258, 1993.

18. Duyao, M., Ambrose, C., Myers, R., Novelletto, A., Persichetti, F., Frontali, M., Folstein, S., Ross, C., Franz, M., Abbott, M., Gray, J., Conneally, P., Young, A., Penney, J., Hollingsworth, Z., Shoulson, I., Lazzarini, A., Falek, A., Koroshetz, W., Sax, D., Bird, E., Vonsattel, J., Bonilla, E., Alvir, J., Bickham Conde, J., Cha, J.-H., Dure, L., Gomez, F., Ramos, M., Sanchez-Ramos, J., Snodgrass, S., de Young, M., Wexler, N., Moscowitz, C., Penchaszadeh, G., MacFarlane, H., Anderson, M., Jenkins, B., Srinidhi, J., Barnes, G., and MacDonald, M. Trinucleotide repeat length instability and age of onset in Huntington's disease. *Nature Genet.* **4**:387–392, 1993.

19. Reyniers, E., Vits, L., de Boulle, K., Van Roy, B., Van Velzen, D., de Graaf, E., Verkerk, A. J. M. H., Jorens, H. Z. J., Darby, J. K., Oostra, B., and Willems, P. J. The full mutation in the FMR-1 gene of male fragile X patients is absent in their sperm. *Nature Genet.* **4**:143–146, 1993.

20. Fu, Y.-H., Pizzuti, A., Fenwick, R. G., Jr., King, J., Rajnarayan, S., Dunne, P. W., Dubel, J., Nasser, G. A., Ashizawa, T., de Jong, P., Wieringa, B., Korneluk, R., Perryman, M. B., Epstein, H. F., and Caskey, C. T. An unstable triplet repeat in a gene related to myotonic muscular dystrophy. *Science* **255**:1256–1258, 1992.

21. Hoogeveen, A., Willemsen, R., Meyer, N., Rooij, K. E., Roos, R. A. C., Ommen, Get-Jan, B. V., and Galjaard, H. Characterization and localization of the Huntington disease gene product. *Hum. Mol. Genet.* **2**:2069–2073, 1993.

22. Li, X. J., Li, S. H., Sharp, A. H., Nucifora, F. C., Jr., Schilling, G., Lanahan, A., Worley, P., Snyder, S. H., and Ross, C. A. A huntington-associated protein enriched in brain with implication for pathology. *Nature* **378**:398–402, 1995.

23. La Spada, A. R., Paulson, H. L., and Fischbeck, K. H. Trinucleotide repeat expansion in neurological disease. *Ann. Neurol.* **6**:814–822, 1994.

24. Mhatre, A. N., Trifiro, M. A., Kaufman, M., Kazemi-Esfarjani, P., Figlewicz, D., Rouleau, G., and Pinsky, L. Reduced transcriptional regulatory competence of the androgen receptor in X-linked spinal and bulbar muscular atrophy. *Nature Genet.* **5**:184–188, 1993.

25. Pieretti, M., Zhang, F., Fu, Y.-H., Warren, S. T., Oostra, B. A., Caskey, C. T., and Nelson, D. L. Absence of expression of the FMR-1 gene in fragile X syndrome. *Cell* **66**:817–822, 1991.

26. Fu, Y. H., Friedman, D. L., Richards, S., Pearlman, J. A., Gibbs, R. A., Pizzuti, A., Ashizawa, T., Perryman, B., Scarlato, G., Fenwick, R. G., Jr., and Caskey, C. T. Decreased expression of myotonin-protein kinase messenger RNA and protein in adult form of myotonic dystrophy. *Science* **260**:235–238, 1993.

27. Sabouri, L. A., Mahadevan, M. S., Narang, M., Lee, D. S. C., Surh, L. C., and Korneluk, R. G. Effect of the myotonic dystrophy (DM) mutation on mRNA levels of the DM gene. *Nature Genet.* **4**:233–238, 1993.

28. Timchenko, L., Monckton, D. G., and Caskey, C. T. Myotonic dystrophy: an unstable CTG repeat in a protein kinase gene. *Semin. Cell Biol.* **6**:13–19, 1995.

29. Waren, S. T. and Nelson, D. L. Advances in molecular analysis of fragile X syndrome. *JAMA* **7**:536–542, 1994.

30. Taylor, A. K., Safanda, J. F., Fall, M. Z., Quince, C., Lang, K. A., Hull, C. E., Carpenter, I., Staley, L. W., and Hagerman, R. J. Molecular predictors of cognitive involvement in female carriers of fragile X syndrome. *JAMA* **271**:507–514, 1994.

31. Pearn, J. Spinal muscular atrophies, in *Principles and Practice of Medical Genetics*, 2nd ed., vol. 1, Emery, A. and Rimoin, A., eds., Churchill Livingston, New York, pp. 565–578, 1990.

32. Baraitson, M. *The Genetics of Neurologic Disorders*, 2nd ed., Oxford University Press, pp. 248–257, 1990.

33. Davies, K. E., Thomas, N. H., Daniels, R. J., and Dubowitz, V. Molecular studies of spinal muscular atrophy. *Neuromuscular Disord.* 1:83–85, 1991.

34. Melki, J., Lefebvre, S., Burglen, L., Burlet, P., Clermont, O., Millasseau, P., Reboullet, S., Benichou, B., Zeviani, M., Le Paslier, D., Cohen, D., Weissenbach, J., and Munnich, A. De novo and inherited deletions of the 5q13 region in spinal muscular atrophies. *Science* 264:1474–1477, 1994.

35. Lefebvre, S., Burglen,, Reboullet, S., Clermont, O., Burlet, P., Viollet, L., Benichou, B., Cruaud, C., Millasseau, P., Zeviani, M., Le Paslier, D., Frezal, J., Cohen, D., Weissenbach, J., Munnich, A., and Melki, J. Identification and characterization of a spinal muscular atrophy-determining gene. *Cell* 80:155–165, 1995.

36. Roy, N., Mahadevan, M. S., McLean, M., Shutler, G., Yaraghi, Z., Farahani, R., Baird, S., Besner-Johnston, A., Lefebvre, C., Kang, X., Salih, M., Aubry, H., Tamai, K., Guan, X., Ioannou, P., Crawford, T. O., de Jong, P. J., Surh, L., Ikeda, J.-E., Komeluk, R. G., and MacKenzie, A. The gene for neuronal apoptosis inhibitory protein is partially deleted in individuals with spinal muscular atrophy. *Cell* 80:167–178, 1995.

37. Hahnen, E., Forkert, R., Marke, C., Rudnikschoneborn, S., Shonling, J., Zerres, K., and Wirth, B. Molecular analysis of candidate genes on chromosome 5q13 in autosomal recessive spinal muscular atrophy. Evidence of homozygous deletions of the SMN gene in unaffected individuals. *Hum. Mol. Genet.* 4:1927–1933, 1995.

38. Rudnik-Schoneborn, S., Rohrig, D., Morgan, G., Wirth, B., and Zerres, K. Autosomal recessive proximal spinal muscular atrophy in 101 sibs out of 48 families: Clinical picture, influence of gender, and genetic implications. *Am. J. Med. Genet.* 51:70–76, 1994.

39. Cobben, J. M., van der Steege, G., Grootscholten, P., de Visser, M., Scheffer, H., and Buys, C. H. C. M. Deletions of the survival motor neuron gene in unaffected siblings of patients with spinal muscular atrophy. *Am. J. Hum. Genet.* 57:805–808, 1995.

40. Wirth, B., Rudnik-Schoneborn, S., Hahnen, E., Rohrig, D., and Zerres, K. Prenatal prediction in families with autosomal recessive proximal spinal muscular atrophy (5q11.2-q13.3): molecular menetics and clinical experience in 109 cases. *Prenat. Diagn.* 15:407–417, 1995.

41. Wang, C. H., Xu, J., Carter, T. A., Ross, B. M., Sugarman, E. A., Allitto, B. A., Penchaszadeh, G. K., Munsat, T. L., and Gilliam, T. C. Analysis of the survival motor neuron (SMN) gene in spinal muscular atrophy families. *Am. Soc. Hum. Genet.* 57:A253, 1995.

42. Gutman, D. H. and Collins, F. von Recklinghausen Neurofibromatosis, in *The Metabolic and Molecular Bases of Inherited Disease*, 7th ed., Scriver C., ed., McGraw-Hill, New York, pp. 677–692, 1995.

43. Barker, D., Wright, E., Nguyen, K., Cannon, L., Fain, P., Goldgar, D., Bishop, D. T., Carey, J., Baty, B., Kivlin, J., Willard, H., Wayne, J. S., Greig, G., Leinwand, L., Nakamura, Y., O'Connell, P., Leppert, M., Lalouel, J.-M., White, R., and Skolnick, M. Gene for von Recklinghausen neurofibromatosis is in the perimcentromeric region of chromosome 17. *Science* 236:1100–1102, 1987.

44. Viskochil, D., White, R., and Cawthon, R. The neurofibromatosis type 1 gene. *Ann. Rev. Neurosci.* 16:183–205, 1993.

45. Upadhyaya, M., Shaw, D. J., and Harper, P. S. Molecular basis of neurofibromatosis type 1 (NF1): mutation analysis and polymorphisms in the NF1 gene. *Hum. Mutat.* 4:83–101, 1994.

46. Johnson, M. R., DeClue, J. E., Felzmann, S., Vass, W. C., Xu, G., White, R., and Lowy, D. R. Neurofibromin can inhibit ras-dependent growth by a mechanism independent of its GTPase-accelerating function. *Mol. Cell. Biol.* **14**:641–645, 1994.

47. McCormick, F. Ras signaling and NF1. *Curr. Opinion Gene. Devel.* **5**:51–55, 1995.

48. Ishioka, C., Ballester, R., Engelstein, M., Vidal, M., Kassel, J., The, I., Bernards, A., Gusella, J. F., and Friend, S. H. A functional assay for heterozygous mutations in GTPase activation protein related domain of the neurofibromin type 1 gene. *Oncogene* **10**:841–847, 1995.

49. Heim, R. A., Kam-Morgan, L. M. W., Binnie, C. G., Corna, D. D., Cayouette, M. C., Farber, R. A., Aylsworth, A. S., Silverman, L. M., and Luce, M. C. Neurofibromatosis 1 (NF1) truncating mutations are dispersed throughout the NF1 gene (abstract). *Am. J. Hum. Gen.* **57(Suppl.)**:A214, 1995.

50. Boder, E. Ataxia-telangiectasia: an overview. Kroc Foundation Series **19**:1–63, 1985.

51. Blaese, R. M. Genetic immunodeficiency syndromes with defects in both T- and B-lymphocyte function, in *The Metabolic and Molecular Bases of Inherited Disease*, 7th ed., Scriver, C., ed., McGraw-Hill, New York, pp. 3901,3902, 1995.

52. Waldmann, T. A., Strober, W., and Blaese, R. M. Immunodeficiency disease and malignancy. *Ann. Intern. Med.* **77**:605,1972.

53. Spector, B. D., Perry, G. S., and Kersey, J. H. Genetically determined immunodeficiency disease and malignancy: report from the immunodeficiency-cancer registry. *Clin. Immunol. Immunopathol.* **11**:12, 1978.

54. Gatti, R. A. Ataxia-telangiectasia. *Dermatol. Clin.* **13**:1–6, 1995.

55. West, C. M., Elyan, S. A., Berry, P., Cowan, R., and Scott, D. A comparison of the radiosensitivity of lymphocytes from normal donors, cancer patients, individuals with ataxia-telangiectasia, and ataxia-telangiectasia heterozygotes. *J. Radiat. Biol.* **68**:197–203, 1995.

56. Swift, M., Morrell, D., Massey, R. B., and Chase, C. L. Incidence of cancer in 161 families affected by ataxia-telangiectasia. *New Engl. J. Med.* **325**:1831–1836, 1991.

57. Easton, D. F. Cancer risks in ataxia-telangiectasia heterozygotes. *J. Radiat. Biol.* **66(Suppl. 6)**:S177–182, 1994.

58. Kojis, T. L., Schneck, R. R., Gatti, R. A., and Sparkes, R. S. Tissue specificity of chromosomal rearrangements in ataxia-telangiectasia. *Hum. Genet.* **83**:347–52, 1989.

59. Kaufman, W. K. Cell cycle checkpoints and DNA repair preserve the stability of the human genome. *Cancer Metastasis Rev.* **14**:31–41, 1995.

60. Jaspers, N. G., Gatti, R. A., Baan, C., Linssen, P. C., and Bootsma, D. Genetic complementation analysis of ataxia-telangiectasia and Nijmegen breakage syndrome: a survey of 50 patients. *Cytogenet. Cell Genet.* **49**:259–263, 1988.

61. Gatti, R. A., Berkel, I., Boder, E., Braedt, G., Charmley, P., Concannon, P., Ersoy, F., Foround, T., Jaspers, N. G. J., Lange, K., Lathrop, G. M., Leppert, M., Nakamura, Y., O'Connell, P., Paterson, M., Salser, W., Sanal, O., Silver, J., Sparkes, R. S., Susi, E., Weeks, D. E., Wei, S., White, R., and Yoder, F. Localization of an ataxia-telangiectasia gene to chromosome 11q22–23. *Nature* **336**:577–580, 1988.

62. Savitsky, K., Bar-Shira, A., Gilad, S., Rotman, G., Ziv, Y., Vanagaite, L., Tagle, D. A., Smith, S., Uziel, T., Sfez, S., Ashkenazi, M., Pecker, I., Frydman, M., Harnik, R., Patanjali, S. R., Simons, A., Clines, G. A., Sartiel, A., Gatti, R. A., Chessa, L., Sanal, O., Lavin, M. F., Jaspers, N. G. J., Malcolm, A., Raylor, R., Arlett, C. F., Miki, T., Weissman, S. M., Lovett, M., Collins, F. S., and Shiloh, Y. A single ataxia telangiectasia gene with a product similar to PI-3 Kinase. *Science* **268**:1749–1753, 1995.

63. Charcot, J. M., Marie, P. Sur une forme particuliere d'atrophie musculaire progressive solvent familiale debutante par les pieds et les jambes et atteigrante plus tard les mains. *Rev. Med.* **6**:97, 1886.

64. Tooth, H. H. *The Peroneal Type of Progressive Muscular Atrophy.* H. K. Lewis, London, 1886.

65. Wise, C. A., Garcia, C. A., Davis, S. N., Zhang, H., Pentao, L., Patel, P. I., and Lupski, J. R. Molecular analysis of unrelated Charcot-Marie-Tooth (CMT) disease patients suggest a high frequency of the CMT1A duplication. *Am. J. Hum. Genet.* **53**:853, 1993.

66. Chance, P. F., Abbas, N., Lensch, M. W., Pentao, L., Roa, B. B., Patel, P. L., and Lupski, J. R. Two autosomal dominant neuropathies results from reciprocal DNA duplication/deletion of a region on chromosome 17. *Hum. Mol. Genet.* **3**:223–228, 1994.

67. Lupski, J. R., Montes de Oca-Luna, R., Slaugenhaupt, S., Pentao, L., Guzzetta, V., Trask, B. J., Saucedo-Cardenas, O., Barker, D. F., Killan, J. M., Garcia, C. A., Chakravarti, A., and Patel, P. I. DNA duplication associated with Charcot-Marie-Tooth disease type 1A. *Cell* **66**:219, 1991.

68. Matsunami, N., Smith, B., Ballard, L., Lensch, M. W., Robertson, M., Albertsen, H., Hanemann, C. O., Muller, H. W., Bird, T. D., White, R., and Chance, P. F. Peripheral myelin protein-22 gene maps in the duplication of chromosome 17p11.2 associated with Charcot-Marie-Tooth 1A. *Nature Genet.* **1**:176, 1992.

69. Nicholson, G. A., Valentijn, L. J., Cherryson, A. K., Kennerson, M. L., Bragg, T. L., DeKroon, R. M., Ross, D. A., Pollard, J. D., Mcleod, J. G., Bolhius, P. A., and Baas, F. A frame shift mutation in the PMP22 gene in hereditary peripheral neuropathy with liability to pressure palsies. *Nature Genet.* **6**:263–266, 1994.

70. Wright, E. C., Goldgar, D. E., Fain, P. R., Barker, D. F., and Skolnick, M. H. A genetic map of human chromosome 17p. *Genomics* **7**:103–109, 1990.

71. Ballabio, A. and Zoghbi, H. Y. Charcot-Marie-Tooth Disease and hereditary neuropathy with liability to pressure palsies, in *The Metabolic and Molecular Basis of Inherited Disease*, 7th ed., McGraw-Hill, New York, pp. 4569–4573, 1995.

72. Chance, P. F., Alderson, M. K., Leppig, K. A., Lensch, M. W., Matsunami, N., Smith, B., Swanson, P. D., Odelberg, S. J., Disteche, C. M., and Bird, T. D. DNA deletion associated with hereditary neuropathy with liability to pressure palsies. *Cell* **72**:143, 1993.

73. Windebank, A. J., Schenone, A., and Dewald, G.W. Hereditary neuropathy with liability to pressure palsies and inherited brachial plexus neuropathy—two genetically distinct disorders. *Mayo Clin. Proc.* **70**:743–746, 1995.

74. Roa, B. B., Garcia, C. A., Suter, U., Kulpa, D. A., Wise, C. A., Mueller, J., Welcher, A. A., Snipes, G. J., Shooter, E. M., Patel, P. I., and Lupski, J. R. Charcot-Marie-Tooth disease type 1A association with a spontaneous point mutation in the PMP22 gene. *New Engl. J. Med.* **329**:96, 1993.

75. Emery, A. E. H. Clinical features, in *Duchenne Muscular Dystrophy*, 2nd ed., Motulsky, A. G., Harper, P. S., Bobrow, M., and Scriver, C., eds. Oxford University Press, New York, pp. 26–41, 1993.

76. Koenig, M., Beggs, A. H., Moyer, M., Scherpf, S., Heindrich, K., Bettecken, T., Meng, G., Muller, C. R., Lindlof, M., and Kaariainen, H. The molecular basis for Duchenne versus Becker muscular dystrophy: correlation of severity with type of deletion. *Am. J. Hum. Genet.* **45**:498, 1989.

77. Monaco, A. P. and Kunkel, L. M. Cloning of the Duchenne/Becker muscular dystrophy locus. *Adv. Hum. Genet.* **17**:61, 1988.

78. Ervasti, J. M. and Campbell, K. P. Membrane organization of the dystrophin-glyco-membrane complex. *Cell* **66**:1121, 1991.

79. Gorecki, D. C., Monaco, A. P., Derry, J. M. J., Walker, A. P., Barnard, E. A., and Barnard, P. J. Expression of four alternative transcripts in brain regions regulated by different promotors. *Hum. Mol. Genet.* **1**:505, 1992.

80. Koenig, M., Hoffman, E. P., Bertelson, C. J., Monaco, A. P., Feener, C., and Kunkel, L. M. Complete cloning of the Duchenne muscular dystrophy (DMD) cDNA and preliminary genomic organization of the DMD gene in normal and affected individuals. *Cell* **50**:509, 1987.

81. Coffey, A. J., Roberts, R. G., Green, E. D., Cole, C. G., Butler, R., Anand, R., Giannelli, F., and Bentley, D. R. Construction of a 2.6-Mb contig in yeast artificial chromosomes spanning the human dystrophin gene using an STS-based approach. *Genomics* **12:**474, 1992.

82. Worton, R. G. and Brooke, M. H. The X-linked muscular dystrophies, in *The Metabolic and Molecular Basis of Inherited Disease,* 7th ed., McGraw-Hill, New York, pp. 4195–4226, 1995.

83. Roberts, R. G., Coffey, A. J., Bobrow, M., Bentley, D. R. Exon structure of the human dystrophin gene. Genomics **16:**536, 1993.

84. Chamberlain, J. S., Gibbs, R. A., Ranier, J. E., Nguyen, P. N., and Caskey, C. T. Deletion screening of the Duchenne muscular dystrophy locus via multiplex DNA amplification. *Nucleic Acids Res.* **16:**11141, 1988.

85. Beggs, A. H., Koenig, M., Boyce, F. M., and Kunkel, L. M. Detection of 98% of DMD/BMD gene deletions by polymerase chain reaction. *Hum. Genet.* **86:**45, 1990.

86. Clements, P. R., Fenwick, R. G., Chamberlain, J. S., Gibbs, R. A., de Andrade, M., Chakroborty, R., and Caskey, C. T. Carrier detection and prenatal diagnosis in Duchenne and Becker muscular dystrophy families, using dinucleotide repeat polymorphisms. *Am. J. Hum. Genet.* **49:**951–960, 1991.

87. Beggs, A. H. and Kunkel, L. M. Improved diagnosis of Duchenne/Becker Muscular Dystrophy. *J. Clin. Invest.* **85:**613–619, 1990.

12

Molecular Mechanisms of Endocrine Disorders

Bruce F. Bower and Carl D. Malchoff

1. INTRODUCTION

Molecular biologic methods and findings have had a major impact in clinical endocrinology. As a result, new concepts of hormone action have developed, major disease mechanisms have been defined, and new diagnostic strategies and therapies have been made possible. This chapter will summarize this rapidly evolving field with particular emphasis on clinical understanding and the application of molecular biologic techniques to clinical endocrine diagnosis. As a result of the pace of development, this chapter and any review will necessarily be selective, and will provide at best a window into a rapid and dynamically evolving area of clinical interest and increasing molecular understanding.

2. HYPOTHALAMIC PITUITARY DISORDERS

A number of independent endocrine disorders involving the hypothalamic–pituitary axis have been defined. These defects include hypothalamic neuronal abnormalities, hypothalamic-posterior pituitary diabetes insipidus syndromes, and heritable growth hormone-deficiency disorders. Included as a result of clinical similarity and molecular insight are both central and nephrogenic variants of diabetes insipidus.

2.1. Kallman's Syndrome (1)

Kallman's syndrome is a familial X-linked disorder of congenital hypogonadotropic hypogonadism, anosmia, or hyposmia, and scattered midline facial defects with occasional unilateral renal aplasia. The disorder arises from a failure of development of neural tracts from the olfactory placode through the cribriform plate to the olfactory bulb. There is associated failure of GnRH neurons to migrate along the olfactory nerves to the hypothalamus. Laboratory findings include hypogonadotropic hypogonadism in the male with low serum testosterone and low serum gonadotrophins, FSH and LH. There are no associated anterior pituitary functional abnormalities. Clinical recognition is achieved by recognition of anosmia/hyposmia in the setting of hypogonadotropic hypogonadism. Diagnostic olfactory gyri aplasia and absent olfactory bulbs may be seen on MRI scan. Testosterone replacement therapy corrects defective male secondary sexual maturation. Fertility is possible with menopausal gonadotrophin replacement therapy.

From: Molecular Diagnostics: For the Clinical Laboratorian
Edited by: W. B. Coleman and G. J. Tsongalis Humana Press Inc., Totowa, NJ

The molecular defect of this syndrome includes variable deletions of the KAL gene located at the Xp22.3 locus of the X chromosome. The presumptive gene product is a 680 amino acid peptide implicated in neuronal migration and axonal growth and guidance.

2.2. Diabetes Insipidus (Familial Hypothalamic Diabetes Insipidus (2)

The clinical manifestations of diabetes insipidus include variable onset of thirst and polyuria typically in the first few months to the first year following birth, often in a setting of a family history of autosomal-dominant central diabetes insipidus. Laboratory findings include elevated serum sodium and osmolality with inappropriately low urine osmolality and failure of increase in plasma arginine vasopressin (AVP) levels following dehydration. Urinary concentration occurs following exogenous desamino-D-arginine vasopressin (DDAVP) administration. The thirst and polyuria are responsive to administration of exogenous intranasal DDAVP.

Molecular defects have been identified in the prepro-arginine vasopressin-neurophysin II (AVP-NPII) secretory complex responsible for single-chain biosynthesis of neurophysin and AVP leading to accumulation and ultimate destruction of hypothalamic magnocellular neurons by accumulation of mutant proteins. The molecular alterations result in several defects in prepro-neurophysin II (not AVP) biosynthesis (Gly57 → Ala, Gly17 → Val; Ala19 → Thr; Glu47 deletion). The disorder is analogous to diabetes insipidus in the Brattleboro rat (autosomal-recessive DI secondary to base deletion in Exon 2 leading to frameshift error in NPII synthesis).

2.3. Familial Nephrogenic Diabetes Insipidus (3)

This is a familial X-linked (male) disorder characterized by neonatal thirst, polyuria, and severe dehydration if not recognized and treated early. The defect is in renal tubule response to antidiuretic hormone (ADH) rather than defective ADH secretion, but may easily be confused clinically with hypothalamic diabetes insipidus. The renal-collecting duct basolateral medullary AVP-R2 receptor, which is normally coupled through a guanosine triphosphate (GTP) transmembrane signaling complex, is defective. The AVP-R1 receptor mediating vascular blood pressure response remains normal. Laboratory findings include an elevated serum sodium and osmolality following dehydration with an inappropriately low urine osmolality. AVP levels are elevated, indicating normal hypothalamic–pituitary response to dehydration. There is absence of urinary concentration following DDAVP administration indicating a defect at the renal tubule level.

The molecular defects are localized to Xq28. There are multiple nonsense, missense, and frameshift mutations in the AVP-R2 receptor gene. Therapy is difficult, and efforts should be made to maintain hydration and high sustained levels of fluid intake. Dehydration should be avoided, particularly during infancy, when recognition of dehydration is clinically difficult and effective water-seeking by infants is not possible.

3. GROWTH AND GROWTH HORMONE (GH) ABNORMALITIES

There are multiple etiologies for growth failure, most of which are nonendocrine in nature. Of the endocrine etiologies of growth failure, several involve GH abnormalities, both growth hormone deficiency and GH resistance.

3.1. Familial Isolated GH (4)

Type IA familial isolated GH deficiency is an autosomal-recessive disorder characterized by profound growth failure. Basal serum GH levels are absent and fail to respond to stimulation with hypoglycemia, arginine infusion, DOPA, or clonidine. Serum insulin-like growth factor (IGF)-I levels are also low. Clinical features include growth failure, hypoglycemia, and micropenis associated with short stature and facial abnormalities, such as large forehead, small nose, retracted nose bridge, and truncal obesity. Laboratory findings include isolated undetectable serum GH levels (Type IA) or low serum GH and IGF-I levels (Type IB, Type II, Type III). The disorders are familial with neonatal onset. Type IA patients who are treated with recombinant GH rapidly develop antibodies to rhGH, requiring discontinuation of therapy. There are several additional variant familial growth hormone deficiency disorders characterized by both inheritance patterns and laboratory variance. Type 1B families have an autosomal-recessive disorder. Serum GH levels are low but detectable, particularly following stimulation, and IGF-I levels are also low. These patients respond to recombinant human growth hormone (rhGH) therapy. Type II families display an autosomal-dominant inheritance pattern with low serum GH and IGF-I levels. Type III is an X-linked disorder. Serum GH and IGF-I levels are also low, but measurable.

Variable deletions in the pituitary h-GH-N growth hormone and associated pituitary sommamotrophin hCS sequences have been identified (5' hGH-N,hCS-L,hCS-A,hGH-V,hGS-B 3'). There are no associated anterior pituitary abnormalities. The molecular defect in these disorders include:

1. Type IA: deletions in hGH-N locus on chromosome 17 secondary to anomalous crossing over between homologous sequences, (5' hGH-N,hCSL,hCS-A,hGH-V,hGS-B 3'), and a G → C transversion at intron IV causing activation of a cryptic splice site and splicing out half of exon IV and a frameshift in exon V;
2. Type II: T → C transition in donor splice site of intron III;
3. Type III: unknown abnormality.

Therapy includes rhGH therapy for Type IB, II, and III disorders. Rapid development of high-titer GH antibodies to rhGH therapy in type IA precludes continued rhGH therapy.

3.2. PIT-I Deficiency (5)

Pit-1 is a 33-kDa, pituitary-specific, transcription factor that is required for anterior pituitary sommatotroph, lactotroph, and thyrotroph differentiation and secretion. Deficiency of Pit-1 results in combined neonatal growth hormone, prolactin, and TSH-β deficiencies leading to short stature and secondary hypothyroidism with pituitary hypoplasia. Adrenocorticotropin (ACTH) and gonadotrophin pituitary function are intact. Clinical and laboratory findings include short stature, neonatal hypothyroidism, and variable mental retardation. GH secretion is unresponsive to DOPA, hypoglycemia, and amino acid stimulation. The decreased serum thyroid-stimulating hormone (TSH) is unresponsive to thyrotropin-releasing hormone (TRH) administration, and decreased serum prolactin is unresponsive to TRH or chlorpromazine administration. Therapy includes both GH (rhGH) and thyroid replacement therapy.

The molecular defect has been identified in the activation domain of this transcription factor as well as POU and Homeo DNA binding domains. These alterations result in the following amino acid substitutions: Arg 172 → Ter; Ala 158 → Pro; Pro 24 → Leu; Arg 143 → Gln; and Arg 271 → Trp.

3.3. GH Resistance Syndrome (Laron's Syndrome) (6)

The clinical manifestations of Laron's syndrome include growth failure, hypoglycemia, micropenis associated with short stature, and facial abnormalities, such as large forehead, small nose, and retracted nose bridge. Truncal obesity and hypoglycemia characteristic of severe neonatal GH deficiency are also characteristic of this syndrome. The disorder results from a defective GH receptor (GHR) protein. Laboratory findings include normal to elevated serum GH levels, but low serum IGF-I levels. In addition, there are low levels of circulating GH binding protein, which has been identified as the soluble extracellular domain of the GHR. There is no response to exogenous GH therapy. Recently, the spectrum of more subtle growth abnormalities secondary to GHR binding, dimerization or transmembrane signaling have been defined.

In classic Laron's syndrome, five molecular defects of the GHR gene have been identified in different families, all resulting in absent GH binding. A T to C transition results in Phe96 being substituted by Ser in the extracellular GHR. Large gene deletions in the extracellular domain of the GHR have also been described. There is no therapeutic response to exogenous rhGH therapy. There is both an anabolic response and clinical growth response to rhIGF-I therapy. In the recently described more subtle GHR disorders, defects include premature stop codons and missense mutations in the GH binding domain and other portions of the GHR. Partial growth response to pharamacologic GH therapy has been suggested (7).

3.4. African Pigmy Short Stature (8)

Short stature in these individuals represents a form of tribal short stature. Serum GH-binding protein (GHBP) levels are borderline low normal in childhood, but fail to rise normally at puberty. At puberty, serum GH-BP levels are only 30% of normal African controls. Laboratory findings include low normal GHBP, which is the result of low levels of IGF-I and failure of normal pubertal increase in IGF-I. There is no known molecular defect and no effective therapy.

3.5. Pituitary Neoplasia—GH-Producing (9)

Pituitary adenomas present with clinical evidence of excess hormone production and/or complications of their mass. Most pituitary tumors are clonal and can develop from the different cell types of the anterior pituitary gland. In general, their etiology is unknown. The exception is GH-producing pituitary tumors. These tumors arise from somatotrophs. In acromegaly, the serum GH concentration cannot be suppressed by a glucose challenge, and there is persistent elevation of circulating IGF-I concentration.

About one-third of GH secreting pituitary tumors have a somatic activating mutation of the α subunit of G_s. This is a GTPase that couples cell membrane receptors to adenylate cyclase. The activating mutations occur at Arg201 and at Gln227. Activating mutations of $G_s\alpha$ actually inhibit the GTPase activity of this protein, so that it remains in its GTP-bound form, which is capable of activating adenylate cyclase. This gives rise to constitutive activation of adenylate cyclase, and the increased cAMP concentration stimulates somatotroph cell division. Should the mutant $G_s\alpha$ occur early in development, then the affected individuals are mosaics and develop the McCune Albright syndrome, of which acromegaly is one clinical feature. The presence of the activating mutation of $G_s\alpha$ does not alter prognosis or direct therapy. Tumor size, concomitant prolactin secretion, and octreotide sensitivity are independent of these mutations.

3.6. Achondroplasia (10)

Chondrodystrophy results in short stature with disproportionate short extremities. Epiphyses are abnormal on radiologic examination. The disorder is the result of an abnormal fibroblast growth factor receptor-3 (FGFR-3) on chromosome 4 (4p16.3). A G → A transition at nucleotide 1138 has been reported in 15/16 patients and a G → C at nucleotide 1138 in 1/16 patients, both resulting in Gly → Arg 380 substitution.

The CpG is a mutational "hot spot" secondary to C methylation/deamination and results in a T → C on the antisense DNA strand and a G → A on the sense strand. Nucleotide 1138 is the most highly mutable nucleotide in the human genome. There is no effective therapy for achondroplasia or any of the related chondrodystrophies.

4. THYROID DISORDERS

Most thyroid disease arises as a result of acquired abnormalities of function, hypothyroidism, or hyperthyroidism, or as a result of benign or malignant neoplasia. Several molecular abnormalities have been described.

4.1. Thyroid-Stimulating Hormone (TSH) Receptor Mutations— Activating Mutations (11)

Activating mutations of the TSH receptor result in neonatal hyperthyroidism in the absence of maternal Graves' disease. Later delayed pediatric and adult recognition of hyperthyroidism may also occur. The disorder results from a gain of function mutation in the sixth transmembrane region of the TSH receptor leading to constitutive activity, increased serum T4 and T3 secretion, and subsequent hyperthyroidism with appropriately suppressed serum TSH levels.

There is a gain of function mutation (TTC → CTC, Phe 631 → Leu) in the sixth transmembrane region of the TSH receptor leading to constitutive activity. An additional Cys 672 → Tyr in a second family has also been documented. In some hyperfunctional thyroid nodules, tissue-specific Ala 623 → Ile and Asp 619 → Gly have also been identified, which lead to autonomous functional thyroid nodules. Therapy of the hyperthyroidism requires surgical thyroidectomy or ^{131}I therapy.

4.2. TSH Receptor Mutations—Inhibiting Mutations (12)

Mutations of the TSH receptor result in elevated serum TSH usually detected on near universal neonatal serum TSH screening for neonatal hypothyroidism. Thyroid function studies are usually normal apparently as a result of the compensatory serum TSH hypersecretion. The molecular abnormality consists of a series of inactivating mutations in exon 6 of the extracellular domain of the TSH receptor. Ile 167 → Asn and Pro 162 → Ala have been identified on paternal and maternal alleles, respectively. The compensated state of thyroid hormone production does not require treatment.

4.3. Generalized Thyroid Hormone Resistance (GTHR) (13,14)

The clinical manifestations of GTHR include variable goiter, growth impairment, and thyroid function abnormality. Variations include selected pituitary resistance with resultant hyperthyroidism and a single case of isolated partial thyroid peripheral resistance. The disorders result in elevated thyroid function studies with inappropriately normal or elevated serum TSH levels.

GTHR results from mutations in the c-*erb*A β thyroid hormone receptor on chromosome 3. A dominant negative effect leads to functional receptor abnormality when only a heterozygote mutant is present, possibly as a result of disruption of dimer needed for binding of the receptor complex to the DNA thyroid response element (TRE) domain. Multiple mutations have been identified in different families with GTHR. These mutations are located in the thyroid binding domain of the receptor. Included are CCT → CAT mutation at 1643 Pro → His (codon 453), CGC → CAC mutation at 1598 Arg → His (codon 438), CAG → CAC mutation at 1305 Gln → His (codon 340), GGT → CGT mutation at 1318 Gly → Arg (codon 345), and GGG → GAG mutation at 1325 Gly → Glu (codon 347). The mutations are usually inherited in a dominant fashion (dominant negative). However, in the original family described the disorder was inherited as a recessive trait owing to a 244–1704 deletion, which led to total absence of the c-*erb*A β receptor.

4.4. Selective Pituitary Thyroid Resistance (13,14)

Selective pituitary TSH resistance is infrequently described. The patients are hyperthyroid as a result of nonsuppressed TSH secretion and unimpaired peripheral thyroid hormone responsiveness. The disorder may result from a possible intrapituitary T4 → T3 conversion defect. Thyroxine (T4) serves as a precursor for the active intracellular thyronine, tri-iodothyronine (T3) derived from enzymatic mono-deiodination of T4. Hyperthyroidism secondary to selective TSH resistance requires therapy of the resultant peripheral hyperthyroidism.

4.5. Thyroid Neoplasms (15)

Thyroid neoplasms may be benign or malignant. Both present as thyroid nodules, and the clinical challenge is to distinguish these two types of neoplasms preoperatively. The etiology of thyroid neoplasms is generally not well understood. Prolonged TSH stimulation and radiation exposure predispose to thyroid neoplasm. Most thyroid neoplasms do not cause hyperthyroidism. It can occur with multinodular goiters and solitary hot thyroid nodules, but rarely with thyroid carcinoma.

About one-third of solitary hot thyroid nodules are caused by somatic activating mutations of the thyrotropin receptor, as has been discussed, and about one-third are caused by activating mutations of the α subunit of G_s. The latter mutations occur at Arg 201 or Gln 227 and are the same mutations that cause GH secreting pituitary tumors, when they occur in somatotrophs. The molecular abnormalities of papillary thyroid carcinoma are largely unknown. There is somatic rearrangement of the papillary thyroid cancer gene (RET) in about one-fourth of papillary thyroid carcinomas, which is presumably etiologic. Genomic activating mutations of RET are etiologic for multiple endocrine neoplasia type 2 (MEN 2). It is, anticipated that analysis of the oncogene and suppressor gene mutations that distinguish benign from malignant neoplasms will be of future clinical utility.

5. CALCIUM DISORDERS

5.1. Hyperparathyroidism (16)

Hyperparathyroidism is often asymptomatic and is discovered when serum calcium is noted to be elevated. Features include kidney stones, osteoporosis, and confusion. The disorder is caused by a parathyroid adenoma in about 85% of subjects, by hyperplasia involving all four glands in about 15% of subjects, and rarely by parathyroid carcinoma. When associated with the syndromes of multiple endocrine neoplasia, the relative frequency of hyperplasia is increased. Hyperparathyroidism is characterized by elevated serum calcium concentrations and increased parathyroid hormone concentrations. It occurs in almost all subjects with MEN 1 and in about 20% of subjects with MEN 2a. The molecular basis of these disorders is understood in only a few cases. In about 5% of parathyroid adenomas, there is a rearrangement of the Prad-1 gene that is now more appropriately termed cyclin D1. Deletions of the retinoblastoma gene have been detected in parathyroid carcinoma. Activating mutations of the RET proto-oncogene occur in MEN 2.

5.2. Jansen-Type Metaphyseal Chondrodysplasia (17)

This is a form of short-limbed dwarfism characterized by high serum calcium, low serum phosphorous, and undetectable parathyroid hormone concentrations. The disorder is the result of constitutive activation of the parathyroid hormone signaling mechanism. Heterozygous activating mutations of the parathyroid hormone-parathyroid hormone-related peptide (PTH-PTHrP) receptor cause this disorder.

5.3. Familial Hypocalciuric Hypercalcemia (FHH) (18)

FHH is a rare dominantly inherited disorder characterized by hypercalcemia, a non-suppressed parathyroid hormone concentration and low urine calcium. It is usually a benign disorder that should be distinguished from primary hyperparathyroidism. FHH cannot be treated by parathyroidectomy.

Parathyroid hormone secretion is regulated by the circulating calcium concentration, which is detected by a calcium sensitive seven transmembrane domain receptor. Mutations that reduce the function of this receptor cause the calcium sensor of the parathyroid glands to be reset to a higher than normal calcium concentration. The decreased urinary excretion of calcium is probably related to the presence of calcium receptors in the kidney. Once the etiologic mutation in a given family is identified, a genetic screening test will identify affected family members.

5.4. Williams Syndrome (19)

Williams syndrome is characterized by a variable combination of congenital heart defects, connective tissue disorders, distinctive facial features, mental retardation, and infantile hypercalcemia. Hemizygosity of the elastin gene at 7q11.23 was identified in 1993 in patients with Williams syndrome. Fluorescence *in situ* hybridization (FISH) is commercially available to detect this disorder.

5.5. Familial Hypoparathyroidism (18,20)

Rarely hypoparathyroidism is inherited as an autosomal-dominant disorder either by itself or associated with thymic aphasia immune deficiencies, and cardiac malformations. The latter is referred to as the DiGeorge syndrome. In both circumstances, the calcium concentrations are low and phosphate concentrations are high. The subject may present with seizures as an infant, and vitamin D therapy is required. Isolated inherited hypoparathyroidism may be caused by an activating mutation of the seven transmembrane domain calcium receptor. These must be identified by DNA sequencing. In the DiGeorge syndrome, there is a deletion of part of chromosome 22. FISH is commercially available to detect this disorder.

5.6. Multiple Endocrine Neoplasia Type 1 (MEN 1) (21)

MEN 1 is characterized by hyperparathyroidism in almost all subjects and variable frequency of other endocrine tumors, including pancreatic tumors, gastrinoma, and pituitary tumors. It is inherited in an autosomal-dominant fashion with nearly complete penetrance. The molecular abnormalities are incompletely understood. It is presumably caused by a tumor suppressor gene that has been localized to 11q13.1. Linkage analysis is available from research laboratories for analysis of large kindreds to predict which members will be affected.

5.7. Multiple Endocrine Neoplasia Type 2 (MEN 2)

This disorder is discussed extensively in the context of DNA analysis with current clinical applications. *See* Section 11.1.

5.8. Pseudohypoparathyrodism (22,23)

Pseudohypoparathyroidism (PHP) Ia is a rare autosomal-dominant disorder characterized by hypocalcemia, elevated parathyroid hormone concentration, short stature, and shortening of the metacarpals and metatarsals. It is caused by decreased activity of the α subunit of G_s. There is not only resistance to parathyroid hormone, but also mild resistance to other hormones, such as thyroid hormone and adrenocorticotropin. An interesting variant of PHP Ia is associated with male sexual precocity owing to peripheral hypergonadism.

Other variants of PHP occur, and their etiology is not well understood. Isolated resistance to parathyroid hormone resistance with normal $G_s\alpha$ activity is called PHP Ib. PHP II is characterized by the low serum calcium, elevated serum PTH concentration, and normal urinary cAMP. Resistance to parathyroid hormone is believed to be distal to the generation of cAMP, but has not yet been localized.

In PHP Ia, multiple mutations of $G_s\alpha$ have been identified. Most commonly these are missense mutations, but can also include deletions. Once the mutation for a given family has been identified, then the disorder can be predicted in other family members. The variant of PHP Ia with peripheral hypergonadism is the result of a mutation that inactivates the GTPase activity of $G_s\alpha$ and renders $G_s\alpha$ unstable at 37°C. Since the testes are maintained at a lower temperature, this $G_s\alpha$ is stable in the testes only and, therefore, activates adenylate cyclase in the Leydig cells. This results in production of testosterone and subsequent peripheral hypergonadism *(23)*. The molecular bases of PHP Ib and PHP II are unknown.

5.9. Vitamin D Resistance (24)

Generalized hereditary vitamin D resistance is an autosomal recessive disorder that presents with partial or total alopecia, elevated concentrations of parathyroid hormone and vitamin D, but with low concentrations of calcium and phosphorous. Rickets develops between the ages 4 to 12 mo. The disorder is caused by abnormalities of the vitamin D receptor, so that it is analogous to other disorders caused by abnormalities of steroid hormone receptors, such as thyroid hormone resistance and androgen resistance. Missense mutations of the vitamin D receptor cause this disorder. These are identified by DNA sequencing. Heterozygote carriers can be identified by similar analyses, but this usually is of limited clinical utility.

6. ADRENAL DISORDERS

Adrenal insufficiency can be caused by mutations of critical enzymes in the steroidogenic pathways. The defect can be as early as the adrenocorticotropin receptor itself or it may be a late step in cortisol synthesis. These disorders are organized roughly in order from the initial step of adrenal stimulation to the final enzymatic step in cortisol production, and finally the effect of cortisol on end organs. Other adrenal disorders result in the actual or apparent increase in aldosterone. The apparent increase in aldosterone is caused by a molecular abnormality in other tissues. Because of the large number of adrenal disorders, this section is not inclusive, but is directed toward some of the more common and more instructive disorders.

6.1. Inherited Autosomal-Recessive ACTH Insensitivity (25)

Adrenal insufficiency caused by resistance to adrenocorticotropin is inherited in an autosomal recessive fashion. ACTH is high and both cortisol and its precursors are low. A variety of mutations in the ACTH receptor sequence have been identified as the cause of this disorder.

6.2. 17α-Hydroxylase/17,20-Lyase Deficiency and 3β-Hydroxysteroid Dehydrogenase Deficiency (26,27)

These rare enzyme deficiencies result in both defective cortisol and gonadal hormone production, since common steroidogenic pathways are involved. Since the deficiencies can be variable, the clinical presentations are diverse. 17α-Hydroxylase/17,20-lyase deficiency is owing to homozygous compound heterozygous mutations in the gene for that enzyme. 3β-Hydroxysteroid dehydrogenase deficiency is the result of mutations in the type II gene for that enzyme.

6.3. 21-Hydroxylase Deficiency (Deficiency of P-450C-21) (28)

This autosomal recessive disorder is the most common form of congenital adrenal hyperplasia and is characterized by virilization in neonates. In the more severe forms, there is significant salt losing, and in the less severe forms (nonclassic form), the disorder may manifest only as androgen excess after puberty. The serum concentration of 17α-hydroxyprogesterone is elevated, since P-450C-21 is responsible for converting this steroid to 11-deoxycortisol. There are two P-450C-21 genes. The P-450C-21A gene is a pseudogene, and the P-450C-21B gene codes for the enzyme. The disorder is caused by deletions, missense mutations, and gene conversions of the P-450C-21 gene. It is currently possible to diagnose the disorder prenatally and institute dexamethasone therapy prior to birth to prevent virilization in the females. The diagnosis can be made by molecular methods. However, these are not essential, since the P-450C-21A gene is tightly linked to the HLA locus. HLA analysis of previous affected individuals and parents allows the clinician to predict which SA allele is linked to the mutant P450C-21A gene.

6.4. 11β-Hydroxylase Deficiency (CYP11B1 or P-450C11 Deficiency) (29)

In this autosomal recessive form of congenital adrenal hyperplasia, there is virilization of female infants and hypertension with hypokalernia. The former is the result of excess androgen production, and the latter owing to overproduction of deoxycorticosterone. Mutations of the CYP 11B1 gene give rise to this disorder.

6.5. Aldosterone Synthetase Deficiency (CYP11B2 Deficiency) (29)

In this autosomal recessive disorder, there is hypotension, hyperkalemia, and in infancy, failure to thrive and hypovolemic shock. Aldosterone concentrations are very low, whereas plasma renin activity is high. The disorder is caused by mutations of aldosterone synthetase (CYP11B2).

6.6. Glucocorticoid Resistance (30,31)

Glucocorticoid resistance is a rare disorder that is characterized by hypercortisolism in the absence of Cushing's syndrome. Patients may present with hypertension and hypokalemia or precocious pseudopuberty. These manifestations are caused by increased adrenal production of mineralocorticoids and androgens, respectively. This disorder is caused by mutations in the glucocorticoid receptor.

6.7. Glucocorticoid Suppressible Aldosteronism (29)

Glucocorticoid suppressible hyperaldosteronism is an autosomal-dominant cause of hypertension. It is caused by increased aldosterone production and often, but not always, is associated with the expected hypokalemia. Aldosterone production can be suppressed by dexamethasone therapy. This disorder is caused by an unequal crossover event, so that aldosterone synthetase (CYP11B2) comes under the control of an ACTH sensitive promoter. The genes for aldosterone synthetase (CYP11B2) and 11 β-hydroxy-lase (CYP11B1) are located close together on the same chromosome and are very similar in structure. Normally the former is under the control of an angiotensin II responsive promoter, whereas the latter is under the control of an ACTH-dependent promoter. When the unequal crossing over event occurs, the aldosterone synthetase gene (CYP11B2) comes under control of the promoter for 11β-hydroxylase (CYP11B1), and aldosterone is made in response to ACTH. Therefore, it is not surprising that aldosterone production can be suppressed by dexamethasone therapy.

6.8. Syndrome of Apparent Mineralocorticoid Excess (32)

In this rare disorder, inherited in an autosomal-dominant fashion, there is volume-dependent hypertension and hypokalemia with suppression of plasma renin activity and aldosterone production. The disorder is caused by decreased activity of the 11β-hydroxysteroid dehydrogenase (11βHSD) enzyme that converts cortisol to cortisone in the kidney tubule. Cortisol, but not cortisone, is a potent stimulator of the mineralocorticoid receptor. The molecular abnormality of this disorder was initially confusing. There was biochemical evidence for abnormal enzyme activity, but the initial molecular analysis suggested that the sequence was normal. It is now understood that there are at least 11βHSD enzymes, and it is the type 2 enzyme that carries mutations in this disorder.

6.9. Liddle's Syndrome (33)

This disorder presents with volume-dependent hypertension and hypokalemia without an identifiable etiologic mineralocorticoid. It differs from the syndrome of mineralocorticoid excess in that hypokalemia is not reversed by spironolactone, which blocks the mineralocorticoid receptor. However, like the syndrome of apparent mineralocorticoid excess, the hypokalemia responds to triamterene. The disorder is caused by mutations in the β subunit of the amiloride-sensitive epithelial sodium channel, which is located in the distal convoluted tubule. This suggests that this subunit serves a regulatory function. When the regulatory function is lost, the channel is activated and sodium is reabsorbed and potassium excreted.

7. TESTICULAR/OVARIAN DISORDERS

7.1. Androgen Resistance (34)

Generalized resistance to androgens is characterized by variable degrees of feminization. There may be complete feminization with female breast development and a female external genitalia, but without internal female organs. Alternatively, the only manifestation of this disorder may be infertility in a phenotypically normal male. An entire gradation of phenotypes has been observed between these two extremes. Testosterone is normal to high and gonadotropins are mildly elevated. The disorder is caused by inherited androgen receptor abnormalities. In general, greater degrees of androgen resistance are associated with more severe defects in the androgen receptor. Since the gene for this receptor is on the X chromosome and since heterozygous women are unaffected, the disorder is X-linked. Since affected males are most often infertile, they cannot pass the disorder on to subsequent generations.

The most common androgen receptor mutations are missense mutations that occur in the ligand binding domain of the molecule and interfere with binding of androgens. Missense mutations also occur in the DNA binding domain of the receptor and interfere with the ability of the activated receptor to modify gene transcription. Occasionally, partial or complete deletion of the androgen receptor gene has been identified. An unusual form of mild androgen resistance occurs in the syndrome of X-linked spinal muscular atrophy and is caused by lengthening of the glutamine polymeric region found in the amino terminus of the molecule.

7.2. Estrogen Resistance (35)

A single male subject with complete estrogen resistance has been identified. This subject presented with severe osteoporosis and failure of epiphyses to close. The disorder in its complete form was caused by a homozygous mutation of the estrogen receptor that left it functionless.

7.3. Hereditary Hypergonadotropic Ovarian Dysgenesis (36)

Occasionally hypergonadotropic ovarian dysgenesis can be inherited in an autosomal-dominant fashion. This disorder was initially linked to chromosome 2p and subsequently shown to be owing to mutations of the follicle stimulating hormone (FSH) receptor. The mutant receptor no longer binds FSH with high affinity and is incapable of stimulating cAMP production.

7.4. Male Familial Precocious Puberty (37)

Families with gonadotropin-independent precocious puberty limited to the male offspring of affected fathers have been known for many years. The precocity is gonadotropin independent in that testosterone is produced in the absence of FSH and luteinizing hormone (LH). The disorder is now recognized to be caused by activation of the LH receptor. This is insufficient to result in female precocity, since both the LH and FSH

receptors must be activated for estrogen production to be stimulated. Missense mutations have been identified in the third intracellular domain of the LH receptor. The
mutant receptor constitutively activates adenylyl cyclase. DNA sequencing is necessary to identify the mutation.

7.5. Sex Reversal Syndromes (38,39)

Rarely phenotypic women will be found to have an XY karyotype. In some, the
short arm of the Y chromosome is missing, and in others there is a mutation of the SRY
gene, which codes for a testis determining factor (tdf) and is located on the short arm of
the Y chromosome. Without an active tdf, the gonads develop into ovaries, not testes.

7.6. McCune-Albright Syndrome (40,41)

This is a sporadic disorder characterized by polyostotic fibrous dysplasia and primary endocrine overactivity. This includes hyperthyroidism, precocious puberty,
Cushing's syndrome, and acromegaly. Although the precocious puberty is a common
presenting feature, most subjects have polyostotic fibrous dysplasia that can be detected
by its classic appearance on radiologic evaluation The endocrine abnormalities are the
result of primary end organ activity. The disorder is caused by activating mutations of
$G_s\alpha$. The mutation presumably occurs in a single cell early in development, so that the
affected subjects are mosaics.

The disorder is caused by the substitution of either His or Cys for Arg at amino acid
201 of $G_s\alpha$. These mutations can be detected by DNA sequencing or restriction enzyme
analysis. Since the subjects are mosaics, affected tissue must be analyzed, because
unaffected tissues, such as skin fibroblasts and mononuclear leukocytes, do not carry
the mutation. The availability of affected tissue limits the molecular diagnosis. If bone
is biopsied, a sample should be saved frozen for DNA analysis. DNA is destroyed by
the usual decalcification procedure utilized to prepare it for pathologic analysis.

8. HYPERLIPEMIA-DYSLIPIDEMIA

The hyperlipemias represent a large, heterogeneous group of disorders characterized by excessive serum cholesterol and triglyceride elevations. Many factors are con-
tributory, and the implications for atherosclerosis are substantial. Several of the
hyperlipemias are related to molecular abnormalities in (apo)lipoproteins, which are
important components of the lipoprotein particles responsible for circulating lipids,
their metabolic targeting, and ultimate clearance and metabolism. This section will
touch on two lipoprotein disorders in which well defined molecular abnormalities give
rise to significant lipid disorders.

8.1. Familial Hypercholesterolemia (FH) (42)

FH is an autosomal-dominant disorder related to a series of apoprotein B receptor
abnormalities. Homozygotes have serum cholesterol concentrations >700 mg/dL, multiple cutaneous and tendon xanthomas, and premature vascular disease often in childhood. Heterozygotes have serum cholesterol of 300–400 mg/dL, tendon xanthoma, and
coronary artery disease in their 30s–50s. Mutations occur in several domains of the low-
density lipoprotein (LDL) apolipoprotein B-100 (apo B-100) receptor located on chromosome 19 p13.1–p13.3. These interfere with clearance of the cholesterol rich LDL apo

B-100 particles, resulting in both failure of clearance of exogenous cholesterol and failure of downregulation of endogenous cholesterol synthesis. Pharmacologic therapy for heterozygotes includes reductase inhibitors, bile sequestrates, nicotinic acid, and diet. Therapy for homozygotes is much more complex and includes ileal bypass surgery, serum LDL apheresis, and liver transplantation. A second less frequent abnormality in apo B-100 itself as opposed to the B-100 receptor produces a similar clinical picture.

Class 1 mutations or null alleles result in absence of the LDL B-100 receptor protein. These consist of multiple stop codons or small deletions, resulting in frameshift mutations and occasional upstream promotor defects. Class 2 mutations or transport-deficient alleles result in defective transport of mutant LDL receptor protein from endoplasmic reticulum (ER) to Golgi site for glycosylation and secretion. Class 3 mutations or binding-deficient alleles result in a mutant LDL receptor that does not bind apo B-100. Class 4 mutations are characterized by internalization defects, which result in defective receptor transport to the cell surface. The receptor binds normally, but fails to localize in coated pits and thus to internalize. In class 5 mutations, the defective receptor–B-100 complex internalizes normally but fails to dissociate in the endosome. The apo B-100 defect is related to a G → A mutation in the B-100 apoprotein, leading to Glu → Arg mutation at amino acid 3500.

8.2. Familial Dyslipidemia, Type III Hyperlipidemia (43)

Atherosclerosis, tendon, and palmar xanthoma secondary to heritable apolipoprotein E polymorphism are characteristic of Type III hyperlipidemia. Elevated serum cholesterol and triglycerides related to remnant triglyceride-rich chylomicra and hepatic very low density lipoprotein (VLDL) particles are among the laboratory findings. Apolipoprotein E (apo E) is a ligand for hepatic clearance by both apo E and apo B-100 receptors. The E3/E3 is the most common phenotype in the population. The E2/E2 results in Type III hyperlipemia, although the gene frequency of 1% suggests that factors in addition to the molecular abnormality are necessary to produce clinical dyslipidemia. Therapy includes diet, nicotinic acid, and fibric acid derivatives (gemfibrozil, clofibrate) to decrease hepatic production of VLDL precursors. There is additional recent interest in the E4/E4 phenotype associated with Alzheimer's disease as a result of increased membrane transport of amyloid-β protein leading to earlier onset of Alzheimer's disease in both sporadic and familial cases.

Three alleles of apo E, E2, E3, and E4 give rise to six phenotypes (E-4/4, E-3/3, E-2/2, E-4/3, E-3/2, E4/2)1. Additional variability occurs related to variable sialylation of apoproteins. The genetic variability is related to the Cys → Arg 112 and Cys → Arg 158 (E2 Cys/Cys, E3 Cys/Arg, E4 Arg/Arg) amino acids.

8.3. Apo C-II Abnormality (43)

Apo C-II, an apolipoprotein that is required for activation of lipoprotein lipase, is required for triglyceride clearance from dietary chylomicra and endogenous VLDL. Patients who are homozygous for an apo C-II abnormality present at an early age with recurrent abdominal pain, eruptive xanthoma, hepatospleomegaly, and profound hypertriglyceridemia. The molecular defects that lead to apo C-II deficiency include missense mutations and amino acid substitutions, donor splice site mutations, and premature stop codons, which prematurely terminate C II synthesis.

9. DIABETES MELLITUS

Diabetes mellitus represents a group of disorders characterized by and sharing hyperglycemia. Approximately 10% of patients have Type I, insulin-dependent diabetes mellitus (IDDM), an autoimmune disorder characterized by progressive loss of pancreatic islet cells and insulin secretion. The majority of the remainder have Type II, noninsulin-dependent diabetes (NIDDM), a more complex disorder with elements of both relative insulin secretory failure as well as cellular resistance to insulin action. A few patients have defined molecular abnormalities leading to diabetes mellitus. Although few in number these patients are quite instructive.

9.1. Diabetes Mellitus, Secondary to Mitochondrial DNA Abnormality (44)

This rare disorder includes hyperglycemia, sensorineural hearing loss, and maternal transmission as a result of mitochondrial DNA as opposed to nuclear DNA abnormality. Clinically the diabetes may be either IDDM or NIDDM. The syndrome mitochondrial myopathy-encephalopathy-lactic acidosis-stroke (MELAS) and ophthalmoplegia, which is common in related mitochondrial disorders, is not seen in patients with this disorder. There is a heteroplasmic A $\rightarrow$ G point mutation in the tRNA gene at nucleotide 3243 in mitochondrial, as opposed to nuclear DNA. Mitochondrial DNA is exposed to a high concentration of oxygen-free radicals generated by oxidative phosphorylation, mutates at 10 times the rate of nuclear DNA, has no introns, and has neither protective histones nor an effective repair system. Insulin replacement therapy is usually necessary to correct the hyperglycemia.

9.2. Maturity-Onset Diabetes of the Young (MODY) (45)

MODY refers to an autosomal-dominant inheritance of Type II NIDDM in a younger population than the typically over age 40 NIDDM population. Clinical onset of hyperglycemia occurs in the second decade. Treatment requires control of hyperglycemia by diet and sulfonylurea therapy. Insulin therapy is usually not necessary, in contrast to the more frequent IDDM at this age. Multiple mutations of the glucokinase gene on chromosome 7, including stop mutations *(3)*, missense mutations leading to amino acid substitutions *(10)* and altered RNA processing *(3)*, have been identified.

9.3. Diabetes Mellitus, Glycogen Synthetase Deficiency (46)

Patients with IDDM, decreased skeletal muscle glycogen content, and decreased glycogen synthetase activity on muscle biopsy respond to conventional therapy for NIDDM. Unknown decrease in glycogen synthetase gene activity is located on chromosome 19 q13.3. The coding region is normal, suggesting a possible decrease in promoter region activity.

9.4. Diabetes Mellitus Secondary to Insulin Receptor Abnormalities (47)

Clinical manifestations include hyperglycemia, insulin resistance with or without phenotypic abnormalities including acanthosis nigricans, polycystic ovary syndrome, connective tissue disorders, and leprechanism. Insulin resistance is secondary to insulin receptor mutations. There is both clinical hyperglycemia and variable insulin resistance to administered insulin, which at times can be extreme. Multiple mutations of the insulin receptor gene have been identified. Loss of the receptor owing to major deletions or stop mutations *(6)*, delayed receptor transport to surface *(3)*, defective insulin binding *(4)*, defective internalization of insulin/insulin receptor complex, defective recycling of insulin receptor to plasma membrane *(1)*, and defective tyrosine kinase and signaling *(4)* have all been described.

9.5. IDDM Secondary to Mutant Insulin Biosynthesis (48)

This is characterized by elevated serum insulin levels as measured by RIA, secondary to several mutant insulin molecules with decreased biologic activity. These mutants include insulins Chicago, Los Angeles, and Wakayama as well as hyperproinsulinemia. There is a resultant hyperglycemia despite hyperinsulinemia as measured by RIA. Hyperglycemia responds readily to exogenous (nonmutant) insulin. Insulin Chicago results from a C → G leading to Leu 25 → Phe substitution in the β chain of human insulin. Insulin Los Angeles results in a Phe 25 → Leu substitution in the β chain. Insulin Wakayama results in a Val 3 → Leu substitution. Hyperproinsulinemia has an Arg 65 → His substitution preventing processing of proinsulin to insulin and C peptide.

9.6. Familial Persistent Hyperinsulinemic Hypoglycemia of Infancy (49)

This syndrome is characterized by neonatal hypoglycemia and hyperinsulinism in the setting of an autosomal-recessive family history of hypoglycemia. Therapy is supportive for hypoglycemia followed by definitive subtotal pancreatectomy. A loss of function mutation in the NBF-2 region of the sulfonylurea receptor gene, analogous to the cystic fibrosis transmembrane regulator (CFTR), leads to persistent insulin secretion despite hypoglycemia. The sulfonylurea receptor gene located on chromosome 11p14–15.1 is a putative subunit of the β cell ATPase potassium channel. Mutations of a 3'-splice site preceding the second nuclear binding fold region, NBF-2, results from a G → A mutation with subsequent 7-, 20-, and 30-bp deletions. Potassium channel activity is decreased, leading to membrane depolarization, the opening of voltage-dependent calcium channels, and increased insulin secretion.

10. OBESITY *(50–52)*

Obesity is a common, multifactorial disorder in developed societies characterized by increased adipose tissue stores. As a result of the increase in body fat stores, there is secondary hyperinsulinemia and often hyperglycemia. Family histories, including twin studies, indicate a strong genetic component to obesity. There has been recent focus on an ob gene product (leptin) identified in normal mice, which is mutated in the ob/ob genetically obese mouse, and a second db/db heritable strain of diabetic obese mice in which the ob gene product is intact, but the ob receptor is deficient. In common obesity in humans, as in the db/db mouse, there is increased circulating leptin produced by adipose tissue. The full clinical significance of this finding is indeterminate at present. The ob/ob gene product, leptin, has been cloned and is under intensive clinical and laboratory evaluation. In both normal and ob/ob mice who are administered the ob gene product, there is decreased calorie intake, increased activity with resultant caloric utilization, and weight loss. In the ob receptor deficient db/db mouse leptin administration has no effect. Clinical trials in humans have just begun.

The β₃-adrenergic receptor is selectively expressed in brown fat, and activation of this receptor increases metabolic rate. A relatively common polymorphism of this receptor has been associated with earlier onset of NIDDM, decreased metabolic rate, obesity, and insulin resistance.

In normal mice, there is a 650-kb DNA sequence on chromosome 6 coding for a 167 amino acid gene product, which is deleted in the genetically obese ob/ob mouse. The comparable human gene is 84% homologous with the mouse ob/ob gene product. The polymorphism of the β_3-adrenergic receptor codes for an arginine in place of a tryptophan at amino acid 64 of this receptor. This can be identified relatively simply by restriction enzyme analysis.

11. CURRENT CLINICAL APPLICATIONS

Most assays for DNA abnormalities remain experimental. They have not been pursued by commercial laboratories for three reasons. The disorders are very rare, identification of the gene abnormality has limited clinical utility, and the gene abnormalities are difficult to identify. Certain disorders represent exceptions and as such are available through commercial laboratories. These include assays of the RET proto-oncogene in multiple endocrine neoplasia type 2A (MEN 2A) and multiple endocrine neoplasia type 2B (MEN 2B), and disorders of apolipoprotein E. The 21-hydroxylase deficiency has been discussed under adrenal disorders. Although the assays remain experimental, an important therapeutic intervention was discussed to prevent virilization of affected newborns. Not discussed here is the classic karyotype analysis, which represents one of the first clinically useful DNA analysis procedures and remains clinically useful. The clinician can often gain access to experimental assays by contacting the appropriate research laboratories. Many of these laboratories are registered with Helix (Seattle, WA, 206-528-2689), which is a national directory of DNA diagnostic laboratories. Helix can provide the names of research laboratories investigating specific disorders.

11.1. MEN 2A and 2B (53)

MEN 2A is an autosomal-dominant disorder characterized by medullary thyroid carcinoma (MTC), bilateral pheochromocytoma, and hyperparathyroidism. The penetrance of MTC is nearly 100% by age 45, but the penetrance of the other manifestations is more variable. Some families may manifest only MTC (fMTC). MEN 2B is characterized by MTC, bilateral pheochromocytoma, marfanoid habitus, mucosal neuromas, and intestinal ganglioneuromatosis. Again MTC is the most common neoplasm.

Both disorders are caused by localized activating mutations of the RET proto-oncogene. Activation of this proto-oncogene gives the cells of affected tissues a greater than normal capacity for cell division. Increased cell division is seen as pathologically as hyperplasia, and gives rise to a greater opportunity for replication errors in other proto-oncogenes and suppressor genes. When enough changes have occurred, a neoplasm develops. The RET proto-oncogene is a tyrosine kinase with extracellular, transmembrane, and intracellular domains (Fig. 1).

Both disorders are identified by the presence of the indicated endocrine tumors in members of a kindred. Hyperparathyroidism is diagnosed by a high serum calcium and high plasma parathyroid hormone concentration. Pheochromocytoma is most frequently diagnosed by the presence of elevated urinary catecholamine metabolites. MTC is diagnosed by elevated basal or stimulated serum calcitonin concentrations.

RET
Proto-Oncogene

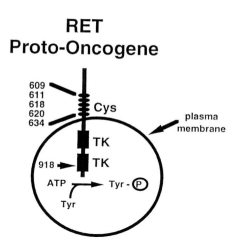

Fig. 1. RET proto-oncogene. A schematic representation of the RET proto-oncogene is shown. This protein resembles tyrosine kinase transmembrane receptors. The majority of the mutations that cause MEN 2A are located at cysteine residues in the extracellular domain near the transmembrane domain. Mutations that cause MEN 2B are in the second tyrosine kinase domain at amino acid residue 918.

About 95% of both MEN 2A and fMTC are caused by germline missense mutations of the RET proto-oncogene at cysteine residues at the following positions: 609, 611, 618, 620, or 634. The first four residues are in exon 10, and residue 634 is in exon 11. In the protein these positions are all in the extracellular domain just adjacent to the transmembrane domain. There seems to be no difference in the mutations leading to MEN 2A and fMTC. In over 90% of cases, MEN 2B is caused by germline mutations, which predict the substitution of a threonine for a methionine at amino acid residue 918 (exon 16), which is located in the putative second tyrosine kinase domain. Since most of the mutations causing these disorders are within a limited region of the molecule, DNA analysis to predict affected individuals is relatively straightforward. The mutation is identified in an affected individual, and a restriction enzyme assay is developed to screen other family members at risk. An example of this analysis from the authors' laboratory is shown in Figs. 2 and 3. A clinically related syndrome of Familial Pheochromocytoma is related to mutations in the von Hippel Lindau gene located on chromosome 3p25–26, not to RET proto-oncogene abnormality *(54)*. The DNA sequence that predicts the substitution of Trp for Cys at amino acid 934 of the RET proto-oncogene is shown in Fig. 2. Figure 3 shows the design of a restriction enzyme analysis for this mutation, which was then used to screen family members. The use of a nearby restriction site that is present in both the wild-type and mutant sequence acts as an internal control. Similar assays are now available in a number of commercial laboratories. Identification of both affected and unaffected family members carries important clinical implications. Those who are unaffected need not undergo routine screening for the development of endocrine neoplasms, and they can be reassured that they will not pass the disorder on to their children. For those that are affected, it is often recommended that total thyroidectomy

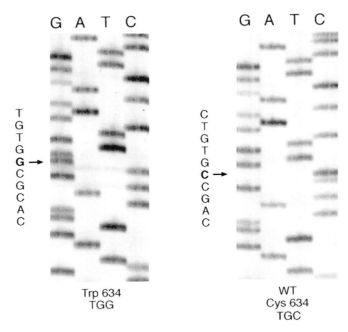

Fig. 2. RET proto-oncogene mutation. This autoradiograph of a DNA sequencing gel shows the region of a C to G substitution in genomic DNA from a subject who is part of a kindred with MEN 2A. The subject is heterozygous for this mutation, which predicts the substitution of a Trp for Cys at position 634 of the RET proto-oncogene.

PCR Template: Genomic DNA from blood
PCR product: 209 bp
Restriction Enzyme: Hha1
Wild Type sequence: 185 bp
Mutant sequence: 129 bp
Heterozygote: 129 bp and 185 bp

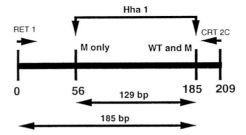

Fig. 3. Restriction enzyme analysis of a RET proto-oncogene mutation. This diagram describes a restriction enzyme analysis that is used to screen family members of the patient described in Fig. 2 for that family's mutation of the RET proto-oncogene.

be performed when the subject is still a child to prevent development of MTC. These individuals must be screened routinely for the development of the other indicated endocrine neoplasm.

ACKNOWLEDGMENTS

C. D. M. is supported by the General Clinical Research Center Grant (NIH 1Mo1RR06192), by NIH Grant R29 DK-42840, and by a grant from the Donaghue Foundation (Hartford, CT).

REFERENCES

1. Rugarli, M. O. and Ballabio, A. Kallman syndrome. From genetics to neurobiology. *JAMA* **270**:2713–2716, 1993.
2. Miller, W. Editorial: molecular genetics of familial central diabetes insipidus. *J. Clin. Endocrinol. Metab.* **77**:592–594, 1993.
3. Rosenthal, W., Seibold, A., Antaramian, A., Lonergan, M., Arthus, M. F., Hendy, G. N., Birnbaumer, M., and Bichet, D. G. Molecular identification of the gene responsible for congenital nephrogenic diabetes insipidus. *Nature* **359**:233–235, 1992.
4. Cogan, J. D., Phillips, J. A., Schenkman, S. S., Milner, R. D., and Sakati, N. Familial growth hormone deficiency: a model of dominant and recessive mutations affecting a monomeric protein. *J. Clin. Endocrinol. Metab.* **79**:1261–1265, 1994.
5. Haugen, B. and Ridgway, E. C. Transcription factor Pit-1 and its clinical implications: from bench to bedside. *Endocrinologist* **5**:132–139, 1995.
6. Amselem, S., Duquesnoy, P., and Goossens, M. Molecular basis of Laron's dwarfism. *Trends Endocr. Metab.* **2**:35–40, 1991.
7. Goddard, A. D., Covello, R. C., Louh, S., Clakson, T., Attie, K. M., Gesundheit, N., Rundle, A., Wells, J. A., and Carlsson, L. M. Mutations of the growth hormone receptor in children with idiopathic short stature. *New Engl. J. Med.* **333**:1093–1098, 1995.
8. Merimee, T. J., Baumann, G., and Daughaday, W. H. Growth hormone binding proteins, II: studies in pygmies and normal statured subjects. *J. Clin. Endocrinol. Metab.* **71**:1183–1188, 1990.
9. Landis, C. A. GTPase inhibiting mutations activate the a chain of Gs and stimulate adenylyl cyclase in human pituitary tumors. *Nature* **340**:692–696, 1989.
10. Rousseau, F., Bonaventure, J., Legeai-Mallet, L., Pelet, A., Rozet, J. M., Maroteaux, P., LeMerer, M., and Munnich, A. Mutations in the gene encoding fibroblast growth factor receptor-3 in achondroplasia. *Nature* **371**:252–254, 1994.
11. Kopp, P., van Sande, J., Parma, J., Duprez, L., Gerber, H., Joss, E., Jameson, J. L., Dumont, J. E., Vassart, G. Congenital hyperthyroidism caused by a mutation in the thyrotropin-receptor gene. *New Engl. J. Med.* **331**:150–154, 1995.
12. Sunthornthevarakul, T., Gottschalk, M., Hayashi, Y., and Refetoff, S. Brief report: resistance to thyrotropin caused by mutations in the thyrotropin-receptor gene. *New Engl. J. Med.* **332**:155–160, 1995.
13. Usala, S. and Weintraub, B. Thyroid hormone resistance syndromes. *Trends Endocr. Metab.* **2**:140–44, 1991.
14. Refetoff, S., Weiss, R. E., and Usala, S. J. The syndromes of resistance to thyroid hormone. *Endocr. Rev.* **14**:284–335, 1993.
15. Farid, N. R., Shi, Y., and Zou, M. Molecular basis of thyroid cancer. *Endocr. Rev.* **15**:202–232, 1994.
16. Arnold, A. Molecular genetics of parathyroid gland neoplasia. *J. Clin. Endocrinol. Metab.* **77**:1108–1111, 1993.
17. Schipani, E., Kruse, K., and Juppner, H. A constitutively active mutant PTH-PTHrP receptor in Jansen-type metaphyseal chondrodysplasia. *Science* **268**:98–100, 1995.
18. Brown, E. M., Pollak, M., Seidman, C., Seidman, J. G., Chou, Y. W., Riccardi, D., and Hebert, S. C. Calcium-ion sensing cell-surface receptors. *New Engl. J. Med.* **333**:234–240, 1995.

19. Jalal, S. M., Crifasi, P. A., Karnes, P. S., and Michels, W. Cytogenetic testing for Williams syndrome. *Mayo Clin. Proc.* **71:**67,68.

20. Driscoll, D. A., Budark, M. L., and Emanuel, B. S. A genetic etiology for Di-George syndrome: consistent deletions and microdeletions of 22ql 1. *Am. J. Hum. Genet.* **50:**924–933, 1992.

21. Larson, C., Shepherd, J., Nakamura, Y., Blomberg, C., Weber, G., Werelius, B., Hayward, N., The, B., Tokino, T., Seizinger, B., Skogseid, B., Oberg, K., and Nordenskjold, M. Predictive testing for multiple endocrine n. eoplasia type 1 using DNA polymorphisms. *J. Clin. Invest.* **89:**1344–1349, 1992.

22. Levine, M. A., Vechio, J. D., and Miric, A. Heterogeneous mutations in the gene encoding the α-subunit of the stimulatory G protein of adenylyl cyclase in Albright hereditary osteodystrophy. *J. Clin. Endocrinol. Metab.* **76:**1560–1568, 1993.

23. Clapham, D. E. Signal transduction. Why testicles are cool. *Nature* **371:**109,110, 1994.

24. Hughes, M., Malloy, P., Kieback, D., Kesterson, R. Pike, J., Feldman, D., and O'Malley, B. Point mutations in the human vitamin D receptor gene associated with hypocalcemic rickets. *Science* **242:**1702–1705, 1988.

25. Weber, A., Toppari, R. D., Harvey, R. C., Klan, C., Shaw, N., Ricker, A. T., Nanto-Salonen, A. T., Vevan, J. S., and Clark, A. J. L. Adrenocorticotropin receptor gene mutations in familial glucocorticoid deficiency: relationships with clinical features in four families. *J. Clin. Endocrinol. Metab.* **80:**65–71, 1995.

26. Yanase, T., Simpson, E. R., and Waterman, M. R. 17α-Hydroxylase/17,20 lyase deficiency: from clinical investigation to molecular definition. *Endocr. Rev.* **12:**91–104, 1992.

27. Mebarki, F., Sanchez, R., Rheaume, E., Laflamme, N., Simard, J., Forest, M. G., Bey-Omar, F., David, M., Labrie, F., and Morel, Y. Nonsalt-losing male pseudo-hermaphroditism due to the novel homozygous N100S mutation in the type II 3b-hydroxysteroid dehydrogenase gene. *J. Clin. Endocrinol. Metab.* **80:**2127–2134, 1995.

28. Mercado, A. B., Wilson, R. C., Cheng, K. C., Wei, J. Q., and New, M. I. Prenatal treatment and diagnosis of congenital adrenal hyperplasia owing to steroid 21-hydroxylase deficiency. *J. Clin. Endocrinol. Metab.* **80:**2014–2020, 1995.

29. White, P. C., Curnow, K. M., and Pascoe, L. Disorders of steroid 1 1β-hydroxylase isozymes. *Endocr. Rev.* 15: 421–438, 1994.

30. Malchoff, D. M., Brufsky, A., Reardon, G., McDermott, P., Javier, E. C., Bergh, C. H., Rowe, D., and Malchoff, C. D. A point mutation of the human glucocorticoid receptor in primary cortisol resistance. *J. Clin. Invest.* **91:**1918–1925, 1993.

31. Karl, M., Lamberts, S. W. J., Detera-Wadleigh, S. D., Encio, I. J., Stratakis, C. A., Hurley, D. M., Accili, D., and Chrousos, G. P. Familial glucocorticoid resistance caused by a splice site deletion in the human glucocorticoid receptor gene. *J. Clin. Endocrinol. Metab.* **76:**683–689, 1993.

32. Stewart, P. M., Murry, B. A., and Mason, J. I. Human kidney 1 1β-hydroxysteroid dehydrogenase is a high affinity nicotinamide adenine dinucleotide-dependent enzyme and differs from the cloned type I isoform. *J. Clin. Endocrinol. Metab.* **79:**480–484, 1994.

33. Shimkets, R. A., Warnock, D. G., Bositis, C. M., Nelson-Williams, C., Hansson, J. H., Schambelan, M., Gill, J. R., Ulick, S., Milora, R. V., Findling, J. W., Canessa, C. M., Rossier, C. B., and Lifton, R. P. Liddle's syndrome: heritable human hypertension caused by mutations in the β subunit of the epithelial sodium channel. *Cell* **79:**407–414, 1994.

34. McPhaul, M. J., Marcelli, M., Zoppi, S., Griffin, J. E., and Wilson, J. D. The spectrum of mutations in the androgen receptor gene that causes androgen resistance. *J. Clin. Endocrinol. Metab.* **76:**17–23, 1993.

35. Smith, E. P., Boyd, J., Frank, G. R., Takahashi, H., Cohen, R., Lubahn, D. B., and Korach, K. S. Estrogen resistance caused by a mutation in the estrogen-receptor gene in a man. *New Engl. J. Med.* **331:**1056–1061, 1994.

36. Homaki, A. H., Dieguez Lucena, J. L., Pakarinen, P., Sistonen, P., Tapanaienen, J., Gromoll, J., Laskikari, R., Sankila, E. M., Lehvaslaiho, H., Engel, A. R., Nieschlag, E., Huhtaniemi, I., and de La Chapelle, A. Mutation of the follicle-stimulating hormone receptor gene causes hereditary hypergonadotropic ovarian failure. *Cell* **82:**959–968, 1995.

37. Shenker, A., Laue, L., Kosugi, S., Merendino, J. J., Minegishi, T., and Cutler, G. B. A constitutively activating mutation of the luteinizing hormone receptor in familial male precocious puberty. *Nature* **365:**652–654, 1993.

38. Jager, R. J., Anvret, M., Hall, K., and Scherer, G. A human XY female with a frame shift mutation in the candidate testis-determining gene SRY. *Nature* **348:**352–354, 1990.

39. Berta, P., Hawkins, J. R., Sinclair, A. H., Taylor, A., Griffiths, B. L., Goodfellow, P. N., and Fellous, M. Genetic evidence equating SRY and the testis-determining factor. *Nature* **348:**448–450, 1990.

40. Weinstein, L., Shenker, A., Gejman, P., Merino, M., Friedman, E., and Spiegel, A. Activating mutations of the stimulatory G protein in the McCune-Albright syndrome. *New Engl. J. Med.* **325:**1688–1695.

41. Malchoff, C. D., Reardon, G., MacGillivray, D., Yamase, H., Rogol, A. D., and Malchoff, D. M. An unusual presentation of McCune-Albright syndrome confirmed by an activating mutation of the $G_s\alpha$-subunit from a bone lesion. *J. Clin. Endocrinol. Metab.* **78:**803–806, 1994.

42. Goldstein, J. L. and Brown, M. S. Familial hypercholesterolemia, in *The Molecular Basis of Inherited Disease*, 6th ed., McGraw Hill, New York, pp. 1215–1250, 1989.

43. Brewer, H. B., Santamarina-Fojo, S., and Hoeg, J. M. Genetic defects in the human plasma apolipoproteins. *Atherosclerosis Rev.* **20:**51–60, 1992.

44. Johns, D. R. Mitochondrial DNA and disease. *New Engl. J. Med.* **333:**638–644, 1995.

45. Frougel, P., Zouali, H., Vionnet, N., Velho, G., Vaxillaire, M., Sun, F., Lesage, S., Stoffel, M., Takeda, J., and Passa P. Familial hyperglycemia due to mutations in glucokinase *New Engl. J. Med.* **328:**697–702, 1993.

46. Vestergaard, H., Bjorbaek, C., Andersen, P. H., Bak, J. F., and Pedersen, O. Impaired expression of glycogen synthetase mRNA in skeletal muscle of NIDDM patients. *Diabetes* **40:**1740–1745, 1991.

47. Bell, G. Molecular defects in diabetes mellitus. *Diabetes* **40:**413–421, 1991.

48. Simon, C., Kwok, M., Steiner, D., Rubenstein, A., and Tager, H. S. Identification of a point mutation in the human insulin gene giving rise to a structurally abnormal insulin (Insulin Chicago). *Diabetes* **32:**872–875, 1983.

49. Thomas, P. M., Cote, G. J., Wohllk, N., Efaddad, B., Mathew, P. M., Rabl, W., Aguilar-Bryan, L., Gagel, R. F., and Bryan, J. Mutations in the sulfonylurea gene in persistent hypoglycemia of infancy. *Science* **268:**426–428, 1995.

50. Pellymounter, M. A., Cullen, M. J., et al. Effects of the obese gene product on body weight regulation in ob/ob mice. *Science* **269:**540–543, 1995.

51. Rohner-Jeanrenaud, F. and Jeanrenaud, B. Obesity, leptin, and the brain. *New Engl. J. Med.* **334:**324,325.

52. Arner, P. The β_3-adrenergic receptor—a cause and cure of obesity. *New Engl. J. Med.* **333:**382,383, 1995.

53. Mulligan, L. M. and Ponder, B. A. J. Multiple endocrine neoplasia Type 2. *J. Clin. Endocrinol. Metab.* **80:**1989–1995, 1995.

54. Ritter, M. M., Frilling, P. A., Crossey, A., Höppner, W., Maher, E. R., Mulligan, L., Ponder, B. A. J., and Engelhardt, D. Isolated familial pheochromocytoma as a variant of von Hippel-Lindau disease. *J. Clin. Endocrinol. Metab.* **81:**1035–1037, 1996.

Molecular Pathogenesis of Cardiovascular Disease

John H. Contois and Juch Chin Huang

1. INTRODUCTION

Cardiovascular disease (CVD) is a major public health problem in many societies. Several types of CVD have a genetic basis or at least a genetic component. It has been estimated that about 50% of the variability of the major risk factors for coronary artery disease (CAD) is genetic. Environmental factors, such as diet, also influence CVD, and may in fact interact with genetic factors to modulate risk. The genes encoding the majority of structural and enzymatic proteins involved in lipid and lipoprotein metabolism have been cloned and characterized, permitting the use of molecular biology techniques to further our understanding of lipid and lipoprotein disorders. Coagulation factors have been implicated in thrombosis and thrombolysis, and a number of mutations and polymorphisms have been described that predispose to vascular disease. The focus of this chapter is to discuss these genetic factors related to atherosclerosis and hemostasis. The laboratory currently plays an important role in the battle against CVD by providing accurate and reliable measurement of lipids, lipoprotein cholesterols, and coagulation factors. With these important new discoveries, it is evident that the laboratory of the future will play a major role in screening, diagnosis, and treatment of familial lipoprotein abnormalities and CVD.

Very few phenotypes related to CVD are entirely determined by a single genetic locus. These monogenic disorders are diseases caused by a single mutant gene and show simple Mendelian patterns of inheritance. The basic biochemical lesions in monogenic disorders related to CVD involve defects in enzymes, receptors, transport proteins, and coagulation factors. The overall population frequency of monogenic disorders is about 10/1000 live births. Interestingly, the most common monogenic disorder (affecting about 1 in 500 individuals) is a defect affecting cholesterol metabolism, familial hypercholesterolemia (FH) *(1)*.

CVD is usually not monogenic, but polygenic and multifactorial. A multifactorial etiology implies the interaction of multiple genes with multiple environmental factors. Some genes act in a cumulative fashion. Individuals with a particular combination of genes acting in concert with environmental factors may or may not express a certain phenotype. Although atherosclerosis and CVD are largely multifactorial, a small percentage of cases are in fact the result of a monogenic component. About 5% of subjects suffering a premature myocardial infarction are heterozygotes for FH, a single-gene

From: Molecular Diagnostics: For the Clinical Laboratorian
Edited by: W. B. Coleman and G. J. Tsongalis Humana Press Inc., Totowa, NJ

Table 1
Major CAD Risk Factors as Identified
by the NCEP Adult Treatment Panel II LDL-C

160 mg/dL (4.2 mmol/L)
HDL-C <35 mg/dL (0.9 mmol/L)
Hypertension
Cigaret smoking
Diabetes
Family history of MI or sudden death prior to 55 yr of age in a male parent
    or sibling and prior to 65 yr of age in a female parent or sibling
Male 45 yr of age
Female 55 yr of age or postmenopausal
Subtract one risk factor if HDL-C [3]60 mg/dL (1.6 mmol/L)

Table 2
Potential Lipid and Lipoprotein Markers for CAD

Elevated triglycerides
Elevated total cholesterol/HDL cholesterol ratio
Elevated apo B/apo A-I ratio
Elevated non-HDL cholesterol
Elevated VLDL cholesterol/plasma triglyceride ratio
Elevated apo B
Elevated lipoprotein(a)
Decreased LDL particle size (pattern B)
Susceptibility of LDL particles to oxidation
Decreased apo A-I
Decreased HDL_2 cholesterol
Decreased LpA-I (HDL particles that contain apo A-I and not apo A-II)
Decreased HDL particle size

disorder affecting binding of low-density lipoprotein (LDL) to the LDL receptor and producing atherosclerosis. However, even in a single-gene disorder, other genetic loci and environmental factors, such as diet, can influence phenotypic expression. The molecular basis of many disorders related to CVD is unclear at present, and this remains an important area for clinical research.

CAD is the predominant form of CVD, and is, in fact, the most common cause of death in both men and women in the United States. Accepted and potential CAD risk factors are listed in Tables 1 and 2, respectively. Atherosclerosis is the underlying condition associated with CAD, stroke, and peripheral vascular disease, but thrombosis appears to be the precipitating event causing acute myocardial infarction (AMI). Atherosclerosis is a progressive disease of the large arteries that begins with the accumulation of cholesterol-laden foam cells and leads to increasingly complex lesions, which can reduce blood flow to major organs. As a consequence of atherosclerosis and thrombosis, 1.5 million Americans suffer an AMI every year, and more than half of these patients will die. The remainder will suffer the debilitating effects of cardiac damage, including tachycardias, cardiogenic shock, reinfarction, heart failure, and sudden cardiac death. Two out of every three AMI survivors

Table 3
Potentially Important Mutations for CAD and MI

Key enzymes and transfer proteins
    Lipoprotein lipase (LL)
    Hepatic lipase (HL)
    Lecithin:cholesterol acyl transferase (LCAT)
    Cholesterol ester transfer protein (CETP)
Lipoprotein receptors
    LDL (apoB/E) receptor
Apolipoproteins

Apo A-I	Apo A-II
Apo B-48	Apo A-IV
Apo B-100	Apo D
Apo C-II	Apo E
Apo C-III	Apo(a)

Hemostasis and coagulation factors

Protein C	Factor VII
Protein S	Antithrombin
Fibrinogen	Heparin cofactor II
Factor V	Factor VIII

Plasminogen activator inhibitor

Table 4
Monogenic Disorders of Plasma Lipoproteins

Apo(a)	Familial lipoprotein(a) excess
Apo A-I	A-I Milano
	Tangier's disease
	Apo A-I deficiency
Apo B	Abetalipoproteinemia
	Familial hypobetalipoproteinemia
	Familial defective apo B-100
Apo C-II deficiency	Multiple mutants
Apo E	Multiple mutants
Enzymes	Lipoprotein lipase deficiency
	Lipoprotein lipase inhibition
	Hepatic lipase deficiency
	Lecithin:cholesterol acyl transferase deficiency
	Fish eye disease
Receptors	Familial hypercholesterolemia
Transfer proteins	Cholesterol ester transfer protein deficiency

will not make a complete recovery; one in five is disabled with heart failure *(2)*. Contrary to popular notion, about half (48%) of AMI cases occur in women.

Most cases of CAD are apparently the result of environmental factors, such as an atherogenic diet, but premature CAD and family history of cardiac death prior to age 65 indicate the presence of a genetic component *(see* Tables 3 and 4). It is clearly established that an elevated plasma cholesterol concentration predisposes an individual to an increased risk of CAD. Lipoprotein metabolism is quite complex, and lipoprotein disorders are related to a variety of factors, including (apo)lipoprotein gene mutations, enzyme activity involved in lipid transport, and lipoprotein receptor binding defects.

2. LIPOPROTEINS

Lipoproteins are specialized complexes that transport cholesterol, triglyceride (TG), and other lipids in the bloodstream. Different classes of lipoproteins share a number of features. They are typically spherical structures that contain varying amounts of lipid and protein, with a core that is predominantly composed of TG and cholesteryl esters (CE), and an outer shell made up of amphipathic lipids, such as phospolipids, free cholesterol, and proteins. These proteins are called apolipoproteins or apoproteins (apo). Lipoproteins have traditionally been classified on the basis of their buoyant density, which is dependent on the proportion of lipid in the lipoprotein. The least dense particles are chylomicrons (CM). CM are made up of TG formed by intestinal cells from dietary lipid sources. These are lipid-rich particles, as large as 1 μ in diameter. These particles are secreted into the lymphatics and enter the bloodstream through the thoracic duct, where they are rapidly catabolized by several tissues, including adipose tissue. The major enzyme involved in CM catabolism is lipoprotein lipase (LPL), an enzyme located on the endothelial surface, that hydrolyzes TG to its constituent fatty acids and other products. The major protein of CM is apo B-48. Without the synthesis of apo B-48 by intestinal cells, CM cannot be formed. The protein apo C-II is also required to activate LPL. CM may also contain apo A-IV, apo C-III, and apo E. Because of the activity of LPL, CM typically have a very short half-life. After the removal of significant amounts of TG through the action of LPL, CMs become smaller, denser particles referred to as CM remnants. The so-called remnant receptor or LDL receptor-related protein (LRP) recognizes apo E and removes these remnant particles from the circulation.

Very low density lipoprotein (VLDL) particles are similar to CM in that they contain predominantly TG. Although CM transports exogenous TG, VLDL transports endogenous TG synthesized and stored in the liver. Similar to CM, VLDLs undergo hydrolysis through the action of LPL into smaller, less dense remnant particles. These remnant particles are further metabolized into LDL or are cleared from the circulation via interaction with the LRP or LDL receptor.

LDL particles contain proportionately more cholesterol than TG and function to supply cholesterol to peripheral tissues. LDL uptake by tissues is mediated by interaction of LDL apo B with its specific cell-surface receptor, the LDL receptor.

High-density lipoproteins (HDLs) are the smallest, densest lipoproteins, and are involved in transport of cholesterol from peripheral tissue and endothelial cells back to the liver for reuse or excretion, so called reverse cholesterol transport. The packaging of cholesterol into the core of the HDL requires the activity of lecithin:cholesterol acyl transferase (LCAT) and an activator, such as apo A-I, or possibly apo A-II or apo A-IV. Exchange of CE and TG between VLDL or LDL and HDL may also help remove cholesterol from the circulation. This process is aided by cholesteryl ester transfer protein (CETP). The uptake of HDL and LDL by the liver appears to be supported by the activity of hepatic lipase (HL), which hydrolyzes CE, TG, and phospholipid. Apo E also appears to be involved in HDL removal by the liver.

Table 5
Hyperlipoproteinemias

Frederickson type	Common name	Known primary disorder
Type I	Chylomicronemia	Familial LPL deficiency apo C-II deficiency
Type IIa	Hypercholesterolemia (increased LDL) (LDL receptor)	Familial hypercholesterolemia Polygenic hypercholesterolemia
Type IIb	Combined hyperlipidemia (increased LDL and/or VLDL)	
Type III	Remnant hyperlipidemia (apo E defect)	Familial dysbetalipoproteinemia
Type IV	Endogenous hyperlipidemia (increased VLDL)	Familial hypertriglyceridemia
Type V	Mixed hyperlipidemia (increased CM and VLDL)	Familial hypertriglyceridemia, familial LPL deficiency apo C-II deficiency

Lipid disorders can be categorized a number of ways. Typically, classification involves cut points based on the concentrations of the major lipids, such as hypercholesterolemia only (240 mg/dL), mild hypertriglyceridemia (200–1000 mg/dL), severe hypertriglyceridemia (1000 mg/dL), and combined hypertriglyceridemia and hypercholesterolemia. These categories overlap with the Frederickson classifications (*see* Table 5). Hypercholesterolemia alone is generally the result of an elevated LDL cholesterol. Combined hypercholesterolemia and hypertriglyceridemia is often caused by elevated levels of VLDL and LDL (type IIb), increased VLDL alone (type IV), or increased CM and VLDL remnant particles (type III). Mild hypertriglyceridemia is generally owing to an increase in VLDL (type IV), whereas severe hypertriglyceridemia is often the result of increased CM alone (type I) or CM and VLDL (type V). Although lipoprotein phenotyping with the Frederickson classification system is useful in classifying lipoprotein abnormalities, a given phenotype does not necessarily correspond to a specific genetic disorder. As knowledge of the genetic basis of dyslipidemias progress, it is likely that lipid and lipoprotein disorders will be increasingly classified by their unique molecular defects.

3. FAMILIAL DISORDERS OF TRIGLYCERIDE METABOLISM

Clinicians usually classify hypertriglyceridemia as moderate or severe. Severe hypertriglyceridemia, classified on the basis of a fasting TG concentration of 1000 mg/dL (type I), is usually the result of CM, and patients with this disorder are at increased risk of pancreatitis. Endogenous hypertriglyceridemia (type IV) is frequently seen in patients with hypertriglyceridemia, but without LPL or apo C-II abnormalities. These patients appear to have increased VLDL production and frequently a defect in CM catabolism. This disorder generally occurs in adulthood, and frequently the patients are obese or diabetic. Elevated TG is clearly associated with CAD risk, but it is unclear whether this association is owing to the correlation of elevated TG with other lipoprotein abnormalities, including a decreased HDL cholesterol concentration. Specific disorders of TG metabolism, both rare and common, are discussed below.

3.1. LPL

LPL resides on the luminal surface of capillary endothelial cells and is responsible for the hydrolysis of di- and triglycerides in CM and VLDL. The human LPL gene has been extensively studied and characterized. It is a relatively large gene located on chromosome 8, and it is composed of 10 exons, which span approx 30 kb. It is expressed mainly in fat and muscle tissue. Numerous mutations at the LPL gene locus have been described. Inheritance of defective LPL genes is associated with severe hypertriglyceridemia (fasting chylomicronemia), pancreatitis, and lipid deposition in macrophages. Patients with LPL deficiency cannot catabolize CM and VLDL. Heterozygotes generally have half-normal LPL activity and moderately elevated serum TG, especially if secondary factors, such as obesity, diabetes, or lipid-increasing medication use, are also involved. Associated lipoprotein disorders may include low HDL cholesterol, cholesterol-enriched VLDL, and small, dense LDL. This disorder usually presents in children and young adults as recurrent abdominal pain and pancreatitis. In adulthood, the disorder is less severe, and is usually the result of partial LPL deficiency. The presentation in adulthood may include pancreatitis and vascular disease.

3.2. Apo C-II Deficiency

A defective apo C-II gene results in the functional equivalent of LPL deficiency, since apo C-II serves as a cofactor for LPL activity. In general, however, hypertriglyceridemia associated with apo C-II deficiency is less severe and occurs later in life. With both LPL and apo C-II deficiency, the accumulation of CM and VLDL occurs in conjunction with a decrease in LDL and HDL. The patient usually presents with type IV hyperlipoproteinemia (increased CM and VLDL).

3.3. Inhibitor of LPL Activity

A single family has been described with chylomicronemia and low postheparin LPL activity, but without any apparent LPL or apo C-II abnormality. The presence of an LPL inhibitor was discovered by adding the suspected plasma to a sample containing normal LPL with a resultant loss in LPL activity. This inhibitor was nondialyzable, heat-stable, sensitive to freeze/thawing, and not associated with plasma lipoproteins *(3)*.

3.4. Hepatic Lipase

HL catalyzes the hydrolysis of TG, phospholipid, and CE primarily in LDL and HDL, which presumably facilitates the uptake of these particles by the liver. HL deficiency usually manifests itself as type III hyperlipoproteinemia, but unlike typical type III HLP, VLDL are not cholesterol enriched and the VLDL cholesterol/plasma TG ratio is normal.

3.5. Familial Combined Hyperlipidemia (FCH) and Familial Hypertriglyceridemia (FHTG)

The vast majority of patients with hypertriglyceridemia do not have one of these relatively rare genetic disorders described above. Instead, they appear to have disorders of TG metabolism associated with more common genetic defects occurring with or without secondary abnormalities, such as obesity. Two genetic disorders, FHTG and FCH, are commonly seen in patients with chylomicronemia and/or endogenous hypertriglyceridemia.

Hypertriglyceridemia often occurs in conjunction with hypercholesterolemia. Often, type III hyperlipoproteinemia (type III HLP), an increase in β-VLDL is the underlying abnormality. The primary abnormality in these patients is typically a defect in apo E. This is discussed in more detail in Section 6. FCH is characterized by the finding of hypercholesterolemia and hypertriglyceridemia within the same kindred, with some members having one or the other or both abnormalities. FCH is present in about 10% of AMI survivors under age 60, using concentrations above the 95th percentile for total cholesterol (TC) and TG as criteria *(4)*. These patients have increased VLDL, LDL, or both, and may also have decreased HDL cholesterol levels as well. Unlike FH, FCH appears in only 10–20% of patients in childhood, and patients usually present with elevated TG and without xanthomas. The primary defect appears to be overproduction of apo B-100, but the molecular defect or defects have not yet been characterized. Secondary factors, such as obesity, hypertension, gout, and diabetes, also appear to contribute to the phenotypic expression of FCH. FCH is at least five times more prevalent than FH, affecting about 1% of the North American population, which makes FCH the most common metabolic cause of premature atherosclerosis.

FHTG is a relatively common disorder characterized by the presence of a fasting TG greater than the 90th percentile in at least two kindred members. It was estimated that 5–15% of CAD kindreds have this disorder *(4)*. Many members of these kindreds also have low HDL cholesterol levels, diabetes, obesity, insulin resistance, and hypertension. The primary genetic defect(s) is not known, but patients have increased hepatic TG secretion and enhanced HDL apo A-I catabolism.

4. FAMILIAL DISORDERS OF LDL METABOLISM

An LDL cholesterol concentration <130 mg/dL is considered desirable, and between 130 and 159 mg/dL borderline high risk for CAD. LDL cholesterol ≥160 mg/dL is considered a high-risk category. Greatly elevated LDL cholesterol levels and family history of elevated LDL cholesterol concentrations and/or history of premature CAD suggest a genetic abnormality. Elevated LDL cholesterol concentrations may involve defects in the LDL receptor or apo B genes.

The apo B gene, located on the short arm of chromosome 2, is 43 kb long with 28 introns and 29 exons. Apo B mRNA contains 14,112 nucleotides, including untranslated regions totaling 429 nucleotides. The protein itself is made up of 4536 amino acids with a mol wt of 513 kDa. A single apo B associates with a single lipoprotein particle. The primary sites of apo B synthesis are liver and intestine. Two forms of apo B exist. Posttranslational processing of the apo B mRNA accounts for the apo B-48 synthesized by the intestine. A C to T substitution at nucleotide 6666 inserts a stop codon into the intestinal apo B mRNA. The intestinal form of apo B, therefore, shares the same N-terminal sequence with the liver form, but is only 48% the size of the liver apo B protein.

The LDL receptor gene, located on the short arm of chromosome 19, spans 45 kb with 18 exons and 17 introns. The receptor binds two apolipoproteins, apo B-100 and apo E. As stated previously, mutations in the LDL receptor gene account for FH.

4.1. FH

Thanks to the pioneering research of Goldstein and Brown, we have a thorough understanding of the role of LDL receptors in normal cholesterol homeostasis and in FH *(5)*. Originally, the metabolic abnormality in FH patients was described as a delayed clearance of LDL apo B. Subsequently, various mutations have been described at the LDL receptor gene locus, which result in a lack of expression or expression of defective LDL receptors. To date, more than 30 separate mutations have been described. Additionally, some patients with phenotypic FH have a defect in the receptor binding domain of apo B. Clinically, the heterozygous FH patient typically presents with an LDL cholesterol concentration >250 mg/dL and xanthomas, but normal TG and HDL cholesterol levels. Individuals heterozygous for an LDL receptor mutation express half the normal number of LDL receptors on their cell surfaces, resulting in a reduced clearance of LDL particles and an increased serum LDL cholesterol concentration. This excess cholesterol deposits in tissues (forming xanthomas) and arterial wall (forming atherosclerotic plaques). The average age at onset of CAD in untreated heterozygous men and women is 45–55 yr. Individuals homozygous for an LDL receptor mutation are very rare (one person in a million), and have little or no functioning LDL receptors and markedly increased LDL cholesterol concentrations (600–1200 mg/dL). They frequently suffer an AMI before the age of 20.

4.2. Polygenic FH

Despite the relatively common prevalence of the FH mutation, only 3% of CAD patients are true FH heterozygotes with LDL receptor defects *(6)*. More commonly, patients present with xanthomas and elevated cholesterol concentrations owing to polygenic factors without any clear genetic defect. A great deal of research in the future will be directed toward delineating and sorting the genetic factors that contribute toward this familial disorder.

4.3. Familial Hyperapobetalipoproteinemia (FHB)

FHB is characterized by apo B concentrations above the 90th percentile in the absence of other lipid abnormalities in the kindred. Genest et al. found this disorder to be present in 5% of the CAD kindreds studied. These authors suggest that FHB is simply a variant of FCH *(6)*.

4.4. Abetalipoproteinemia

This rare disorder is characterized by fat malabsorption, acanthocytosis, anemia, retinopathy, and progressive neurological disease, and results from the absence of apo B-containing lipoproteins, including CM, VLDL, and LDL. Plasma levels of TG and cholesterol are dramatically decreased, and plasma TG fails to increase after ingestion of a fatty meal. Cholesterol delivery to peripheral tissues is apparently mediated by HDL particles containing apo E. However, the uptake of cholesterol by cells is insufficient to support steroid biosynthesis. The genetic defect has not yet been elucidated, but appears to involve microsomal triglyceride transfer protein (MTP) *(7)*. Recent studies have identified mutant alleles for MTP by restriction fragment length polymorphism (RFLP) and direct sequencing techniques in abetalipoproteinemic patients. The apo B gene is apparently normal, but lipoprotein secretion is inhibited.

4.5. Familial Hypobetalipoproteinemia

This disorder is characterized by abnormally low levels of cholesterol and apo B, but usually without the classical symptoms associated with abetalipoproteinemia. In the heterozygous state, total cholesterol concentration ranges from 40–180 mg/dL with a mean of 90 mg/dL; TG concentration is normal. Unlike abetalipoproteinemia, the ratio of free to esterified cholesterol is normal. It is likely that different mechanisms are responsible for phenotypic expression of hypobetalipoproteinemia in different kindreds. In many cases, hypobetalipoproteinemia is owing to various mutations in the apo B gene that result in a truncated form of the protein. Most of these mutations are single nucleotide deletions or transitions that introduce a premature stop codon *(7)*. Clinical manifestations range from essentially asymptomatic to severe. Severe hypobetalipoproteinemia may be clinically indistinguishable from abetalipoproteinemia. Apo B-37 is an example of a truncated apo B associated with low levels of LDL cholesterol, normal TG, and mild fat malabsorption. HDLs were noted to contain apo B. The defect results from a deletion in the apo B gene, which produces a premature stop codon *(8)*. Various other truncated forms of apo B have been reported that appear to influence both LDL and HDL cholesterol concentrations.

A specific hypobetalipoprotein disorder that results from the specific deletion of apo B-48 is known as CM retention disease. This disorder is associated with low plasma concentrations of LDL and HDL, fat malabsorption, growth retardation, and malnutrition. Some patients have acanthocytosis and neurological symptoms.

4.6. Familial Defective Apo B-100

Unlike the apo B mutations described above, familial defective apo B-100 is associated with an elevated LDL cholesterol concentration. The mutation is a single base transition that results in the substitution of glutamine for arginine at position 3500. This mutation occurs in the LDL receptor binding domain of the protein, and results in reduced binding of LDL to its receptor. Clinically, these patients are similar to FH heterozygotes, with elevated LDL cholesterol, xanthomas, and premature CAD.

4.7. LDL Particle Size

LDL particle size is another genetic factor of interest as a potential marker for CAD risk. Studies have shown that LDL size is heterogeneous and patients with CAD tend to have lower mol-wt particles than control subjects. At least seven discrete LDL size bands have been documented by electrophoresis, with most individuals having a single, dominant band (size) with smaller adjacent bands. Austin et al. have dichotomized LDL particle size electrophoretic patterns into pattern A (large LDL) and pattern B (small, dense LDL); pattern B LDL was associated with CAD *(9)*. LDL particle size pattern was highly heritable. LDL particle size is highly correlated with other lipid and nonlipid risk factors, including TG, and appears to be metabolically interrelated with other familial lipid disorders.

5. FAMILIAL DISORDERS OF HDL METABOLISM

A low HDL cholesterol concentration is considered a major risk factor for CAD, but relatively little is known about the genetic control of HDL cholesterol levels. Several inborn errors of metabolism affect HDL levels, including apo A-I deficiency, LCAT deficiency, and fish eye disease. Population studies suggest that about 50% of HDL cholesterol variability is genetic *(10)*. The genetic variability is largely polygenic. The common mutations affecting HDL cholesterol concentration have not yet been identified, although certain loci, including the apo A-I, apo C-III, apo A-IV, and LCAT genes, are candidates.

The apo A-I gene is 1863 bp long with three introns and four exons. The protein is synthesized as a preproprotein that undergoes intracellular cleavage to proapo A-I and extracellular hydrolysis to the mature protein with a mol wt of 28,000 Dalton. Apo A-I synthesis is essential for the formation of HDL particles. Certain mutations in the apo A-I gene have profound effects on HDL cholesterol levels and risk of CAD.

5.1. Apo A-I Deficiency

Apo A-I deficiency is a rare disorder involving at least three genetic loci. Two sisters were described with a deficiency of apo A-I and apo C-III, which are coded for by loci on the same gene complex. Both had barely detectable concentrations of HDL cholesterol and both developed atherosclerosis at a young age. An unrelated patient with a different mutation in the apo A-I/C-III gene complex (type 2) also had atherosclerosis and heart failure by age 45. An additional mutation (type 3) was detected in an individual with corneal clouding and premature CAD. All these patients had HDL cholesterol concentrations between 0 and 7 mg/dL and all had premature CAD. Type 1 apo A-I deficiency is caused by an inversion in the apo A-I/C-III gene complex; the genetic defect responsible for types 2 and 3 has not been elucidated.

5.2. Apo A-I Polymorphism

A number of apo A-I variants have been described based on isoelectric focusing techniques. With the exception of apo A-I$_{Milano}$, none has been consistently associated with alterations in HDL cholesterol concentrations. Apo A-I$_{Milano}$ was discovered in a large kindred from an Italian village and is characterized by a low HDL cholesterol concentration, but apparently no increased risk of atherosclerosis. The primary gene defect results in a cysteine for arginine substitution at amino acid 173, which changes the physical properties of an amphipathic, helical region involved in lipid binding.

5.3. Tangier Disease

Tangier disease is also a rare apo A-I deficiency state, but it differs from the others in certain respects. Clinically, the patients present with hyperplastic, orange tonsils, splenomegaly, and neuropathy. HDL are completely absent, and CM are present in fasting plasma. CE accumulate in tissues throughout the body. There does not appear to be a striking predisposition to premature vascular disease among these patients. The precise genetic defect is unknown, although it does involve the homozygous expression of mutant autosomal allele *(11)*.

5.4. Familial Hypoalphalipoproteinemia

The apo A-I deficiency states described above are rare, whereas familial hypoalphalipoproteinemia is common. This disorder is distinguished clinically by an HDL cholesterol concentration less than the 10th percentile of normal. It was reported that hypoalphalipoproteinemia is present in 4% of CAD kindreds *(4)*. The exact molecular defect is not yet known. It has been suggested that FCH, FHTG, FHB, and familial hypoalphalipoproteinemia may be variants of the same disorder *(4)*.

5.5. LCAT Deficiency

Familial disorders of LCAT are rare. These disorders result from a failure of LCAT to esterify cholesterol in plasma. Clinically, the patients present with corneal opacities, anemia, and in many cases, proteinuria and renal failure. Interestingly, abnormalities involve all lipoprotein classes. The disorder results from a functionally defective enzyme, low levels of normal enzyme, or complete absence of enzyme.

The LCAT gene is located on chromosome 16 and contains six exons. The enzyme is a glycoprotein with a mol wt of 63,000 Dalton, and contains regions with homology to both pancreatic and lingual lipase. LCAT is synthesized in the liver and circulates as a complex with HDL and/or CETP. It is primarily activated by apo A-I. Heterozygotes are apparently healthy, but LCAT mass and activity are reduced. Heterogeneity exists among the mutations that have been documented. Ultimately, unesterified cholesterol accumulates in tissues, leading to dysfunction. Premature atherosclerosis develops in many patients with familial LCAT deficiency.

Familial partial LCAT deficiency, also known as fish eye disease, is associated with a decrease in plasma HDL cholesterol concentration to <10% of normal. Unlike LCAT deficiency, which affects all lipoproteins, patients with partial LCAT deficiency have normal levels of esterified cholesterol in VLDL and LDL, but decreased levels of esterified cholesterol in HDL. These patients have corneal opacities, which are said to resemble the eyes of boiled fish—hence the common name.

5.6. CETP Deficiency

CETP deficiency is a rare disorder that has been reported in only a few families. The molecular defect appears to be a point mutation in the CETP gene that prevents normal mRNA processing. Patients are unable to transfer TG and CE between lipoproteins, and have increased HDL cholesterol levels. Although an elevated HDL cholesterol concentration is protective, the transfer of CE from HDL to VLDL and LDL is thought to contribute to reverse cholesterol transport. Therefore, it is unclear whether lack of CETP influences CAD risk.

6. APO E POLYMORPHISM

Apo E is a 299 amino acid polypeptide found in CM, VLDL, and HDL. The gene was localized to chromosome 19, closely linked to the apo CI/CII gene complex, and found to consist of four exons and three introns spanning 3597 nucleotides. The structural gene for apo E is polymorphic, with three alleles inherited in a codominant fashion accounting for three isoforms and six common phenotypes. Apo E isoforms interact differently with specific lipoprotein receptors to alter circulating lipid levels. Specific apo E phenotypes or genotypes have been implicated in type III HLP, CAD, stroke, and late-onset Alzheimer's disease.

The three common isoforms E2, E3, and E4 differ in their amino acid sequence at positions 112 and 158. Apo E3, the most common isoform with a population frequency of 77%, contains cysteine at position 112 and arginine at position 158. Apo E2 contains cysteine at both these positions, and apo E4 contains arginine at both positions. These

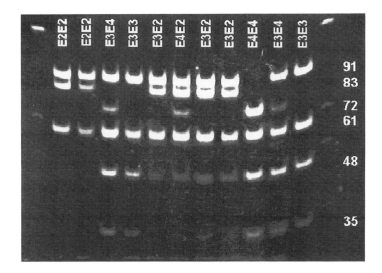

Fig. 1. Polyacrylamide gel electrophoresis of common apo E genotypes. Each lane represents a different genotype as labeled (top). Molecular sizes of restriction fragments, in base pairs (right). (Courtesy of G. J. Tsongalis, Hartford Hospital.)

mutations influence lipoprotein binding to receptors and circulating levels of cholesterol and TG. Apo E-containing lipoproteins bind to the LDL receptor and the LRP. Apo E4 binds to these receptors with equal or slightly greater affinity than apo E3, whereas apo E2 binds with only 2% of the affinity of apo E3. Apo E4 imparts a tendency for moderately elevated plasma levels of total and LDL cholesterol, whereas apo E2 gives a predisposition for lower LDL cholesterol levels relative to apo E3. Both apo E2 and E4 are associated with higher plasma TG concentrations. Polyacrylamide gel electrophoresis of apo E genotypes is shown in Fig. 1.

Type III HLP is a plasma lipid disorder characterized by the presence of xanthomas, elevated plasma cholesterol and TG concentrations, and an accumulation of CM and VLDL remnant particles. The majority of patients with type III HLP are homozygous for the apo E2 allele. Apo E2 homozygosity is present in about 1% of the population, but type III HLP occurs in only one in 1000–5000 individuals *(12)*. Other factors, such as FCH, hypothyroidism, and diabetes, appear to be involved in the full expression of type III HLP. Complete absence of apo E in humans also leads to a form of type III HLP. Three kindreds with apo E deficiency have been described with type III HLP and premature atherosclerosis.

The association of the apo E4 allele with an increased risk of CAD has been clearly documented in a number of studies. Although much of the risk associated with this allele is attributed to its LDL elevating effect, two studies show that apo E phenotype remains significantly associated with CAD even after adjusting for lipid and lipoproteins in a multivariate model. The data linking the apo E2 allele with CAD is less clear. An increased risk of CAD was observed in Japanese subjects and in American subjects participating in the Multiple Risk Factor Intervention Trial. However, other studies report no significant association between apo E2 and CAD (for review, *see* ref. *13*).

7. FAMILIAL LIPOPROTEIN(A) EXCESS

Lipoprotein(a)—Lp(a)—is a unique LDL-like particle with an added apolipoprotein, apo(a), covalently linked to apo B. Elevated levels of Lp(a) are associated with an increased risk of atherosclerosis, CAD, and stroke. Lp(a) cholesterol may promote atherosclerosis by delivering cholesterol to the arterial intima in much the same way as LDL cholesterol. Apo(a) has close homology with plasminogen, and there is evidence to suggest that this homology results in competitive inhibition of the fibrinolytic properties of plasminogen, which in turn results in a predisposition for thrombotic complications. Lp(a) may also promote vascular smooth muscle cell proliferation. Population studies have clearly identified Lp(a) as a strong, independent risk factor for CAD.

Apo(a) is a heterogenous protein with variable numbers of a repeating protein domain, kringle 4, which accounts for a variable mol wt of 280–800 kDa. The apo(a) gene contains a DNA sequence with 91% homology to kringle 5 of plasminogen and multiple repeats of a sequence with 75–85% homology to kringle 4 of plasminogen. The number of kringle 4 repeats is genetically determined and is inversely proportional to circulating Lp(a) concentration. The gene coding for apo(a) is located on the long arm of chromosome 6, in close proximity to the plasminogen gene. The polymorphism in kringle 4 repeats is believed to be the result of internal recombination. There is not yet agreement on the exact number of apo(a) alleles in the general population; estimates range from 9–24, depending on the technology used for identification.

8. HEMOSTASIS

The integrity of the hemovascular system is dependent on the balance between thrombosis (coagulation) and thrombolysis (anticoagulation, fibrinolysis). Under normal physiological conditions, coagulant and anticoagulant mechanisms are balanced in favor of anticoagulation, whereas at sites of vascular lesions, the anticoagulant system is downregulated to favor coagulation. Defects (acquired or genetic) that disturb this balance will lead to an increased risk of thrombosis. The aim of this section is threefold. The first aim is to provide a general overview of hemovascular regulation. Second, we wish to summarize important factors and mechanisms (factor VII, fibrinogen, and plasminogen activator inhibitor) that relate to familial arterial thrombosis. Finally, we wish to summarize significant factors and mechanisms (antithrombin III, factor V, protein C, and protein S) that are associated with familial venous thrombosis.

8.1. Overview of Thrombosis and Thrombolysis

The hemovascular regulatory system (coagulation vs anticoagulation) involves activation of zymogens to active enzymes either by conformational change or by converting enzymes in a complex cascade. As shown in Fig. 2, there are three pathways in the coagulation system: the intrinsic pathway, including factors VIII, IX, XI, and XII; the extrinsic pathway, including factors TF and VII; and the common pathway, involving factor X, prothrombin, and fibrinogen *(14)*. When vascular injury occurs, thrombin activates factors V and VIII, stimulates platelet aggregation, and converts fibrinogen to fibrin to form a blood clot. The anticoagulation system (Fig. 3) is regulated by antithrombin III (AT-III), protein C, and fibrinolysis pathways *(14)*. In the AT-III pathway, factors XII_a, XI_a, and IX_a of the extrinsic coagulation pathway ($_a$ refers to active

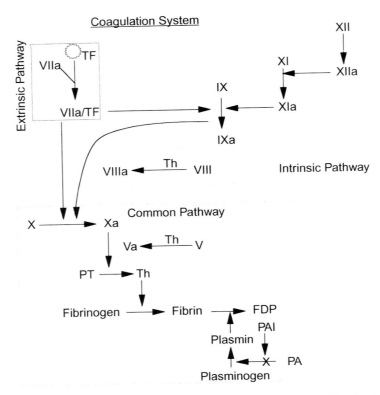

Fig. 2. The coagulation system is subdivided into three pathways. The intrinsic pathway includes factors VIII, IX, XI, and XII. The extrinsic pathway includes tissue factor (TF) and factor VII. The common pathway includes factors V, X, prothrombin (PT), fibrinogen, plasminogen, plasminogen activator inhibitor (PAI), plasminogen activator (PA), and thrombin (Th). The arrow indicates the direction of the reaction. "X" indicates an inhibitory reaction and "a" refers to active form.

form) and thrombin of the common coagulation pathway are inactivated. In the protein C pathway, factor VIII_a of the extrinsic coagulation pathway and factor V_a of the common coagulation pathway are inactivated by the combined effect of activated protein C (APC) and protein S. Fibrinolysis is regulated by I2-antiplasmin (inhibiting fibrin degradation), plasminogen activators (activating plasmin formation), and plasminogen activator inhibitor (PAI, inhibiting plasmin formation). For a detailed review, *see* Tuddenham and Cooper *(15)*.

8.2. Arterial Thrombotic Disease

PAI-1, factor VII, and fibrinogen have been implicated as risk factors for arterial thrombotic disease *(16)*. Fibrinogen is a 340-kDa glycoprotein synthesized in the liver. Plasma concentration of fibrinogen rises sharply in response to inflammation and trauma. It is made up of three pairs of individual polypeptide chains I, J, and K. Each polypeptide chain is coded by a separate gene, located in the distal third of the long arm of chromosome 4. A number of genetic polymorphisms in the fibrinogen gene cluster have been reported. Two common polymorphisms, C to T substitution at nucleotide

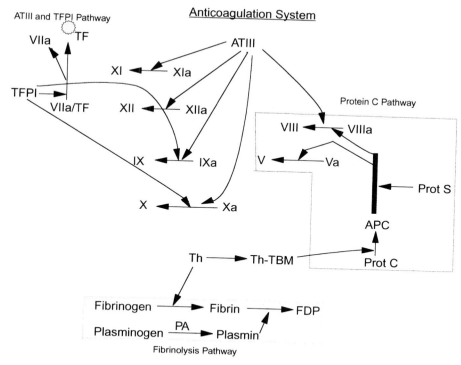

Fig. 3. The anticoagulation system is subdivided into three pathways. The antithrombin III (ATIII) and tissue factor pathway inhibitor (TFPI) pathway includes factors VII, VIII, IX, X, XI, XII, and thrombin (Th). "a" Refers to active form. The protein C pathway includes thrombomodulin (TBM), protein C (Prot C), activated protein C (APC), and protein S (Prot S). The fibrinolysis pathway includes fibrinogen, plasminogen, plasminogen activator (PA), and fibrin degradation products (FDP).

148 and G to A substitution at nucleotide 455, appear to be in complete linkage disequilibrium in the European population studied, with a frequency of 0.19 for the two rare alleles, T^{148} and A^{455}. In another study, the effect of genotype on plasma fibrinogen concentration was much more pronounced in smokers than nonsmokers. Individuals with the TA genotype had higher mean plasma fibrinogen level than individuals with the CG genotype. The difference in fibrinogen level among genotypes may be explained by the variation in gene transcription through differential effects of transcription factor binding. The C/T^{148} polymorphism affects the binding of hepatic nuclear proteins to the promoter region of J-fibrinogen. The G/A^{455} polymorphism affects the binding of liver nuclear proteins. Data from the Northwick Park Study showed an overall 1 SD variation in the population distribution of fibrinogen of 0.6 g/L, whereas the mean difference between genotype groups varied between 0.33 and 0.6 g/L *(16)*. Individuals with elevated levels of fibrinogen were at increased risk of AMI. These data suggest that fibrinogen genotype may have a significant effect on risk of arterial thrombosis and AMI through its effect on plasma fibrinogen level. However, the effect is difficult to quantitate accurately because of the interactions between fibrinogen genotype and other risk factors, such as smoking.

Factor VII is a 50-kDa vitamin K-dependent glycoprotein synthesized in the liver. A study by Mede et al. showed a 45% increase in AMI risk when factor VII coagulation activity was 1 SD above the mean *(16)*. The factor VII gene is located on chromosome 13, and a common genetic polymorphism, Arg for Gln substitution at residue 353, was identified in the coding region. It was estimated that 20% of the population is heterozygous for this allele. Arg^{353} homozygotes had the highest plasma concentrations of factor VII, whereas Gln^{353} homozygotes had the lowest concentration of factor VII. The substitution of Arg to Gln may influence the interaction between factor VII and lipid surfaces, or factor VII secretion, resulting in decreased factor VII concentration in Gln^{353} homozygotes. Carriers of the Gln^{353} allele may therefore be afforded protection from arterial thrombotic disease. Data from Green and Humphires show a 25–50% increased risk of AMI in patients with increased plasma factor VII concentration *(16)*. The difference in factor VII concentration was much greater in the tertile with the highest concentration of triglyceride, suggesting that Arg^{353} homozygotes with elevated triglyceride levels may be at increased risk of disease.

PAI-1 is synthesized in the liver and endothelial cells. Platelets contain about 90% of the total amount of immunoreactive PAI-1 present in blood. PAI-1 concentration is believed to be the major determinant of fibrinolytic activity, and high PAI-1 concentration is associated with various thrombotic disorders. The PAI-1 gene is located on chromosome 7. Its genetic polymorphisms include a two-allele *Hin*dIII RFLP, an eight-allele dinucleotide (CA) repeat, and a four G/five G (G_4/G_5) polymorphism at nucleotide 675. CA repeats and *Hin*dIII RFLP occur in regions of the gene that are probably not directly related to PAI-1 function. However, the G_4/G_5 polymorphism appears to play a functional role. The G_5 allele contains an additional protein binding site that is not present in the G_4 allele. Dawson et al. showed that homozygosity for the G_4 allele was associated with increased plasma PAI-1 concentrations. The data suggest that homozygosity for the G_4 allele may contribute to reduced fibrinolysis and, therefore, an increased risk of thrombotic disease. Since the PAI-1 G_4/G_5 genotype may affect PAI-1 levels more strongly in an acute-phase situation, it is possible that genotype may be a determinant of risk in such conditions as restenosis after angioplasty or in patients with diabetes, although it may be less predictive for risk of a first AMI.

Fibrinogen, factor VII, and PAI-1 are three independent risk factors for arterial thrombotic diseases. Data suggest that it may be more predictive to determine an individual's genotype, rather than simply measuring protein level, in assessing future risk of arterial thrombosis. Individuals identified by simple genetic tests could be targeted for more frequent monitoring and given appropriate advice on lifestyle changes (low-fat diets, smoking cessation, and exercise) that would reduce subsequent risk of disease. Future research should address these issues.

8.3. Venous Thrombosis

Individuals with defects in the genes encoding the hemostatic regulatory factors AT-III, protein C, protein S, and factor V are at highest risk for familial venous thrombosis *(17)*. AT-III is a 58-kDa glycoprotein synthesized in the liver that strongly binds heparin. The gene is located on the long arm of chromosome 1 with 10 Alu repetitive sequences. Three polymorphisms appear to be informative: the *Nhe*I RFLP (20 or 9/11 kb, frequency 0.64 and 0.36, respectively), *Dde*I RFLP

(127 or 53/74 bp, frequency 0.83 and 0.17, respectively), and a variable number of tandem repeats in Alu 8 (ATT)$_n$. AT-III deficiencies are usually inherited in an autosomal-dominant fashion.

There are two types of AT-III deficiency. Type I is classified by an equal reduction in AT-III mass and activity, whereas type II is characterized by a higher AT-III mass than activity. The majority of type I deficiencies are caused by short deletions and insertions of 1–2 bp. Most type II deficiencies are caused by a single base-pair substitution. Symptomatic familial AT-III deficiency occurs at a frequency of 1 in 2000–5000 in the general population *(15,17)*. However, asymptomatic type IIC deficiency (heparin binding defects) may occur as frequently as 1 in 350. About 3% of patients presenting with recurrent venous thrombosis have an inherited deficiency of AT-III. About 40 different missense mutations in the AT-III gene responsible for AT-III deficiency and recurrent thrombosis have been characterized. By age 50, 85% of heterozygous individuals will have at least one thromboembolic episode. The median age for onset of symptoms is approx 24 yr. Recurrent thrombosis occurs in 60% of these patients. The search for mutations in the AT-III gene has been performed either by sequencing all seven exons, by single-strand conformational polymorphism (SSCP) screening analysis, or by the Hydrolink heteroduplex detection procedure.

Protein C is a 62-kDa glycoprotein synthesized in the liver. The protein is activated by thrombomodulin (TBM), a high-affinity endothelial receptor for thrombin. The protein C gene (PROC) is located on the long arm of chromosome 2. In vitro mutagenesis studies have shown that Gla residues at positions 6, 7, 19, and 20 are important for the anticoagulant properties of activated protein C (APC). A number of DNA polymorphisms are known within and outside the coding region of the gene. Polymorphisms inside the coding region include an A/T substitution at nucleotide 25 and silent substitutions within codons Arg 87, Ser 99, Lys 156, and Asp 214. Polymorphisms outside the coding region include *Msp*I and *Apa*I RFLPs located 7 kb 5' of the gene and a second *Msp*I RFLP in intron 8. Two types of protein C deficiency are described. Type 1 is the most prevalent and is classified by reduced protein C activity and mass. In type 2, there is only a loss of protein C activity. PROC gene defects include nonsense and missense mutations, as well as some deletions. Protein C deficiency is found in 2–5% of patients with thromboembolic disease. The prevalence may be as high as 10–15% when only young patients with recurrent thrombosis are considered *(18)*. Heterozygous protein C deficiency is thought to have a prevalence of between 1 in 16,000 and 36,000 in the general population. Homozygous protein C deficiency was first described as a cause of neonatal purpura fulminans, resulting in rapid death owing to massive venous thrombosis. Severe protein C deficiency may also be caused by compound heterozygosity for two nonidentical gene lesions. The search for mutations in the PROC gene has been performed by sequencing all nine exons, by screening with SSCP, or by denaturing gradient gel electrophoresis.

Protein S is a 72-kDa glycoprotein synthesized in liver, endothelial cells, testicular Leydig cells, platelets, and megakaryocytic cell lines. It is a vitamin K-dependent protein, but is not a member of the serine proteinase family. The free form of protein S is a cofactor for APC, but 60% is bound to C4b binding protein and is inactive *(15)*. The

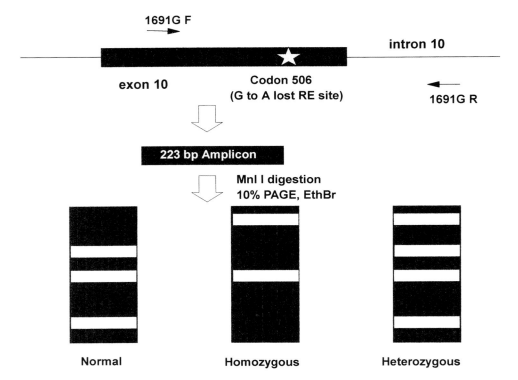

Fig. 4. RFLP analysis of factor V (codon 506) mutation. The genomic DNA is amplified by PCR with a primer pair (1691G F and 1691G R), the 223-bp amplicon is digested with *Mnl*I restriction enzyme, and fragments are separated on a 10% polyacrylamide gel and stained with ethidium bromide. Normal DNA will have three DNA fragments (37, 82, and 104 bp). Homozygotes will show two DNA fragments (82 and 141 bp). Heterozygotes will have four DNA fragments (37, 82, 104, and 141 bp).

protein S gene (PROS) is located on chromosome 3. Protein S deficiency appears to be less common than protein C deficiency; however, in cohorts of venous thrombosis patients, it was found to be as equally prevalent as protein C deficiency *(18)*. There are three types of protein S deficiency *(17)*. Type 1 is defined by a decreased total and free protein S concentration, whereas type 2 is defined by reduced protein S function. Type 3 is characterized by a low free protein S, but normal total protein S concentration. Five percent of patients with a history of thrombotic disease exhibit heterozygous protein S deficiency. Molecular analysis of protein S deficiency is still in its infancy, and currently, genetic analysis relies on PCR and sequencing of all 15 exons because of the low yield of mRNA associated with type 1 deficiency. Examples of mutations that have been identified include Cys 22/Stop, 82 T deletion, G to A transition at nucleotide 5 of intron 10 (splice site mutation), A to T transversion at codon 636 (Stop/Tyr), one T insertion at nucleotide 25, premature stop codon at nucleotide 4, a 5.3 kb deletion in exon 13, and a deletion in the middle of the coding sequence. These are all type I deficiencies. A G/A transition at nucleotide 5 of intron E has been identified, associated with type III deficiency.

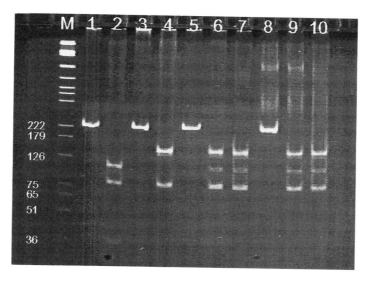

Fig. 5. Polyacrylamide gel of restriction fragments for factor V. Lanes 1, 3, 5, and 8 are undigested amplicons (223 bp). Lanes 2, 4, 6, and 9 are amplicons digested with *Mnl*I for 2 h at 37°C. Lanes 7 and 10 are amplicons after overnight digestion with *Mnl*I. Lane 2 is a normal DNA pattern. Lane 4 is a homozygous pattern. Lanes 6 and 9 are heterozygous patterns. The 37-bp fragment is not as obvious as in normal DNA because of the decrease in DNA after digestion. (Courtesy of G. J. Tsongalis, Hartford Hospital.)

Factor V is a 286-kDa asymmetric glycoprotein. The factor V gene is located on chromosome 1. Recently, a codon 506 mutation (Arg to Gln) of the factor V gene was identified as a cause of APC resistance *(19)*. The mutation affects the cleavage of factor V_a, which inactivates factor V, leading to a hypercoagulable state *(20)*. The codon 506 mutation appears to be the most common inherited factor recognized thus far predisposing to venous thrombosis. The mutation can be detected by PCR, RFLP, and *Mnl*I digestion (Fig. 4). The mutation destroys an *Mnl*I restriction enzyme recognition site in the amplified DNA. From the electrophoretic pattern (Fig. 5), the wild-type or normal factor V will show three bands (37, 82, and 104 bp), the homozygote will show two bands (82 and 141 bp), and the heterozygote will show four bands (37, 82, 104, and 141 bp). Studies show that up to 87% of patients with venous thrombosis and 7% of healthy individuals carry the codon 506 mutation. The relative risk of venous thrombosis associated with the codon 506 mutation is sevenfold for heterozygous individuals and 80-fold for homozygous individuals *(21)*. Among the factors described, the codon 506 mutation of the factor V gene is probably the most common cause of familial venous thrombosis.

9. CONCLUSIONS

With molecular genetic techniques, we can identify a spectrum of gene mutations that give rise to both venous and arterial thrombosis, familial lipid disorders, and atherosclerosis. However, the major challenge facing us is to relate specific gene lesions to the probability, severity, and frequency of atherosclerosis, thrombotic episodes, CVD, and other negative outcomes.

REFERENCES

1. Beaudet, A. L., Scriver, C. R., Sly, W. S., Valle, D., Cooper, D. N., McKusick, V. A., and Schmidke, J. Genetics and biochemistry of variant human phenotypes, in *The Metabolic Basis of Inherited Disease*, Scriver, C. R., Beaudet, A. L., Sly, W. S., Valle, D., eds., McGraw Hill, New York, pp. 3–53, 1989.
2. Bazunga, M. The use of angiotensin converting enzyme inhibitors in asymptomatic patients with left ventricular dysfunction after myocardial infarction. *Conn. Med.* **59**:663–666, 1995.
3. Brunzell, J. D. Familial lipoprotein lipase deficiency and other causes of the chylomicronemia syndrome, in *The Metabolic Basis of Inherited Disease*, Scriver, C. R., Beaudet, A. L., Sly, W. S., Valle, D., eds., McGraw Hill, New York, pp. 1165–1180, 1989.
4. Schaefer, E. J. Familial lipoprotein disorders and premature coronary artery disease. *Med. Clin. North Am.* **78**:21–39, 1994.
5. Brown, M. S. and Goldstein, J. L. A receptor-mediated pathway for cholesterol homeostasis. *Science* **232**:34–47, 1986.
6. Genest, J. J., Jr., Martin-Munley, S. S., McNamara, J. R., Ordovas, J. M., Jenner, J., Myers, R. H., Silberman, S. R., Wilson, P. W. F., Salem, D. N., and Schaefer, E. J. Familial lipoprotein disorders in patients with premature coronary artery disease. *Circulation* **85**:2025–2033, 1992.
7. Knecht, T. P. and Glass, C. K. The influence of molecular biology on our understanding of lipoprotein metabolism and the pathobiology of atherosclerosis. *Ad. Genet.* **32**:141–198, 1995.
8. Kane, J. P. and Havel, R. J. Disorders of the biogenesis and secretion of lipoproteins containing the B apolipoprotein, in *The Metabolic Basis of Inherited Disease*, Scriver, C. R., Beaudet, A. L., Sly, W. S., and Valle, D., eds., McGraw Hill, New York, pp. 1139–1164, 1989.
9. Austin, M. A., Breslow, J. L., Hennekens, C. H, Buring, J. E., Willett, W. C., and Krauss, R. M. Low-density lipoprotein subclass patterns and risk of myocardial infarction. *JAMA* **260**:1917–1921, 1988.
10. Breslow, J. L. Familial disorders of high density lipoprotein metabolism, in *The Metabolic Basis of Inherited Disease*, Scriver, C. R., Beaudet, A. L., Sly, W. S., and Valle, D., eds., McGraw Hill, 1989.
11. Assman, G., Schmitz, G., and Brewer, H. B., Jr. Familial high density lipoprotein deficiency, in *The Metabolic Basis of Inherited Disease*, Scriver, C. R., Beaudet, A. L., Sly, W. S., and Valle, D., eds. McGraw Hill, New York, pp. 1251–1266, 1989.
12. Mahley, R. W. and Rall, S. C., Jr. Type III hyperlipoproteinemia (dysbetalipoproteinemia): the role of apolipoprotein E in normal and abnormal lipoprotein metabolism, in *The Metabolic Basis of Inherited Disease*, Scriver, C. R., Beaudet, A. L., Sly, W. S., and Valle, D., eds., McGraw Hill, New York, pp. 1267–1282, 1989.
13. Contois, J. H., Anamani, D. E., and Tsongalis, G. J. The underlying molecular mechanism od apolipoprotein E polymorphism: relationships to lipid disorders, cardiovascular disease, and Alzheimer's disease. *Clin. Lab. Med.* **16**:105–123, 1996.
14. Rosenberg, R. D. and Aird, W. C. Thrombosis, in *Molecular Cardiovascular Medicine*, Haber, E., ed., Scientific American, New York, pp. 115–132, 1995.
15. Tuddenham, E. G. D. and Cooper, D. N. *The Molecular Genetics of Haemostasis and its Inherited Disorders*, section V. Oxford University Press, 1994.
16. Green, F. and Humphries, S. E. Genetic determinants of arterial thrombosis. *Baillière's Clin. Haemotol.* **7**:675–692, 1994.
17. Cooper, D. N. The molecular genetics of familial venous thrombosis. *Baillière's Clin. Haematol.* **7**:637–673, 1994.
18. Dahlbäck B. Inherited thrombophilia: resistance to activated protein C as a pathogenic factor of venous thromboembolism. *Blood* **85**:607–614, 1995.

19. Bertina, R. M., Koeleman, B. P. C., Koster, T., Rosendaal, F. R., Driven, R. J., deRonde, H., van der Velden, P. A., and Reitsma, P. H. Mutation in blood coagulation factor V associated with resistance to activated protein C. *Nature* **369**:64–67, 1995.
20. Dahlbäck B. Molecular genetics of thrombophilia: factor V gene mutation causing resistance to activated protein C as a basis of the hypercoagulable state. *J. Lab. Clin. Med.* **125**:566–571, 1995.
21. Rosendaal, F. R., Koster, T., Vandenbroucke, J. P., and Reitsma, P. H. High risk of thrombosis in patients homozygous for factor V Leiden (activated protein C resistance). *Blood* **85**:1504–1508, 1995.

SUGGESTED READING

Breslow, J. L. Lipoprotein transport gene abnormalities underlying coronary heart disease susceptibility. *Ann Rev Med.* **42**:357–371, 1991.

Hobbs, H. H., Russell, D. W., Brown, M. S., and Goldstein, J. L. The LDL receptor locus in familial hypercholesterolemia: mutational analysis of a membrane protein. *Ann. Rev. Genet.* **24**:133–170, 1990.

Humphries, S. E. The genetic contribution to the risk of thrombosis and cardiovascular disease. *Trends Cardiovasc. Med.* **4**:8–17, 1994.

Kwiterovich, P. O., Jr. Genetics and molecular biology of familial combined hyperlipidemia. *Curr. Opinion Lipidology* **4**:133–143, 1993.

Nassar, B. A. Familial defective apolipoprotein B-100: a cause of hypercholesterolemia and early coronary heart disease. *Can. Med. Assoc. J.* **148**:579–580, 1993.

Sing, C. F. and Moll, P. P. Genetics of atherosclerosis. *Ann. Rev. Genet.* **24**:171–187, 1990.

14

Molecular Mutations in Human Neoplastic Disease

Application of Nucleic Acid Technology in Assessment of Familial Risk, Diagnosis, and Prognosis of Human Cancers

William B. Coleman and Gregory J. Tsongalis

1. INTRODUCTION

Cancer represents a significant health problem worldwide. The successful curative treatment of almost every form of this disease depends on early diagnosis, and in the case of solid tumors, surgical resection with or without adjuvant therapy. Intensive research efforts during the last two decades have increased our understanding of carcinogenesis and have identified a genetic basis for the multistep nature of cancer development *(1–3)*. In several human tumor systems, specific genetic alterations have been shown to correlate with well defined histopathologic stages of tumor development and progression *(4,5)*. Although the significance of molecular mutations to the etiological mechanisms of tumor development has been debated, a causal role for such genetic lesions is now commonly accepted for a number of human tumors. Thus, genetic lesions represent an integral part of the processes of neoplastic transformation and tumor progression, and as such represent potentially valuable markers for cancer detection and staging *(6–9)*. Through the application of specific and sensitive nucleic acid methodologies, the clinical laboratory of the future will be able to effectively screen populations at high risk for the development of cancer, potentially impacting the early detection and diagnosis of human cancers. In addition, development of new molecular diagnostic assays will expand the ability of clinicians to accurately stage tumor development, monitor progression of metastatic disease, and evaluate therapeutic outcome, facilitating the application of effective intervention strategies in the treatment of human tumors.

2. CANCER AS A MULTISTEP GENETIC DISEASE

Cancer represents a unique form of genetic disease, characterized by the accumulation of multiple somatic mutations in a population of cells undergoing neoplastic transformation *(1–3,10)*. Various types of genetic alterations are associated with neoplastic development and tumor progression, including gene amplifications, deletions, rearrangements, and point mutations *(3)*. Statistical analyses of age-specific mortality rates

From: Molecular Diagnostics: For the Clinical Laboratorian
Edited by: W. B. Coleman and G. J. Tsongalis Humana Press Inc., Totowa, NJ

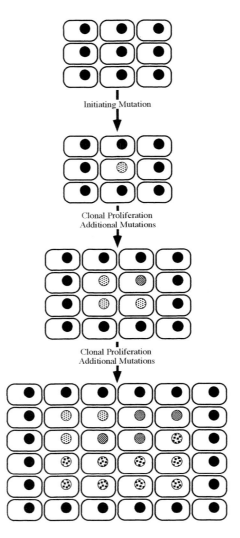

Fig. 1. Clonal selection and proliferation of cell populations in neoplastic development. ●, normal epithelial cell; ⊜, epithelial cell harboring a single genetic lesion; ◉, epithelial cell harboring two genetic lesions; ⊗, epithelial cell with multiple genetic lesions.

for different forms of human cancer predict that three to eight mutations are required for the genesis of most clinically diagnosable tumors *(11)*. In accordance with this prediction, tumors grow by a process of clonal expansion driven by mutation *(1,10)*. In this model, the first mutation leads to limited expansion of progeny of a single cell, and each subsequent mutation gives rise to a new clonal outgrowth with greater proliferative potential (Fig. 1). The idea that carcinogenesis is a multistep process is supported by morphologic observations of the transitions between premalignant (benign) cell growths and malignant tumors. In some tumor systems (such as colon), the transition from benign to malignant can be easily documented and occurs in discernible stages, including benign adenoma, carcinoma *in situ*, invasive carcinoma, and eventually local

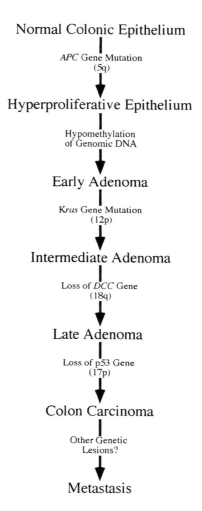

Fig. 2. Colorectal carcinogenesis: the paradigm for mutation driven multistage tumor development. (The information contained in this schematic was adapted from refs. *4, 5,* and *28*)

and distant metastasis *(12)*. These definable stages of tumor progression, along with their underlying genetic lesions, reflect degrees of tumor behavior that impact on clinical outcome (Fig. 2). This observation suggests that molecular analysis of specific genetic targets could aid in the proper staging of tumors and the accurate prediction of the response of specific tumors to postoperative therapy. In addition, some of the genetic alterations associated with neoplastic transformation can be identified in precancerous lesions, suggesting the possibility of premorphologic diagnosis of developing tumors and early clinical intervention. In cases of familial or inherited cancers, identification of specific genetic alterations in affected individuals will facilitate the screening of other family members that are potentially at high risk for cancer development. This will allow the implementation of early treatment regimens in affected individuals or chemopreventative regimens in high-risk individuals prior to evidence of tumor development. It is of great importance to recognize that the accumulation of

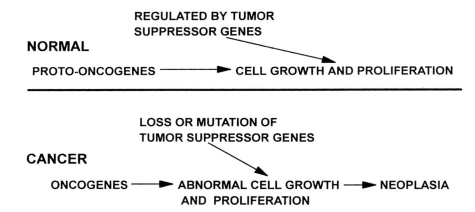

Fig. 3. Interactions between cellular proto-oncogenes and tumor suppressor genes in normal and neoplastic cells.

multiple genetic alterations, and not necessarily the order in which these changes accumulate, determines tumor progression. From a clinical perspective, the process of accumulation of genetic alterations and molecular mutations, over time, during neoplastic transformation and tumor progression provides a window of opportunity for early detection, diagnosis, and intervention *(7–9)*. However, the selection of appropriate molecular markers will depend on the nature and temporal occurrence of the various genetic alterations that govern the establishment of a particular tumor type, and the relationship between these genetic alterations and the histopathological features of the developing tumor.

3. MOLECULAR TARGETS AND MECHANISMS OF MUTATION IN CARCINOGENESIS

Numerous genetic targets have been implicated in the etiology of human tumors, including oncogenes *(13,14)*, tumor suppressor genes *(15,16)*, and others. Oncogenes were the first type of gene associated with the malignant process. Oncogenes represent activated forms of normal cellular genes, termed proto-oncogenes, that are normally expressed in proliferative cells. Proto-oncogene activation can reflect either abnormal regulation of gene expression (owing to gene amplification or deregulated transcription), or expression of a mutated form of the gene with altered biologic activity *(3,13,14)*. Cells that express activated oncogenes do not respond normally to the usual controls over cell cycle progression, resulting in the uncontrolled growth of affected cells through the activation of positive mechanisms governing cell proliferation (Fig. 3).

A second type of gene associated with cancer is the so-called antioncogene, or more commonly, the tumor suppressor gene. Tumor suppressor genes function in a recessive manner, and generally mutations in tumor suppressor genes result in loss of function. Nonetheless, mutations resulting in gain of function have been documented for some tumor suppressor genes *(17)*. Tumor suppressor genes normally function in the negative regulation of cell-cycle progression and cell proliferation *(18,19)*. Thus, inactivation of tumor suppressor gene function can result in the uncontrolled proliferation of cells through the loss of negative regulatory pathways (Fig. 3). Of note is the observation that unlike proto-oncogenes that may be activated through very specific point mutations *(20)*, tumor suppressor genes can be inactivated through various forms of mutational alteration over large areas of the gene coding sequence *(21,22)*.

In recent years, several other groups of genes have been identified that represent critical components of the normal mechanisms governing cell proliferation and homeostasis and have been associated with development of neoplastic disease, but may or may not fit neatly into the general classifications of oncogene or tumor suppressor gene. These include genes encoding proteins involved in DNA repair mechanisms, which ensure the fidelity of the human genome, and numerous genes associated with the complex signal transduction pathways, which regulate cell-cycle progression. The ability to repair damaged DNA is fundamental to all biological processes, since damaged sites can be converted to permanent mutations during DNA replication. Susceptibility to carcinogenesis is related to the ability of a cell to metabolize genotoxic carcinogens and to repair damaged DNA *(23)*. DNA damage is repaired through several pathways, including enzymatic reversal repair, nucleotide excision repair, and postreplication repair *(24)*. Acquired or familial deficiency for one or more of the enzyme activities associated with DNA repair can predispose individuals to development of cancer resulting directly or indirectly from an accumulation of genetic alterations in proto-oncogenes and/or tumor suppressor genes *(25)*.

The normal control mechanisms governing cell cycle progression involve a large number of proteins, including the cyclins, cyclin-dependent kinases, and cyclin-dependent kinase inhibitors *(26,27)*. The levels of expression of the cyclin proteins and cyclin-dependent kinases have been shown to be regulated during the cell cycle, with transient expression of specific proteins at specific time-points in the cell-cycle *(26)*. Transit of cells through the various cell cycle checkpoints requires the presence of sufficient levels of these regulator proteins. The escape of cells from the normal controls over cell-cycle progression can be accomplished through any of several possible mechanisms, including overexpression or constitutive expression of cell-cycle regulatory proteins and loss of expression of genes encoding inhibitors of cyclin activity *(27)*. Cells that transit the cell cycle in an uncontrolled manner may accumulate mutations because of the inappropriate replication of damaged DNA. Thus, molecular alterations affecting the activity of cyclins or the cyclin-dependent kinases could alter the normal cell-cycle regulation, contributing to carcinogenesis through indirect mutational mechanisms related to increased cell proliferation and inappropriate DNA synthesis *(25)*.

4. COLORECTAL CARCINOMA: A GENETIC MODEL OF HUMAN TUMOR DEVELOPMENT AND PROGRESSION

A tumor progression model describing the genetically defined stages of colorectal tumorigenesis has been established *(4,5,28)*, and has come to represent the paradigm for multistep tumor development. The genetic model for colorectal carcinogenesis *(4)* suggests that:

1. Tumors arise as a result of mutational activation of proto-oncogenes and mutational inactivation of tumor suppressor genes;
2. Alteration of at least four or five genes is required for development of a malignant tumor; and
3. The total accumulation of genetic alterations and not their relative order of appearance determine the biological behavior of the developing tumor.

Table 1
Criteria for Identifiaction of Familial Cancer Genes[a]

Mutations must be found in the constitutional DNA of affected patients, as well as in the tumors of these patients.

Germline transmission of the mutated gene should be demonstrable on examination of the constitutional DNA of parents, offspring, or other first-degree relative; the mode of inheritance should conform to autosomal-dominant.

Segregation of the mutated gene within the family pedigree should be linked to cancer susceptibility among family members.

Technical artifacts must be excluded by repetition and through the use of different tissue sources in the preparation of DNA.

The mutation should be observed in multiple family pedigrees to eliminate the possibility of a linked polymorphism within any single kindred, and the mutation should not be detected among control populations.

Mutations of the same gene should occur in appropriate sporadic cancers.

[a]Adapted from ref. *112*.

In colorectal tumor development mutations of the K-*ras* proto-oncogene and the APC gene occur in early lesions, whereas alterations of the p53 and DCC tumor suppressor genes represent late molecular events occurring in advanced tumors (Fig. 2). Approximately 50% of colorectal carcinomas and colorectal adenomas >1 cm in size harbor *ras* gene mutations *(29)*. The occurrence of *ras* gene mutations in early colorectal lesions suggests that alteration of this gene may represent an initiating event in the development of a large percentage of colorectal tumors. Conversely, 70–80% of colorectal carcinomas demonstrate allelic losses at 17p and 18q *(5)*, and significant numbers of tumors exhibited p53 tumor suppressor gene mutations in addition to 17p chromosome deletions *(30)*. Epigenetic alterations have also been documented in colorectal carcinogenesis, including global hypomethylation of the genomic DNA of tumors early in progression *(31)*. Accumulation of genetic alterations is associated with histologic progression through the dysplasia-carcinoma continuum. Greater than 90% of early adenomas demonstrate one or zero alterations, 25 and 49% of intermediate and late adenomas (respectively) demonstrate at least two alterations, and >90% of carcinomas exhibit two or more alterations *(4)*.

5. FAMILIAL CANCERS

That familial clustering of specific cancers occurs supports a role for some common heritable factor among cancer-prone families (Table 1). Several familial cancer syndromes have been characterized through the study of rare families in which individual members are affected by either the same type of cancer or a variety of cancer types with an early age of onset and a pattern consistent with a hereditary mechanism. Several candidate cancer susceptibility genes have been identified (Table 2). When these genes are altered in the germline of an individual, that individual carries a higher risk for the development of neoplastic disease. Whereas the number of families affected by such familial cancer syndromes is low, the underlying susceptibility genes that provide the genetic basis for cancer predisposition are important in the development of the corresponding sporadic cancers or in cancers that are not associated with germline mutations.

Table 2
Tumor Suppressor Genes Associated with Familial Cancers

Gene	Location	Tumor predisposition	Protein function
APC	5q21	Adenomatous polyposis coli	Cytoplasmic protein, function unknown
ATM	11q22-23	Ataxia telangiectasia	Mitogenic signal transduction, mediator of response to DNA damage
BRCA1	17q21	Breast carcinoma, ovarian carcinoma	Function unknown
BRCA2	13q12-13	Breast carcinoma (female and male)	Function unknown
hMLH1	3p21-23	HNPCC	DNA mismatch repair
hPMS1	2q31-33	HNPCC	DNA mismatch repair
hPMS2	7q22	HNPCC	DNA mismatch repair
MSH2	2p22	HNPCC, sporadic colorectal carcinoma	DNA mismatch repair
NF1	17q11	Neurofibrosarcoma, schwanoma, glioma, pheochomocytoma	Protein with anti-*ras* activity
NF2	22q12	Vestibular schwanoma, meningioma	Cytoskeleton binding protein
p15^{INK4B}	9p21	Melanoma?	Cyclin-dependent kinase 4 inhibitor
p16^{INK4}	9p21	Melanoma?	Cyclin-dependent kinase 4 inhibitor
p53	17p13	Rhabdomyosarcoma, breast carcinoma	Nuclear transcription factor, mediator of cell cycle arrest and DNA repair responses
RB1	13q14	Retinoblastoma, osteosarcoma	Nuclear protein, negative regulator of cell-cycle progression
WT1	11p13	WAGR syndrome, nephroblastoma	Nuclear transcription factor
WT2	11p15.5	Wilms' tumor, rhabdomyosarcoma	Function unknown
VHL	3p25	Von-Hippel-Lindau syndrome, hemangioblastoma, renal cell carcinoma	Membrane protein, function unknown

5.1. Retinoblastoma

Retinoblastoma is a rare malignant tumor of the retina in infants and is the result of mutations in the RB tumor suppressor gene *(32)*. Approximately 40% of retinoblastoma cases are familial in origin where one mutant allele of the RB gene is inherited and a second somatic mutation is later acquired in the other RB allele. Familial retinoblastoma is characterized by multiple and bilateral tumors. Nonhereditary or sporadic retinoblastoma, which accounts for approx 60% of all cases, results from somatic mutation of both RB alleles. In these cases, there is usually only a single unilateral tumor. The early age of onset and characteristic bilaterality of familial retinoblastoma was explained by Knudson in 1971 *(33)*. Knudson's model proposed a "two-hit" molecular mechanism for tumor development. In this model, individuals displaying a genetic predisposition for developing retinoblastoma (inherited or otherwise) had acquired a germline mutation in one RB allele, which constituted the first "hit." The second "hit" represented an acquired somatic mutation inactivating the one remaining normal RB allele. The accumulation of two hits eliminated RB tumor suppressor gene function in affected cells that then proliferate to form retinoblastomas. Consistent with this model, individuals who inherit the first hit are more likely to develop a tumor, and tumor onset is more likely to occur early in life. Normal individuals are statistically less likely to accumulate the required number of hits, and thereby are less likely to form a tumor. In addition, the late onset of sporadic tumors reflects the probabilistic nature of spontaneous somatic mutations at a specific genetic locus.

5.2. Li-Fraumeni Syndrome

In a detailed study of four families in which siblings or cousins were affected by rhabdomyosarcoma, Li and Fraumeni described what appeared to be an inherited predisposition to cancer development *(34)*. Within these extended families there was an unusually high incidence of early onset cancers, including breast cancer, soft tissue sarcomas, brain tumors, and leukemias *(34)*. Followup studies of members in these four families revealed new cancers in previously unaffected individuals, and a number of individuals developed second primary tumors *(35)*. In both cases, the patterns and types of cancers that developed were similar to that in the original study, supporting the idea of genetic susceptibility *(36)*. Segregation analysis among the individuals in these families demonstrated that the distribution of cancers was compatible with a rare autosomal gene with an approximate frequency of 0.00002 and a penetrance of 50% by age 30 yr and 90% by age 60 yr *(37)*. The cancer susceptibility gene in Li-Fraumeni syndrome was subsequently suggested to be the p53 tumor suppressor gene *(38)*. Germline mutations of the p53 gene were found in affected individuals of Li-Fraumeni syndrome families in studies conducted by several laboratories *(38,39)*. However, the p53 tumor suppressor gene is not affected in all Li-Fraumeni syndrome families *(40)*. The genetic basis for the cancer-prone phenotype in Li-Fraumeni families without p53 mutations is not known. However, it has been suggested that the p53 protein function among individuals in this particular group of families is compromised by virtue of interactions with other cellular proteins *(41)*, such as the MDM2 gene product, which negatively regulate p53 function *(42)*.

5.3. Hereditary Colon Cancers

Genetic susceptibility to colorectal cancer can occur in association with familial adenomatous polyposis coli (FAP), or in the absence of FAP in a condition termed hereditary nonpolyposis colorectal cancer (HNPCC), also known as Lynch syndrome *(43)*. Genes associated with each of these conditions have been identified and characterized, and have been determined to play important roles in sporadic colorectal tumors.

The APC gene is responsible for FAP, and has been implicated in the development of sporadic colorectal cancers *(44)*. The APC gene is located on chromosome 5q21 and has been cloned and sequenced *(45,46)*. Mutational alteration of the APC gene over a large area of the coding region results in inactivation of the gene product. The mechanism of inactivation frequently involves the generation of frameshift or nonsense mutations, which lead to the production of truncated APC protein products. A correlation between the location of mutations in the APC coding sequence and the FAP phenotype has been observed *(47)*. Germline mutations between codons 1250 and 1464 are associated with profuse polyps, whereas mutations occurring in other regions are associated with sparse polyps. In addition, it has been suggested that certain truncated forms of the APC protein can interact with wild-type protein, giving rise to a dominant negative inhibition of APC function *(48)*.

HNPCC is characterized by the occurrence of predominantly right-sided colorectal carcinoma with an early age of onset and an increased risk for the development of certain extracolonic cancers, including cancers of the endometrium, stomach, urinary tract, and breast *(49,50)*. HNPCC is thought to account for <10% of colorectal cancers. However, precise determination of the contribution of HNPCC to colorectal cancer is difficult because of heterogeneity in the clinical features of the syndrome. Genetic linkage studies demonstrated a close linkage of the disease to anonymous microsatellite markers on chromosome 2 without allelic deletion in two large HNPCC kindreds *(51)*. Tumors associated with HNPCC exhibit a unique form of genomic instability, which represents a unique mechanism for a genome-wide tendency for replication errors, and is termed the replication error phenotype (RER). The RER phenotype was first described in a subset of patients with colorectal carcinoma *(52–54)*, and was shown to occur frequently in patients with HNPCC *(52,55)*. The molecular defect responsible for the RER phenotype in hereditary colon cancer involves genes that encode proteins required for normal mismatch repair *(56–60)*. These genes are mutated in the germline of the majority of individuals with HNPCC. Expression of the RER phenotype occurs early in colorectal tumorigenesis *(61)*, suggesting a causative role for this type of genetic instability in the formation of tumors of the colon. The RER phenotype is typically detected as instability in microsatellite repeat sequences. Changes in size of microsatellite length in tumor vs normal DNA from the same individual can involve mono-, di-, tri-, and tetranucleotide repeats *(54)*. Although the expansion of microsatellite repeat sequences is used as the main criteria for identification of the RER phenotype, the molecular defect responsible for the phenotype is likely to cause point mutational alterations of DNA sequences in addition to alterations in microsatellites *(62)*.

5.4. Familial Breast and Ovarian Cancer

Hereditary predisposition to breast cancer is a causal factor in approx 5–10% of all cases. Recently, two genes, termed BRCA1 *(63)* and BRCA2 *(64)*, have been implicated in the etiology of familial breast cancer, and a third breast cancer susceptibility gene has been suggested to exist *(65)*. The BRCA1 gene has also been implicated in a hereditary predisposition to the development of ovarian cancer *(66)*. Approximately half of all families displaying a dominant predisposition to breast cancer and 80–90% of families in which multiple cases of breast and ovarian cancer occur have been suggested to harbor germline mutations in the BRCA1 gene *(67)*. These mutations are highly penetrant, conferring a risk of about 90% of either breast or ovarian cancer by age 70. The actual frequencies of occurrence of breast and ovarian cancers vary among families. Epidemiological evidence suggests a model in which the majority of families are strongly predisposed to breast cancer, but have only a moderately increased risk of ovarian cancer, with the remaining families displaying an equally strong predisposition to both breast and ovarian cancer *(66)*. In type 1 breast/ovarian cancer syndrome, the life-time risk of developing breast cancer is very high (80–90%) and there is a moderate risk of life-time development of ovarian cancer (30%). In type 2 breast/ovarian cancer syndrome, the life-time risk for breast cancer is somewhat lower (approx 70%), whereas the risk for ovarian cancer is increased to approx 85%.

Mutations in the BRCA1 gene have been identified over a large area of the coding sequence of the gene, and a large percentage of the identified mutations result in truncated BRCA1 protein products with abnormal function or complete loss of function *(68,69)*. Gayther and colleagues evaluated germline BRCA1 gene mutations with respect to breast and ovarian cancer frequencies among affected family members *(70)*. These investigators found that mutations in the 3' one-third of the coding sequence of the BRCA1 gene were associated with a lower proportion of ovarian cancers, suggesting a connection between the location of the mutation and the chances for developing either breast or ovarian cancer *(70)*.

Like BRCA1, the BRCA2 gene has been shown to be linked to early onset familial breast cancers *(71)* and to be mutated in the germline of families with a high rate of breast cancers *(64)*. However, unlike BRCA1, the BRCA2 gene has been shown to be mutated in rare cases of male breast cancer and is not associated with hereditary ovarian cancer *(64)*. All of the mutations identified in the BRCA2 gene to date represent small deletions that result in frameshifts *(64)*.

5.5. Familial Melanoma

Approximately 8–12% of all cases of cutaneous melanoma are related to an inherited predisposition *(72)*. Individuals at high risk are often identified as having dysplastic nevus syndrome, a highly penetrant autosomal-dominant disorder characterized by predisposition to development of malignant melanoma *(73)*. A variety of studies have contributed to the suggestion that genes on chromosomes 1, 6, 7, and 10 (and to a lesser extent 2, 3, and 11) are involved in the etiology of malignant melanoma *(72)*. Genetic linkage studies implicate at least two familial melanoma loci which are located at 1p36 and 9p21 *(74,75)*. The candidate 9p21 gene is the MTS1 (or CDKN2, or CDK4I) tumor suppressor gene that encodes the p16 cyclin-dependent kinase inhibitor that negatively regulates CDK4 *(76)*. This gene is mutated in 75% of all cell lines established from sporadic metastatic melanomas *(76,77)*. However, analysis of several kindreds has failed to associate germline mutations of this gene with the occurrence of melanoma consistently among these families *(78–80)*. Thus, other genes located at 9p21 may be involved with the development of this tumor. An alternative mechanism for inactivation of normal cell-cycle progression control pathways in melanoma has been suggested by Dracopoli and colleagues, who have described a mutation in the CDK4 gene that gives rise to a protein product that cannot be regulated by normal p16 protein *(81)*. These observations combine to suggest that abrogation of the p16-CDK4 regulatory pathway, through the mutational alteration of either gene, represents a critical step in the pathogenesis of malignant melanoma. Viable candidate genes have not been identified on the other chromosomes implicated in melanoma progression, although there is evidence to suggest that progression of the tumor involves genes that regulate apoptosis and cell adhesion *(72)*.

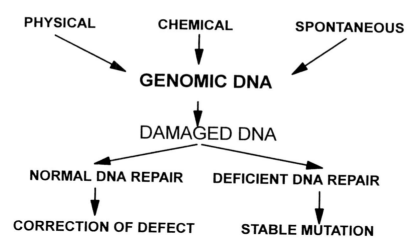

Fig. 4. DNA damage, mutation, and repair in cancer development. The DNA of the cellular genome is subject to endogenous and environmentally induced structural damage that can lead to errors in replication and the generation of stable DNA mutations. The proper functioning of DNA repair processes ensures that damaged sites in the genome are repaired prior to DNA replication, whereas, faulty DNA repair mechanisms promote the generation of stable DNA mutations.

5.6. Inherited DNA Repair Deficiency Syndromes

Several rare genetic disorders have been identified in humans that involve dysfunctional DNA repair pathways (Fig. 4). These disorders include xeroderma pigmentosum, Cockayne's syndrome, trichothiodystrophy, ataxia telangiectasia, Bloom's syndrome, and Fanconi's anemia. Of these disorders, xeroderma pigmentosum, ataxia telangiectasia, Bloom's syndrome, and Fanconi's anemia predispose affected individuals to the development of various malignancies when exposed to specific DNA-damaging agents. Patients with xeroderma pigmentosum display hypersensitivity to ultraviolet light and increased incidence of several types of skin cancer, including basal cell carcinoma, squamous cell carcinoma, and malignant melanoma *(82)*. Ataxia telangiectasia is an autosomal-recessive disorder characterized by cerebellar ataxia, oculocutaneous telangiectasiases, immune defects, and predisposition to malignancy. Ataxia telangiectasia affects between 1 in 40,000 and 1 in 200,000 individuals worldwide *(83)*. Patients with ataxia telangiectasia exhibit hypersensitivity to ionizing radiation and chemical agents, and are predisposed to the development of B-cell lymphoma, chronic lymphocytic leukemias *(83)*, and affected women demonstrate an increased risk of developing breast cancer *(84)*. Patients with Fanconi's anemia demonstrate sensitivity to DNA cross-linking agents and are predisposed to malignancies of the hematopoietic system, particularly acute myelogenous leukemia. Patients with Bloom's syndrome demonstrate an increased incidence of several forms of cancer, including leukemia, skin cancer, and breast cancer *(85)*.

The molecular basis for several of these genetic DNA repair deficiencies has been partially determined through genetic complementation analyses. Each complementation group identified represents a different genetic defect that eliminates a specific functional aspect of a DNA repair pathway. Seven complementation groups have been identified in xeroderma pigmentosum *(82)*, four complementation groups have been identified in ataxia telangiectasia *(86)*, and four complementation groups have been identified in Fanconi's anemia *(87)*. The molecular defect in Bloom's syndrome has been suggested to involve faulty regulation of DNA repair processes rather than faulty DNA repair enzymes *(85)*. Candidate genes for each of the xeroderma pigmentosum complementation groups have now been cloned. Each of these genes encode proteins involved with various aspects of DNA nucleotide excision repair, including proteins that function in the recognition of DNA damage, and factors that couple the processes of transcription and repair *(82)*. Recently, a candidate ataxia telangiectasia susceptibility gene (termed ATM) has been identified, cloned, and characterized *(88)*. The ATM gene product is similar to several mammalian phosphotidylinosital kinases that are involved in mitogenic signal transduction, meiotic recombination, and cell cycle control *(88)*.

5.7. Other Genetic Syndromes Associated with Increased Cancer Risk

Several syndromes have been described that are characterized by congenital anomalies with varying phenotypic features and increased risk of specific forms of cancer. von Recklinghausen neurofibromatosis or neurofibromatosis type 1 (NF 1) is one of the most common autosomal-dominant disorders of humans, occurring with a frequency of 1 in 2500 to 1 in 5000 individuals. NF 1 is characterized by benign skin lesions (cafe au lait spots), lisch nodules of the iris, and multiple benign cutaneous and soft tissue neurofibromata *(89)*. Individuals with NF 1 are at high risk for the development of tumors of the central nervous system, malignant peripheral nerve sheath tumors, rhabdomyosarcoma, and leukemias. The genetic basis for NF 1 has been determined to be a tumor suppressor gene located on 17q *(89)*. Multiple endocrine neoplasia type 2 (MEN 2) is characterized by medullary thyroid carcinoma, bilateral pheochromocytoma, and hyperparathyroidism. MEN 2 and familial medullary thyroid carcinoma are caused by germline mutations of the RET proto-oncogene *(90)*. Wilms' tumor or nephroblastoma is a pediatric kidney neoplasm that can develop as a sporadic tumor or in the setting of genetic predisposition. Genetically predisposed individuals include those affected by the WAGR syndrome (characterized by Wilms' tumor, aniridia, genitourinary malformations, and mental retardation), Denys-Drash syndrome (characterized by intersexual disorders, nephropathy, and Wilms' tumor), or the Beckwith-Weidemann syndrome (characterized by macroglossia, organomegaly, hemihypertrophy, neonatal hypoglycemia, and various embryonal tumors) *(91)*. Initially, this pediatric tumor was thought to be owing to the sole deletion of the WT1 tumor suppressor gene, located on human chromosome 11p13. It has since been recognized that Wilms' tumor constitutes a contiguous genetic syndrome whereby several genes, responsible for the various phenotypes of WAGR, Denys-Drash, and Beckwith-Weidemann syndromes, located in the same region of chromosome 11 are mutated or deleted *(91)*.

6. MOLECULAR MUTATIONS IN HUMAN TUMORIGENESIS: IMPLICATIONS FOR THE EARLY DETECTION AND DIAGNOSIS OF HUMAN CANCER

Exploitation of genetic alterations for the early diagnosis of cancer prior to clinical manifestation should increase the survival of patients by allowing intervention at a time when lesions are either localized and most amenable to surgical resection, or not yet even morphologically diagnosable. Several technical considerations must be given to the appropriateness of a genetic test for early detection of precancers. These include:

1. The genetic target or targets for a specific cancer type;
2. The appropriate source of DNA for testing;
3. The nature of the mutational spectra for specific genetic targets observed in specific cancers; and
4. The sensitivity of the detection methodology.

The appropriate molecular targets for diagnostic procedures depends on the specific cancer subtype, and the known genetic alterations associated with its initiation and progression to clinical detection. A significant component of this consideration is the frequency with which a specific target is mutated during the transformation process. Following the identification of an appropriate genetic target, a source of patient DNA must be obtained for use in the testing procedure. Desirable sources for preparation of DNA include those that can be obtained with minimal invasion of the patient. Once the DNA sample enters the molecular biology laboratory, it is necessary to consider the expected mutational spectrum with respect to where in the overall structure of the gene mutations are likely to be found. Genes that are typically mutated at a few hot-spot codons are preferable targets to genes that can be activated or inactivated through any of a number of mutations over a wide area of the gene sequence. The economic feasibility of the diagnostic procedure will depend greatly on this consideration. Assays that detect rare mutations (mutation frequency $>1 \times 10^{-6}$) may be too sensitive to be generally useful in clinical diagnosis *(7)*. Such tests have the potential to detect mutations that are fixed in a small number of cells prior to clonal expansion and clinical progression. Thus, a significant rate of false positives could occur, resulting in the inappropriate clinical screening or intervention. The ultimate goal for the development of effective molecular screening techniques is the identification of molecular alterations prior to the onset of clinical symptoms or even morphologic manifestations, such that patients identified in this manner could then be evaluated at regular intervals for the appearance of lesions that are curable by surgical resection. In addition, effective screening strategies may facilitate the identification of candidates for chemoprevention strategies.

6.1. Early Detection of Colorectal Cancer

Traditional screening methods for colorectal cancer through the use of stool guaiac tests remain controversial, with many false-positive and false-negative results *(92)*. With the establishment of the early genetic alterations in the development of colorectal cancer, it became evident that these changes could serve as markers for early detection of developing neoplasms. This led to the discovery that *ras* gene mutations could be identified in DNA isolated from stool samples obtained from patients with colorectal cancer using a PCR-based method *(93)*. Subsequently, Tobi et al. *(94)* developed an enriched PCR method for detection of K-*ras* gene mutations in high-risk patients prior to the development of colorectal cancer. In their study, mutations in codon 12 of K-*ras* were detected in approx 40% of high-risk patients *(94)*. Application of these methods may facilitate the identification of patients with developing colorectal neoplasms prior to the emergence of a tumor that can be identified using conventional methods (i.e., endoscopy, barium enema, stool guaiac). Given that most colon cancers progress through the adenoma-carcinoma sequence, early detection will facilitate surgical intervention when adenomas are small and localized without high-grade dysplasia or carcinoma *in situ*, potentially impacting long-term patient survival.

Familial adenomatus polyposis is an inherited disease characterized by multiple colorectal tumors. Traditional diagnosis relies on detection of numerous colorectal polyps during young adulthood. Identification of the FAP locus at 5q21 and subsequent cloning of the APC gene *(44–46)* have provided the opportunity for genetic testing for this disease. However, the APC gene represents a difficult target for use in molecular diagnostics, because it can be inactivated through mutational alteration at a number of sites within its coding sequence, which encompasses more than 8500 bp of DNA *(45,46)*. Based on the observation that mutations in the APC gene frequently give rise to truncated gene products, Kinzler and colleagues developed a strategy for identification of mutations based on examination of APC proteins synthesized in vitro and allele-specific expression of endogenous APC transcripts *(95)*. The protein assay revealed altered (truncated) APC products in 82% of patients evaluated. In patients that did not demonstrate aberrantly sized APC protein, the allele-specific expression assay showed reduced expression from one allele, suggesting mutational alteration of the affected allele. When applied in combination, these procedures were able to identify germline mutations in the APC gene in 87% of patients evaluated *(95)*. This methodology should enable the diagnosis of FAP before the establishment of benign colorectal polyps and improve the management of these patients with respect to preventive measures prior to the development of colorectal tumors. The application of potential pharmacologic treatments for polyposis might be more effective if initiated prior to the appearance of polyps *(95)*.

6.2. Early Detection of Lung Carcinoma

Sidransky and colleagues have examined the occurrence of *ras* and p53 gene mutations in primary lung carcinomas and corresponding sputum samples obtained from the same patients prior to clinical diagnosis of their tumors *(96)*. In their study, 10/15 tumors contained either a *ras* or p53 gene mutation. Using a PCR-based assay, the same molecular mutations were identified in sputum samples corresponding to 8/10 cases. Each of these sputum samples was cytologically negative for diagnosis of carcinoma. The applied technique was shown to be quite sensitive in that the molecular mutation was detected in the sputum sample of a patient more than 1 yr prior to the clinical diagnosis of lung carcinoma. This method combines PCR amplification of the target gene with plaque screening of bacteriophage clones of the amplified DNA product using mutant or wild-type sequence-specific oligonucleotide probes. Subsequently, mutant gene sequences were confirmed through DNA sequence analysis. Validation of the specificity of this methodology was indicated in that five control lung tumors that contained no K-*ras* or p53 gene mutations were negative by PCR cloning and plaque screening *(96)*. In addition, 6/8 patients who initially tested positive for mutation were found to test negative in sputum samples obtained following the complete surgical resection of their tumor. The authors suggest that sensitive molecular analyses can detect potentially diagnostic molecular mutations in cytologically negative sputum samples prior to the clinical detection of lung cancer by radiological methods, presenting the possibility that chemoprevention strategies could be employed in clinical intervention *(96)*.

6.3. Early Detection of Pancreatic Cancer

The K-*ras* proto-oncogene is activated by point mutation in 72–100% of primary pancreatic adenocarcinomas *(97)*. Thus, evaluation of mutations in the K-*ras* gene may facilitate the early diagnosis of pancreatic tumors. Bernaudin and colleagues developed a rapid screening method for K-*ras* mutations in fine-needle aspirates and evaluated the potential of K-*ras* mutations in the diagnosis of pancreatic adenocarcinoma *(98)*. In their method, regions of the K-*ras* gene were PCR-amplified using sequence-specific oligonucleotide primers, and a unique restriction site was introduced into the amplified products of a codon 12 mutant K-*ras* gene by virtue of the sequence-specific oligonucleotide primers utilized. Subsequently, products of mutant and wild-type K-*ras* genes were distinguished by restriction digestion and RFLP analysis. Using this methodology, a mutation present in only 1% of the cells within a specimen could be detected. Mutations of the K-*ras* gene were detected in 11/12 (92%) pancreatic adenocarcinomas using PCR/RFLP, suggesting that evaluation of K-*ras* mutations could facilitate diagnosis of pancreatic tumors *(98)*. In a similar study, Pradayrol and colleagues utilized PCR/RFLP to evaluate K-*ras* mutations in DNA obtained from samples of pancreatic juice collected during endoscopic retrograde pancreatography of patients prior to clinical diagnosis *(99)*. The results of this later study suggested that evaluation of K-*ras* mutations in samples of pancreatic juice is useful in the differential diagnosis of neoplastic and nonneoplastic pancreatic disease *(99)*. Further, these investigators demonstrated that K-*ras* mutations can be detected in the pancreatic juice many months (18–40 mo) prior to the clinical manifestation of pancreatic cancer *(99)*. Other studies have also demonstrated the potential for early detection of pancreatic cancers by evaluation of K-*ras* gene mutations in gastric aspirates and stool specimens *(100,101)*.

7. MOLECULAR MUTATIONS IN HUMAN TUMORIGENESIS: IMPLICATIONS FOR THE PREDICTION OF CLINICAL OUTCOME OF HUMAN CANCER

In a large number of cancer cases, patients present with an established primary tumor that can be detected and diagnosed using conventional clinical techniques, and all too often patients present with relatively advanced neoplastic disease involving both primary and metastatic lesions. Carcinomas of the lung and pancreas, as noted above, typify this presentation. Management of early stage tumors generally involves surgery with or without adjuvant therapies (radiation or chemotherapy). However, advanced stages of neoplastic disease are not simply managed and represent a formidable challenge for the clinician. With respect to patients with advanced disease, clinicians must choose an appropriate course of treatment, given the available options, that is most likely to result in patient benefit, be that goal palliation of symptoms or attempted cure. As a component of patient benefit, clinicians must consider patient quality of life, which necessitates that harsh treatment strategies with potential adverse side effects not be employed in cases in which the potential for therapeutic success is low. Numerous studies have now demonstrated that evaluation of specific molecular lesions within a specific tumor subtype can provide clues regarding the appropriate treatment course. That is, tumors harboring specific gene mutations may be unresponsive to certain forms of treatment, which is manifest as lack of response to radiation or drug treatment. In this case, knowledge of the gene mutation would allow the clinician to discount the use of certain treatment modalities that hold little promise of long-term patient benefit. Alternatively, the presence of specific gene mutations within a tumor may be indicative of a poor prognosis that is contrary to the predicted outcome based on conventional prognostic indicators. In these cases, the clinician will be able to dictate a more aggressive treatment regimen, with a higher probability of long-term patient benefit.

7.1. Prediction of Clinical Outcome in Colorectal Carcinoma

The genetic alterations associated with colorectal carcinoma have been established *(4,5)*. Several groups have examined the value of these progression-associated genetic alterations in the prediction of clinical outcome. Smith and colleagues analyzed p53 tumor suppressor gene mutations in colorectal cancer patients and correlated the presence of specific mutations with clinical aggressiveness, patient response to postoperative therapy, and patient survival *(102)*. In this study, patients found to possess a point mutation in the p53 gene showed a significantly poorer prognosis than those without one. In a similar study, Hamelin and colleagues observed a strong correlation between the presence of p53 gene mutations and short survival among colorectal cancer patients *(103)*. Among patients with a mutated p53 gene, the occurrence of the point mutation within the highly conserved regions of the gene demonstrated a significant association with lymph node dissemination and an increased risk for the development of distant metastasis, and patients possessing a mutation in codon 175 of the p53 gene demonstrated the poorest prognosis of all patients *(102)*. In addition, the response of patients to palliative therapy was determined to be markedly dependent on the p53 mutation status of the primary tumor; none of the patients with p53 gene mutation survived to the 40 mo followup among those receiving palliative postoperative therapy, whereas only one patient without p53 gene mutation died during the same interval *(102)*. These authors suggest that knowledge of the p53 mutation status and the nature of specific lesions is required to predict accurately the clinical course of the disease and the response of patients to postoperative therapeutic options *(102)*.

Hamilton and colleagues have examined the prognostic value of allelic losses at 18q in colorectal cancers *(104)*. Alterations at this chromosomal site generally represent late events preceding metastasis *(4,5)*. Thus, the authors hypothesized that allelic loss at 18q may be indicative of rapidly progressing cancers irrespective of the clinicopathological diagnosis *(104)*. The experimental approach involved PCR-mediated amplification of chromosome-specific polymorphic microsatellite markers along chromosome 18q. Patients with stage II disease and no 18q loss exhibited a significantly better prognosis than patients with stage II disease and 18q loss (5-yr survival rates of 93 and 54% respectively). In patients with stage III disease, those with 18q loss had a 5-yr survival of 38 vs 52% for those without 18q loss. The authors observed that the prognosis of stage II patients with 18q loss was comparable to that of stage III patients without 18q loss *(104)*. Patients with stage III disease are frequently treated more aggressively than stage II patients, with routine clinical intervention involving both surgery and adjuvant therapy *(105)*. Thus, evaluation of stage II patients for 18q allelic loss may identify a subset of patients that would benefit from aggressive clinical intervention *(104)*.

7.2. Prediction of Clinical Outcome in Breast Carcinoma

Mutations of the p53 tumor suppressor gene are variably but frequently observed in breast carcinoma (15–40%), suggesting that mutation of this gene is important in the genesis of this tumor type. The observation that patients with Li-Fraumeni syndrome exhibit an increased risk for development of breast tumors supports this suggestion. Several studies have examined the prognostic significance of p53 mutations in breast tumors. Kovach and colleagues determined that breast cancer patients with mutated p53 exhibit a shorter time to tumor recurrence and a shorter overall survival than patients who do not possess a mutated p53 gene *(106)*. Further, these investigators demonstrated that both missense-type mutations (point mutation and in-frame microdeletions) and null mutations (hemizygous nonsense and frameshift mutations) were associated with poor prognosis *(106)*. Thorlacius et al. *(107)* found that p53 mutations occurred in approx 17% of breast carcinomas examined, but that patients with mutated p53 exhibited significantly greater mortality rates than patients without detected p53 mutations. In a recent study, Sommer and colleagues *(108)* found that detection of p53 gene mutations was associated with a high probability of tumor recurrence and death in affected patients. These authors suggest that evaluation of p53 gene mutations in breast carcinomas could serve to identify patients who lack conventional indicators of poor prognosis, but are at high risk for recurrence and early death *(108)*. This subset of patients may benefit from aggressive adjuvant therapy following surgical resection of the primary tumor.

8. CONSIDERATIONS FOR THE APPLICATION OF MOLECULAR TECHNIQUES IN CANCER SCREENING

Because of the public health threat cancer poses, investigators have been searching for clues to better understand carcinogenesis. The "War on Cancer" declared over 25 years ago by the Nixon Administration is far from over, and many believe it has only just begun. Although numerous genes have been identified that are associated with both sporadic and familial tumors, the diagnostic and prognostic relevance of many of these remains to be proven. The fact that cancer itself arises because of many different alterations to the cellular genome presents a diagnostic dilemma for the clinical laboratory. Furthermore, the inconsistent presence of specific gene mutations in individual tumors of a single type represents a formidable problem to the application of molecular diagnostics in cancer screening.

For familial or inherited cancers, family members can be screened for predisposing risks if identification of a mutant gene or marker sequence associated with that type of tumor has been established in the germline of the affected individual. Even in these cases, which seem to be relatively straightforward, the data must be interpreted and handled very cautiously. As we have learned from the search for mutations in the BRCA1 gene in familial cases of breast cancer, this type of laboratory testing has opened a Pandora's box with respect to ethical, legal, and technical issues never before imagined. Determining one's predisposition to development of a sporadic tumor and the associated diagnostic/prognostic issues will continue to challenge the laboratory in an unprecedented fashion. Since the definitive diagnosis of cancer is dependent on histological evaluation of tissues by a pathologist, the College of American Pathologists has published a summary of clinically relevant prognostic markers in solid tumors *(109–111)*. The general conclusions for solid tumors, such as breast, colon, and prostate cancers, supported the fact that many biological markers are currently available. However, with respect to many of them, considerable technical advances need to be made for routine analysis in the clinical laboratory and clinical data evaluated to determine the relevance of any particular marker to patient management. As an evolving area of clinical research, future studies should identify new markers for predisposition and prognostication testing as well as confirm the efficacy of existing potential markers.

ACKNOWLEDGMENTS

We wish to thank Andrew Ricci, Jr. (Department of Pathology and Laboratory Medicine, Hartford Hospital) for critically reviewing this manuscript and making helpful suggestions.

REFERENCES

1. Foulds, L. The natural history of cancer. *J. Chronic Dis.* **8**:2–37, 1958
2. Weinberg, R. A. Oncogenes, antioncogenes, and the molecular bases of multistep carcinogenesis. *Cancer Res.* **49**:3713–3721, 1989.
3. Bishop, J. M. Molecular themes in oncogenesis. *Cell* **64**:235–248, 1991.
4. Fearon, E. R. and Vogelstein, B. A genetic model for colorectal tumorigenesis. *Cell* **61**:757–767, 1990.
5. Vogelstein, B., Fearon, E. R., Hamilton, S. R., Kern, S. E., Leppert, M., Nakamura, Y., White, R., Smits, M. M., and Bos, J. L. Genetic alterations during colorectal tumor development. *New Engl. J. Med.* **319**:525–532, 1988.
6. Sidransky, D., Boyle, J., Koch, W., and van der Riet, P. Oncogene mutations as intermediate markers. *J. Cell. Biochem. Suppl.* **17F**:184–187, 1993.
7. Sidransky, D. Molecular screening—How long can we afford to wait? *J. Natl. Cancer Inst.* **86**:955–956, 1994.
8. Mao, L. and Sidransky, D. Cancer screening based on genetic alterations in human tumors. *Cancer Res.* **54**:1939S–1940S, 1994.
9. Sidransky, D. Molecular markers in cancer: can we make better predictions? *Int. J. Cancer* **64**:1–2, 1995.
10. Nowell, P. The clonal evolution of tumor cell populations. *Science* **194**:23–38, 1976.
11. Renan, M. J. How many mutations are required for tumorigenesis? Implications from human cancer data. *Mol. Carcinog.* **7**:139–146, 1993.
12. Sugarbaker, J. P., Gunderson, L. L., and Wittes, R. E. Colorectal cancer, in *Cancer: Principles and Practice of Oncology*, De Vita, V. T., Hellman, S., and Rosenberg, S. A., eds., Lippincott, Philadelphia, pp. 800–815, 1985.
13. Anderson, M. W., Reynolds, S. H., You, M., and Maronpot, R. M. Role of proto-oncogene activation in carcinogenesis. *Environ. Health Perspect.* **98**:13–24, 1992.
14. Cooper, G. M. *Oncogenes*, 2nd ed., Jones and Bartlett Publishers, Boston, 1995.
15. Marshall, C. J. Tumor suppressor genes. *Cell* **64**:313–326, 1991.
16. Friend, S. p53: a glimpse at the puppet behind the shadow play. *Science* **265**:334–335, 1994.
17. Zambetti, G. P. and Levine, A. J. A comparison of the biological activities of wild-type and mutant p53. *FASEB J.* **7**:855–865, 1993.
18. Hollingsworth, R. E., Hensely, C. E., and Lee, W. H. Retinoblastoma protein and the cell cycle. *Curr. Opinion Genet. Dev.* **3**:55–62, 1993.
19. Perry, M. E. and Levine, A. J. Tumor-suppressor p53 and the cell cycle. *Curr. Opinion Genet. Dev.* **3**:50–54, 1993.

20. Bos, J. L. *ras* Oncogenes in human cancer: a review. *Cancer Res.* **49**:4682–4689, 1989.
21. Hollstein, M., Sidransky, D., Vogelstein, B., and Harris, C. C. p53 mutations in human cancers. *Science* **253**:49–53, 1991.
22. Greenblatt, M. S., Bennett, W. P., Hollstein, M., and Harris, C. C. Mutations in the p53 tumor suppressor gene: clues to cancer etiology and molecular pathogenesis. *Cancer Res.* **54**:4855–4878, 1994.
23. Spitz, M. R. and Bondy, M. L. Genetic susceptibility to cancer. *Cancer* **72**:991–995, 1993.
24. Friedberg, E. C. *DNA Repair.* Freeman, New York, 1985.
25. Coleman, W. B. and Tsongalis, G. J. Multiple mechanisms account for genomic instability and molecular mutation in neoplastic transformation. *Clin. Chem.* **41**:644–657, 1995.
26. Pines, J. Cyclins and their associated cyclin-dependent kinases in the human cell cycle. *Biochem. Soc. Trans.* **21**:921–925, 1993.
27. Cordon-Cardo, C. Mutation of cell cycle regulators. Biological and clinical implications for human neoplasia. *Am. J. Pathol.* **147**:454–560, 1995.
28. Kinzler, K. W. and Vogelstein, B. The colorectal cancer gene hunt: current findings. *Hosp. Pract.* **27**:37–44, 1992.
29. Bos, J. L., Fearon, E. R., Hamilton, S. R., Verlaan-de Vries, M., van Boom, J. H., van der Eb, A. J., and Vogelstein, B. Prevalence of ras gene mutations in human colorectal cancers. *Nature* **327**:293–297, 1987.
30. Baker, S. J., Fearon, E. R., Nigro, J. M., Hamilton, S. R., Preisinger, A. C., Jessup, J. M., van Tuinen, P., Ledbetter, D. H., Barker, D. F., Nakamura, Y., White, R., and Vogelstein, B. Chromosome 17 deletions and p53 gene mutations in colorectal carcinomas. *Science* **244**:217–221, 1989.
31. Feinberg, A. P., Gehrke, C. W., Kuo, K. C., and Ehrlich, M. Reduced genomic 5-methylcytosine content in human colonic neoplasia. *Cancer Res.* **48**:1159–1161, 1988.
32. Lee, W.-H, Bookstein, R., Hong, F., Young, L.-H., Shew, J.-Y., and Lee, E. Y.-H. P. Human retinoblastoma susceptability gene: cloning, identification, and sequence. *Science* **235**:1394–1399, 1987.
33. Knudson, A. G. Mutation and cancer: a statistical study of retinoblastoma. *Proc. Natl. Acad. Sci. USA* **68**:820–823, 1971.
34. Li, F. P and Fraumeni, J. F., Jr. Soft-tissue sarcomas, breast cancer, and other neoplasms. A familial syndrome? *Ann. Intern. Med.* **71**:747–752, 1969.
35. Li, F. P, Fraumeni, J. F., Jr., Mulvihill, J. J., Blattner, W. A., Dreyfus, M. G., Tucker, M. A., and Miller, R. W. A cancer family syndrome in 24 kindreds. *Cancer Res.* **48**:5358–5362, 1988.
36. Li, F. P and Fraumeni, J. F., Jr. Prospective study of a family cancer syndrome. *JAMA* **247**:2692–2694, 1982.
37. Lustbader, E. D., Williams, W. R., Bondy, M. L., Strom, S., and Strong, L. C. Segregation analysis of cancer families of childhood soft-tissue-sarcoma patients. *Am. J. Hum. Genet.* **51**:344–356, 1992.
38. Malkin, D., Li, F. P., Strong, L. C., Fraumeni, J. F., Nelson, C. E., Kim, D. M., Kessel, J., Gryka, M. A., Bischoff, F. Z., Tainsky, M. A., and Friend, S. Germ line mutations in a familial syndrome of breast cancer, sarcomas, and other neoplasms. *Science* **250**:1233–1238, 1990.
39. Srivastava, S., Zou, Z., Pirollo, K., Blattner, W., and Chang, E. H. Germ-line transmission of a mutated p53 gene in a cancer-prone family with Li-Fraumeni syndrome. *Nature* **348**:747–749, 1990.
40. Birch, J. M., Hartley, A. L., Tricker, K. J., Prosser, J., Condie, A., Kelsey, A. M., Harris, M., Jones, P. H. M., Binchy, A., Crowther, D., Craft, A. W., Eden, O. B., Evans, D. G. R., Thompson, E., Mann, J. R., Martin, J., Mitchell, E. L. D., and Santibanez-Koref, M. F. Prevalence and diversity of constitutional mutations in the p53 gene among 21 Li-Fraumeni families. *Cancer Res.* **54**:1298–1304, 1994.

41. Birch, J. M. Familial cancer syndromes and clusters. *Br. Med. Bull.* **50**:624–639, 1994.

42. Momand, J., Zambetti, G. P., Olson, D. C., George, D., and Levine, A. J. The mdm-2 oncogene product forms a complex with the p53 protein and inhibits p53-mediated transactivation. *Cell* **69**:1237–1245, 1992.

43. Lynch, H. T., Lanspa, S., Smyrk, T., Boman, B., Watson, P., and Lynch, J. Hereditary nonpolyposis colorectal cancer (Lynch syndromes I and II). Genetics, pathology, natural history, and cancer control, part I. *Cancer Genet. Cytogenetics* **53**:143–160, 1991.

44. Nishisho, I., Nakamura, Y., Miyoshi, Y., Miki, Y., Ando, H., Horii, A., Koyama, K., Utsunomiya, J., Baba, S., Hedge, P., Markham, A., Krush, A. J., Peterson, G., Hamilton, S. R., Nilbert, M. C., Levy, D. B., Bryan, T. M., Preisinger, A. C., Smith, K. J., Su, L., Kinzler, K. W., and Vogelstein, B. Mutations of chromosome 5q21 genes in FAP and colorectal cancer patients. *Science* **253**:665–669, 1991.

45. Groden, J., Thliveris, A., Samowitz, W., Carlson, M., Gelbert, L., Albertson, H., Joslyn, G., Stevens, J., Spiro, L., Robertson, M., Sargent, L., Krapcho, K., Wolff, E., Burt, R., Hughes, J. P., Warrington, J., McPherson, J., Wasmuth, J., Le Paslier, D., Abderrahim, H., Cohen, D., Leppert, M., and White, R. Identification and characterization of the familial adenomatous polyposis coli gene. *Cell* **66**:589–600, 1991.

46. Kinzler, K. W., Nilbert, M. C., Su, L. K., Vogelstein, B., Bryan, T. M., Levy, D. B., Smith, K. J., Preisinger, A. C., Hedge, P., McKechnie, D., Finniear, R., Markham, A., Groffe, J., Boguski, M. S., Altschul, S. F., Horii, A., Ando, H., Miyoshi, Y., Miki, Y., Nishisho, I., and Nakamura, Y. Identification of a chromosome 5q21 gene that is mutated in colorectal cancers. *Science* **251**:1366–1370, 1991.

47. Nagase, H., Miyoshi, Y., Horii, A., Aoki, T., Ogawa, M., Utsunomiya, J., Baba, S., Sasuki, T., and Nakamura, Y. Correlation between the location of germ-line mutations in the APC gene and the number of colorectal polyps in familial adenomatous polyposis patients. *Cancer Res.* **52**:4055–4057, 1992.

48. Su, L., Johnson, K. A., Smith, K. J., Hill, D. E., Vogelstein, B., and Kinzler, K. W. Association between wild type and mutant APC gene products. *Cancer Res.* **53**:2728–2731, 1993.

49. Vasen, H. F. A., Offerhaus, G. J. A., den Hartog Jager, F. C. A., Menko, F. H., Nagengast, F. M., Griffioen, G., van Hogezand, R. B., and Heintz, A. P. M. The tumour spectrum in hereditary non-polyposis colorectal cancer: a study of 24 kindreds in the Netherlands. *Int. J. Cancer* **46**:31–34, 1990.

50. Mecklin, J.-P. and Jarvinen, H. J. Tumor spectrum in cancer family syndrome (hereditary nonpolyposis colorectal cancer). *Cancer* **68**:1109–1112, 1991.

51. Peltomaki, P., Aaltonen, L. A., Sistonen, P., Pykkanen, L., Mecklin, J. P., Jarvinen, H., Green, J. S., Jass, J. R., Weber, J. L., Leach, F. S., Petersen, G. M., Hamilton, S. R., de la Chapelle, A., and Vogelstein, B. Genetic mapping of a locus predisposing to human colorectal cancer. *Science* **260**:810–812, 1993.

52. Aaltonen, L. A., Peltomaki, P., Leach, F. S., Sistonen, P., Pylkkanen, L., Mecklin, J.-P., Jarvinen, H., Powell, S. M., Jen, J., Hamilton, S. R., Petersen, G. M., Kinzler, K. W., Vogelstein, B. and de la Chapelle, A. Clues to the pathogenesis of familial colorectal cancer. *Science* **260**:812–816, 1993.

53. Thibodeau, S. N., Bren, G., and Schaid, D. Microsatellite instability in cancer of the proximal colon. *Science* **260**:816–819, 1993.

54. Ionov, Y., Peinado, M. A., Malkhosyan, S., Shibata, D. and Perucho, M. Ubiquitous somatic mutations in simple repeated sequences reveal a new mechanism for colonic carcinogenesis. *Nature* **363**:558–561, 1993.

55. Aaltonen, L. A., Peltomaki, P., Mecklin, J.-P., Jarvinen, H., Jass, J. R., Green, J. S., Lynch, H. T., Watson, P., Tallqvist, G., Juhola, M., Sistonen, P., Hamilton, S. R., Kinzler, K. W., Vogelstein, B. and de la Chapelle, A. Replication errors in benign and malignant tumors from hereditary nonpolyposis colorectal cancer patients. *Cancer Res.* **54**:1645–1648, 1994.

56. Fishel, R., Lescoe, M. K., Rao, M. R. S., Copeland, N. G., Jenkins, N. A., Garber, J., Kane, M. and Kolodner, R. The human mutator gene homolog *MSH2* and its association with hereditary nonpolyposis colon cancer. *Cell* **75**:1027–1038, 1993.

57. Leach, F. S., Nicolaides, N. C., Papadopoulos, N., Liu, B., Jen, J., Sistonen, P., Aaltonen, L. A., Nystrom-Lahti, M., Guan, X.-Y., Zhang, J., Meltzer, P. S., Yu, J.-W., Kao, F.-T., Chen, D. J., Cerosaletti, K. M., Fournier, R. E. K., Todd, S., Lewis, T., Leach, R. J., Naylor, S. L., Weissenbach, J., Mecklin, J.-P., Jarvinen, H., Petersen, G. M., Hamilton, S. R., Green, J., Jass, J., Watson, P., Lynch, H. T., Trent, J. M., de la Chapelle, A., Kinzler, K. W., and Vogelstein, B. Mutations of a *mutS* homolog in hereditary nonpolyposis colorectal cancer. *Cell* **75**:1215–1225, 1993.

58. Bronner, C. E., Baker, S. M., Morrison, P. T., Warren, G., Smith, L. G., Lescoe, M. K., Kane, M., Earabino, C., Lipford, J., Lindbloom, A., Tannergard, P., Bollag, R. J., Godwin, A. R., Ward, D. C., Nordenskjold, M., Fishel, R., Kolodner, R., and Liskay, R. M. Mutation in the DNA mismatch repair gene homologue hMLH1 is associated with hereditary non-polyposis colon cancer. *Nature* **368**:258–261, 1994.

59. Nicolaides, N. C., Papadopoulos, N., Liu, B., Wel, Y.-F., Carter, K. C., Ruben, S. M., Rosen, C. A., Haseltine, W. A., Fleischmann, R. D., Fraser, C. M., Adams, M. D., Venter, J. C., Dunlop, M. G., Hamilton, S. R., Petersen, G. M., de la Chapelle, A., Vogelstein, B., and Kinzler, K. W. Mutations of two PMS homologues in hereditary nonpolyposis colon cancer. *Nature* **371**:75–80, 1994.

60. Papadopoulos, N., Nicolaides, N. C., Wei, Y.-F., Ruben, S. M., Carter, K. C., Rosen, C. A., Haseltine, W. A., Fleishmann, R. D., Fraser, C. M., Adams, M. D., Venter, J. C., Hamilton, S. R., Petersen, G. M., Watson, P., Lynch, H. T., Peltomaki, P., Mecklin, J.-P., de la Chapelle, A., Kinzler, K. W., and Vogelstein, B. Mutation of a mutL homolog in hereditary colon cancer. *Science* **263**:1625–1629, 1994.

61. Shibata, D., Peinado, M. A., Ionov, Y., Malkhosyan, S., and Perucho, M. Genomic instability in repeated sequences is an early somatic event in colorectal tumorigenesis that persists after transformation. *Nature Genet.* **6**:273–281, 1994.

62. Parsons, R., Li, G.-M., Longley, M. J., Fang, W.-H., Papadopoulos, N., Jen, J., de la Chapelle, A., Kinzler, K. W., Vogelstein, B., and Modrich, P. Hypermutability and mismatch repair deficiency in RER$^+$ tumor cells. *Cell* **75**:1227–1236, 1993.

63. Miki, Y., Swensen, J., Shattuck-Eidens, D., Futreal, P. A., Harshman, K., Tavtigian, S., Liu, Q., Cochran, C., Bennett, M., Ding, W., Bell, R., Rosenthal, J., Hussey, C., Tran, T., McClure, M., Frye, C., Hattier, T., Phelps, R., Haugen-Strano, A., Katcher, H., Yakumo, K., Golami, Z., Shaffer, D., Stone, S., Bayer, S., Wray, C., Bogden, R., Dayananth, P., Ward, J., Tonin, P., Narod, S,A., Bristow, P., Norris, P., Helvering, L., Morrison, P., Rosteck, P., Lai, M., Barrett, C., Lewis, C., Neuhausen, S., Cannon-Albright, L., Goldgar, D., Wiseman, R., Kamb, A., and Skolnick, M. A strong candidate for the breast and ovarian cancer susceptibility gene BRCA1. *Science* **266**:67–71, 1994.

64. Wooster, R., Bignell, G., Lancaster, J., Swift, S., Seal, S., Mangion, J., Collins, N., Gregory, S., Gumbs, C., Micklem, G., Barfoot, R., Hamoudi, R., Patel, S., Rice, C., Biggs, P., Hashim, Y., Smith, A., Connor, F., Arason, A., Gundmundsson, J., Ficenec, D., Kelsell, D., Ford, D., Tonin, P., Bishop, D. T., Spurr, N. K., Ponder, B. A. J., Eeles, R., Peto, J., Devilee, P., Cornelisse, C., Lynch, H., Narod, S., Lenoir, G., Egilsson, V., Barkadottir, R. B., Easton, D. F., Bentley, D. R., Futreal, P. A., Ashworth, A., and Stratton, M. R. Identification of the breast cancer susceptibility gene BRCA2. *Nature* **378**:789–792, 1995.

65. Sobol, H., Neuhausen, S. L., and Eisinger, F. Evidence for a third breast-cancer susceptibility gene. *Lancet* **344**:1151,1152, 1994.

66. Easton, D. F., Ford, D., Bishop, D. T., and the Breast Cancer Linkage Consortium. Breast and ovarian cancer incidence in BRCA1-mutation carriers. *Am. J. Hum. Genet.* **56**:265–271, 1995.

67. Easton, D. F., Bishop, D. T., Ford, D., Cockford, G. P., and the Breast Cancer Linkage Consortium. Genetic linkage analysis in familial breast and ovarian cancer. *Am. J. Hum. Genet.* **52:**718–722, 1993.

68. Shattuck-Eidens, D., McClure, M., Simard, J., Labrie, F., Narod, S., Couch, F., Hoskins, K., Weber, B., Castilla, L., Erdos, M., Brody, L., Friedman, L., Ostermeyer, E., Szabo, C., King, M.-C., Jhanwar, S., Offit, K., Norton, L., Gilewski, T., Lubin, M., Osborne, M., Black, D., Boyd, M., Steel, M., Ingles, S., Haile, R., Lindblom, A., Olsson, H., Borg, A., Bishop, D. T., Solomon, E., Radice, P., Spatti, G., Gayther, S., Ponder, B., Warren, W., Stratton, M., Liu, Q., Fujimura, F., Lewis, C., Skolnick, M. H., and Goldgar, D. E. A collaborative survey of 80 mutations in the BRCA1 breast and ovarian cancer susceptibility gene: implications for presymptomatic testing and screening. *JAMA* **273:**535–541, 1995.

69. Futreal, P. A., Liu, Q., Shattuck-Eidens, D., Cochran, C., Harshman, K., Tavtigian, S., Bennett, L. M., Haugen-Strano, A., Swensen, J., Miki, Y., Eddington, K., McClure, M., Frye, C., Weaver-Feidhaus, J., Ding, W., Gholami, Z., Soderkvist, P., Terry, L., Jhanwar, S., Berchuck, A., Inglehart, J. D., Marks, J., Ballinger, D. G., Barrett, J. C., Skolnick, M. H., Kamb, A., and Wiseman, R. BRCA1 mutations in primary breast and ovarian carcinomas. *Science* **266:**120–122, 1994.

70. Gayther, S. A., Warren, W., Mazoyer, S., Russell, P. A., Harrington, P. A., Chiano, M., Seal, S., Hamoudi, R., van Rensburg, E. J., Dunning, A. M., Love, R., Evans, G., Easton, D., Clayton, D., Stratton, M. R., and Ponder, B. A. J. Germline mutations of the BRCA1 gene in breast and ovarian cancer families provide evidence for a genotype-phenotype correlation. *Nature Genet.* **11:**428–433, 1995.

71. Wooster, R., Neuhausen, S., Mangion, J., Quirk, Y., Ford, D., Collins, N., Nguyen, K., Seal, S., Tran, T., Averill, D., Fields, P., Marshall, G., Narod, S., Lenoir, G., Lynch, H. T., Feunteun, J., Devilee, P., Cornelisse, C., Menko, F., Daley, P., Ormiston, W., McManus, R., Pye, C., Lewis, C., Cannon-Albright, L., Peto, J., Ponder, B. A. J., Skolnick, M., Easton, D., Godgar, D., and Stratton, M. Localization of a breast cancer susceptibility gene, BRCA2, to chromosome 13q12–13. *Science* **265:**2088–2090, 1994.

72. Albino, A. P. Genes involved in melanoma susceptibility and progression. *Curr. Opinion Oncol.* **7:**162–169, 1995.

73. Bale, S. J., Chakravarti, A., and Greene, M. H. Cutaneous malignant melanoma and familial dysplastic nevi: evidence for autosomal dominance and pleiotropy. *Am. J. Hum. Genet.* **38:**188–196, 1986.

74. Cannon-Albright, L., Goldgar, D., Meyer, L., Lewis, C., Anderson, D., Fountain, J., Hegi, M., Wiseman, R., Petty, E., and Bale, A. Assignment of a locus for familial melanoma, MLM, to chromosome 9p13–p22. *Science* **258:**1148–1152, 1992.

75. Goldstein, A., Dracopoli, N., Engelstein, M., Fraser, M., Clark, W. Jr., Tucker, M. Further evidence for a locus for cutaneous malignant melanoma-dysplastic nevus (CMM/DN) on chromosome 1p, and evidence for genetic heterogeneity. *Am. J. Hum. Genet.* **52:**537–550, 1993.

76. Kamb, A., Gruis, N. A., Weaver-Feldhaus, J., Lui, Q., Harshman, K., Tavtigian, S. V., Stockert, E., Day, R. S., Johnson, B. E., and Skolnick, M. H. A cell cycle regulator potentially involved in genesis of many tumor types. *Science* **264:**436–440, 1994.

77. Nobori, T., Miura, K., Wu, D. J., Lois, A., Takabayashi, K. and Carson, D. A. Deletions of the cyclin-dependent kinase-4 inhibitor gene in multiple human cancers. *Nature* **368:**753–756, 1994.

78. Hussussian, C. J., Strvewing, J. P., Goldstein, A. M., Higgins, P. A. T., Ally, D. S., Sheahan, M. D., Clark, W. H., Jr., Tucker, M. A., and Dracopoli, N. C. Germline p16 mutations in familial melanoma. *Nature Genet.* **8:**15–21, 1994.

79. Kamb, A., Shattuck-Eidens, D., Eeles, R., Liu, Q., Gruis, N. A., Ding, W., Hussey, C., Tran, T., Miki, Y., Weaver-Feldhaus, J., McClure, M., Aitken, J. F., Anderson, D. E., Bergman, W., Frants, R., Goldgar, D. E., Green, A., MacLennan, R., Martin, N. G., Meyer, L. J., Youl, P., Zone, J. J., Skolnick, M. H., and Cannon-Albright, L. A. Analysis of the p16 gene (CDKN2) as a candidate for the chromosome 9p melanoma susceptibility locus. *Nature Genet.* **8:**22–26, 1994.

80. Ohta, M., Nagai, H., Shimizu, M., Rasio, D., Berd, D., Mastrangelo, M., Singh, A. D., Shields, J. A., Shields, C. A., Croce, C. M., and Heubner, K. Rarity of somatic and germline mutations of the cyclin dependent kinase 4 inhibitor gene, CDK4I, in melanoma. *Cancer Res.* **54:**5269–5272, 1994.

81. Zuo, L., Weger, J., Yang, Q., Goldstein, A. M., Tucker, M. A., Walker, G. J., Hayward, N., and Dracopoli, N. C. Germline mutations in the p^{16INK4a} binding domain of CDK4 in familial melanoma. *Nature Genet.* **12:**97–99, 1996.

82. Cleaver, J. E. and Kraemer, K. H. Xeroderma pigmentosum and Cockayne sundrome, in *The Metabolic and Molecular Bases of Inherited Disease*, 7th ed., Scriver, C. R., Beaudet, A. L., Sly, W. S., and Valle, D., eds., McGraw-Hill Inc., New York, pp. 4393–4419, 1995.

83. Boder, E. Ataxia-telangiectasia: an overview, in *Ataxia-telangiectasia: Genetics, Neuropathology, and Immunology of a Degenerative Disease of Childhood*, Gatti, R. A. and Swift, M., eds., Liss, New York, pp. 1–63, 1985.

84. Swift, M., Morrell, D., Massey, R. B., and Chase, C. L. Incidence of cancer in 161 families affected by ataxia-telangiectasia. *New Engl. J. Med.* **325:**1831–1836, 1991.

85. German, J. and Passarge, E. Bloom's syndrome. XII. Report from the Registry for 1987. *Clin. Genet.* **35:**57–69, 1989.

86. Gatti, R. A. Localizing the genes for ataxia telangiectasia: a human model for inherited cancer susceptibility. *Adv. Cancer Res.* **56:**77–104, 1991.

87. Digweed, M. Human genetic instability syndromes: single gene defects with increased risk of cancer. *Toxicol. Lett.* **67:**659–681, 1993.

88. Savitsky, K., Bar-Shira, A., Gilad, S., Rotman, G., Ziv, Y., Vanagaite, L., Tagle, D. A., Smith, S., Uziel, T., Sfez, S., Ashkenazi, M., Pecker, I., Frydman, M., Harnik, R., Patanjali, S. R., Simmons, A., Clines, G. A., Sartiel, A., Gatti, R. A., Chessa, L., Sanal, O., Lavin, M. F., Jaspers, N. G. J., Taylor, A. M. R., Arlett, C. F., Miki, T., Weissman, S. M., Lovett, M., Collins, F. S., and Shiloh, Y. A single ataxia telangiectasia gene with a product similar to PI-3 kinase. *Science* **268:**1749–1753, 1995.

89. Gutmann, D. H. and Collins, F. S. von Recklinghausen neurofibromatosis, in *The Metabolic and Molecular Bases of Inherited Disease*, 7th ed., Scriver, C. R., Beaudet, A. L., Sly, W. S., and Valle, D., eds., McGraw-Hill, New York, pp. 677–696, 1995.

90. Carlson, K. M., Dou, S., Chi, D., Scavarda, N., Toshima, K., Jackson, C. E., Wells, S. A., Jr., Goodfellow, P. J., and Donis-Keller, H. Single missense mutation in the tyrosine kinase catalytic domain of the RET protooncogene is associated with multiple endocrine neoplasia type 2B. *Proc. Natl. Acad. Sci. USA* **91:**1579–1583, 1994.

91. Haber, D. A. and Housman, D. E. Wilms tumor, in *The Metabolic and Molecular Bases of Inherited Disease*, 7th ed., Scriver, C. R., Beaudet, A. L., Sly, W. S., and Valle. D., eds., New York: McGraw-Hill, pp. 665–676, 1995.

92. Levin, B. Colorectal cancer screening. *Cancer* **72:**1056–1060, 1993.

93. Sidransky, D., Tokino, T., Hamilton, S. R., Kinzler, K. W., Levin, B., Brost, P., and Vogelstein, B. Identification of ras oncogene mutations in the stool of patients with curable colorectal tumor. *Science* **256:**102–105, 1992.

94. Tobi, M., Luo, F.-C., and Ronai, Z. Detection of K-ras mutation in colonic effluent samples from patients without evidence of colorectal carcinoma. *J. Natl. Cancer Inst.* **86:**1007–1010, 1994.

95. Powell, S. M., Petersen, G. M., Krush, A. J., Booker, S., Jen, J., Giardiello, F. M., Hamilton, S. R., Vogelstein, B., and Kinzler, K. W. Molecular diagnosis of familial adenomatous polyposis. *New Engl. J. Med.* **329:**1982–1987, 1993.

96. Mao, L., Hruban, R. H., Boyle, J. O., Tockman, M. and Sidransky, D. Detection of oncogene mutations in sputum precedes diagnosis of lung cancer. *Cancer Res.* **54:**1634–1637, 1994.

97. Almoguera, C., Shibata, D., Forrester, K., Martin, J., Arnheim, N., and Perucho, M. Most human carcinomas of the exocrine pancreas contain mutant c-K-*ras* genes. *Cell* **53:**549–554, 1988.

98. Urban, T., Ricci, S., Grange, J.-D., Lacave, R., Boudghene, F., Breittmayer, F., Languille, O., Roland, J., and Bernaudin, J.-F. Detection of c-Ki-*ras* mutation by PCR/RFLP analysis and diagnosis of pancreatic adenocarcinomas. *J. Natl. Cancer Inst.* **85:**2008–2012, 1993.

99. Berthelemy, P., Bouisson, M., Escourrou, J., Vaysse, N., Rumeau, J. L., and Pradayrol, L. Identification of K-ras mutations in pancreatic juice in the early diagnosis of pancreatic cancer. *Ann. Intern. Med.* **123:**188–191, 1995.

100. Tada, M., Omata, M., Kawai, S., Saisho, H., Ohto, M., Saiki, R. K., and Sninsky, J. J. Detection of ras gene mutations in pancreatic juice and peripheral blood of patients with pancreatic adenocarcinoma. *Cancer Res.* **53:**2472–2474, 1993.

101. Caldas, C., Hahn, S. A., Hruban, R. H., Redston, M. S., Yeo, C. J., and Kern, S. E. Detection of K-ras mutations in stool of patients with pancreatic adenocarcinoma and pancreatic ductal hyperplasia. *Cancer Res.* **54:**3568–3573, 1994.

102. Goh, H.-S., Yao, J., and Smith, D. R. p53 point mutation and survival in colorectal cancer patients. *Cancer Res.* **55:**5217–5221, 1995.

103. Hamelin, R., Laurent-Puig, P., Olschwang, S., Jego, N., Asselain, B., Remvikos, Y., Girodet, J., Salmon, R. J., and Thomas, G. Association of p53 mutations with short survival in colorectal cancer. *Gastroenterology* **106:**42–48, 1994.

104. Jen, J., Kim, H., Piantadosi, S., Liu, Z.-F., Levitt, R. C., Sistonen, P., Kinzler, K. W., Vogelstein, B., and Hamilton, S. R. Allelic loss of chromosome 18q and prognosis in colorectal cancer. *New Engl. J. Med.* **331:**213–221, 1994.

105. Gastrointestinal Tumor Study Group. Prolongation of the disease-free interval in surgically treated rectal carcinoma. *New Engl. J. Med.* **312:**1465–1472, 1985.

106. Saitoh, S., Cunningham, J., De Vries, E. M. G., McGovern, R. M., Schroeder, J. J., Hartmenn, A., Blaszyk, H, Wold, L. E., Schaid, D., Sommer, S. S., and Kovach, J. S. p53 gene mutations in breast cancers in midwestern US women: null as well as missense-type mutations are associated with poor prognosis. *Oncogene* **9:**2869–2875, 1994.

107. Thorlacius, S., Borresen, A.-L., and Eyfjord, J. E. Somatic p53 mutations in human breast carcinomas in an Icelandic population: a prognostic factor. *Cancer Res.* **53:**1637–1641, 1993.

108. Kovach, J. S., Hartmann, A., Blaszyk, H., Cunningham, J., Schaid, D., and Sommer, S. S. Mutation detection by highly sensitive methods indicates that p53 gene mutations in breast cancer can have important prognostic value. *Proc. Natl. Acad. Sci. USA* **93:**1093–1096, 1996.

109. Henson, D. E., Fielding, L. P., Grignon, D. J., Page, D. L., Hammond, M. E., Nash, G., Pettigrew, N. M., Gorstein, F., and Hutter, R. V. P. College of American Pathologists Conference XXVI on clinical relevance of prognostic markers in solid tumors: summary. *Arch. Pathol. Lab. Med.* **119:**1109–1112,1995.

110. Fielding, L. P. and Pettigrew, N. College of American Pathologists Conference XXVI on clinical relevance of prognostic markers in solid tumors: report of the colorectal cancer working group. *Arch. Pathol. Lab. Med.* **119:**1115–1121, 1995.

111. Grignon, D. J. and Hammond E. H. College of American Pathologists Conference XXVI on clinical relevance of prognostic markers in solid tumors: report of the prostate cancer working group. *Arch. Pathol. Lab. Med.* **119:**1122–1126, 1995.

112. Wright, P. A. and Wynford-Thomas, D. Mutations in familial cancer. *J. Pathol.* **172:**167–170, 1994.

Molecular Genetics and the Diagnosis of Hematological Malignancies

William N. Rezuke and Evelyn C. Abernathy

1. INTRODUCTION

The hematological malignancies can be broadly categorized into the malignant lymphomas, which include the two major categories, non-Hodgkin's lymphoma (NHL) and Hodgkin's disease, the acute and chronic lymphoid leukemias, which may be of B- or T-cell type, acute myelogenous leukemia, the myelodysplastic syndromes, and the myeloproliferative disorders. The goal of this chapter is to focus on the hematopathological approach to the diagnosis of the various hematological disorders with emphasis on those disorders in which molecular genetic methods, specifically Southern blotting and polymerase chain reaction (PCR), are most commonly employed.

In general, precise diagnosis of hematological malignancies often requires a multiparameter approach that correlates traditional hematoxylin-and-eosin-stained tissue sections or Wright-stained smears with a variety of special studies. These special studies may include any combination of cytochemical and histochemical stains, immunopathological studies, molecular genetic techniques, and cytogenetic techniques. Although many of these studies are quite sensitive and specific, final interpretation of any study must always be made in the context of traditional morphological findings.

2. THE LYMPHOID MALIGNANCIES: NHL AND ACUTE AND CHRONIC LYMPHOID LEUKEMIAS

The lymphoid malignancies are a heterogenous group of disorders that occur as a result of neoplastic transformation of B- and T-lymphocytes at different stages of B- and T-cell development. The wide variety of lymphoid malignancies reflects the varying stages of lymphocyte development and the complexity of the immune system. The clinical and pathological characteristics of the lymphoid malignancies are summarized in a comprehensive manner in the recently proposed Revised European American Lymphoma (REAL) classification (1).

Our understanding of the immune system and ability to diagnose and classify lymphoid malignancies improved significantly in the 1980s. This was largely because of the development of immunopathological methods that employ a wide variety of monoclonal antibodies (MAbs) to study cell-surface antigens (2) (Figs. 1A,B). Traditional morpho-

From: Molecular Diagnostics: For the Clinical Laboratorian
Edited by: W. B. Coleman and G. J. Tsongalis Humana Press Inc., Totowa, NJ

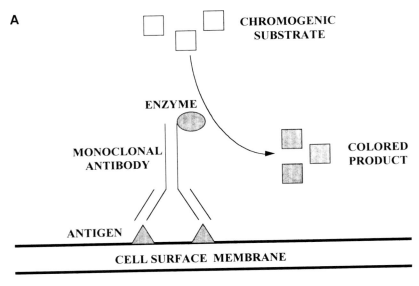

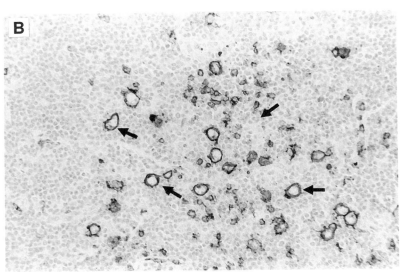

Fig. 1. Immunopathological detection of cell surface antigens. **(A)** Diagram illustrating the basic principle of immunopathological methods. An enzyme is linked to an MAb, which recognizes a specific cell-surface membrane antigen. A chromogenic substrate is added and is enzymatically converted to a colored product, which is visualized microscopically. **(B)** A case of lymphocyte predominance Hodgkin's disease showing immunoreactivity in RS variants for CD20 (arrows), a B-cell antigen that is characteristically positive in this disease. LSAB immunoperoxidase, ×500.

logical findings in conjunction with immunopathological studies are now the cornerstone of diagnosis in lymphoid malignancies. In the mid-1980s, the availability of molecular genetic methods further enhanced our ability to diagnose and classify lymphoid malignancies *(3)*. These methods are extremely powerful tools, and are used in select situations.

The major application of molecular genetic methods in the evaluation of lymphoid neoplasms involves the determination of B- and T-cell clonality. These methods are considered to be the "gold standard" for determining clonality and are utilized primarily when clonality cannot be determined immunopathologically. For B-cell neoplasms, clonality can often be determined immunopathologically by demonstrating the presence of monoclonal surface immunoglobulin *(2)*. For T-cell malignancies, there is no immunopathological equivalent to monoclonal surface immunoglobulin, although aberrant loss of T-cell antigen expression is considered to be presumptive evidence of T-cell malignancy *(2)*. Thus, in T-cell malignancies, molecular genetic studies for the determination of clonality are especially important.

Other applications of molecular genetic methods to the assessment of lymphoid malignancies include determination of B- or T-cell lineage, detection of chromosomal translocations, and detection of minimal residual disease. The latter is becoming increasingly important in evaluating patients before and after bone marrow transplantation *(4)*. The detection of a specific chromosomal translocation may help define a specific type of malignancy. For example, the detection of a clonal *bcl*-2 rearrangement indicates the presence of a chromosomal translocation involving chromosomes 14 and 18, t(14;18), which is commonly associated with NHLs of follicular center-cell origin, and the detection of a clonal *bcl*-1 rearrangement indicates the presence of a t(11;14), which is common to NHLs of mantle cell origin *(5)*.

2.1. Normal B-Cell Development

According to current concepts of the normal humoral immune system, all B-lymphocytes arise from pluripotent stem cells in the bone marrow and then subsequently migrate to secondary lymphoid organs, such as lymph node follicles and Peyer's patches in the GI tract. The stages of B-cell differentiation in the bone marrow occur largely independent of the presence of antigen, whereas the stages of differentiation in secondary lymphoid organs require the presence of antigen for transformation *(6)*.

Figure 2 shows the normal stages of B-cell development that occur in an orderly fashion, beginning with a progenitor B-cell, which matures to a terminally differentiated plasma cell. A variety of recognized changes occur at different maturational stages both at the molecular level and with regard to the presence of specific cellular antigens. At the molecular level, the genes that code for the immunoglobulin heavy- and light-chain proteins undergo sequential rearrangements early in B-cell development (Fig. 2). Initially, the immunoglobulin μ heavy chain located on chromosome 14q32 rearranges and is followed by κ light-chain rearrangement on chromosome 2p12 and λ light-chain rearrangement on chromosome 22q11 *(7)*. Subsequent transcription and translation of the μ heavy-chain gene result in the appearance of cytoplasmic μ heavy-chain protein, which defines the pre-B-cell stage of development. The immature, mature, and activated B-cell stages are characterized by the presence of an intact surface immunoglobulin receptor, which consists of two heavy- and two light-chain proteins (Fig. 3A). As illustrated in Fig. 2, a variety of cellular antigens can be detected at different stages of B-cell development, and the majority are referred to by cluster designation (CD) numbers.

The earliest antigens expressed on B-cells are terminal deoxynucleotidyl transferase (TdT) and HLA-Dr. Neither of these antigens are B lineage specific. B-cell associated

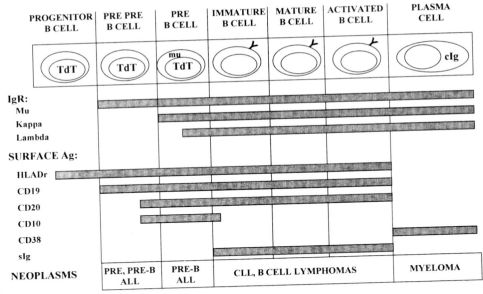

Fig. 2. Normal stages of B-cell development. *See text* for discussion. TdT, terminal deoxynucleotidyl transferase; μ, cytoplasmic μ heavy chain; cIg, cytoplasmic immunoglobulin; IgR, immunoglobulin rearrangements; sIg, surface immunoglobulin.

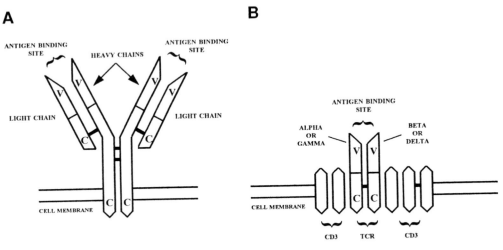

Fig. 3. Schematic diagram of immunoglobulin and T-cell receptors. **(A)** The immunoglobulin protein is a heterodimer composed of two heavy and two light chains, each of which has variable V and constant C regions. **(B)** The T-cell receptor (TCR) is also a heterodimer composed of either one α and one β chain or one γ and one δ chain. Each of the TCR proteins has variable V and constant C regions. CD3 is a complex of five proteins associated with the TCR.

antigens CD19, CD20, and CD10 are subsequently expressed. As a B-cell matures to a terminally differentiated plasma cell, the majority of B-cell associated antigens are lost and the CD38 antigen appears.

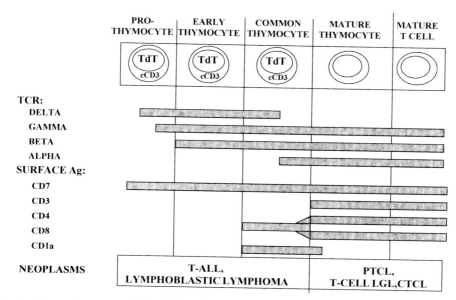

Fig. 4. Normal stages of T-cell development. *See text* for discussion. TdT, terminal deoxynucleotidyl transferase; cCD3, cytoplasmic CD3; TCR, T-cell receptor rearrangements; Ag, antigen.

The fundamental theory of lymphoid neoplasia is that disorders of lymphoid cells represent cells arrested at various stages in the normal differentiation scheme *(8)*. For example, pre-B-cell acute lymphocytic leukemia mimics normal pre-B-cells showing expression of TdT, HLA-Dr, CD10, CD19, CD20, and cytoplasmic μ heavy chains (Fig. 2). Other examples of neoplastic counterparts to normal precursors include chronic lymphocytic leukemia/small lymphocytic lymphoma at the mature B-cell stage, follicular center-cell lymphoma at the activated B-cell stage, and multiple myeloma at the plasma cell stage.

2.2. Normal T-Cell Development

T-lymphocytes also arise from pluripotent stem cells in the bone marrow. In contrast to B-cell development, in which the earliest stages of maturation occur in the bone marrow, progenitor T-cells migrate from the bone marrow to the thymus, where the early stages of T-cell development occur *(9)*. Subsequently, mature T-cells circulate in the peripheral blood and seed peripheral lymphoid tissues, which include paracortical areas of lymph nodes and periarteriolar sheaths of the spleen.

Figure 4 shows the normal stages of T-cell development in the thymus, which, analogous to B-cell development, occur in an orderly fashion. T-lymphocytes possess a surface membrane protein complex referred to as the T-cell receptor, which is structurally similar to the immunoglobulin receptor *(10)* (Fig. 3B). The genes that code for the T-cell receptor undergo sequential rearrangements early in T-cell development. There are four T-cell receptor genes (α, β, γ, and δ), which code for two types of T-cell receptors that exist as heterodimers—the α-β receptor and the γ-δ receptor. The majority of T-cells (98–99%) possess the α-β receptor, with the remaining 1–2% possessing the γ-δ receptor *(10)*. The α and δ chain genes are located on chromosome 14q11, the β chain gene on chromosome 7q34, and the γ chain gene on chromosome 7p15 *(7)*. The first T-cell receptor gene to rearrange is δ, which is followed sequentially by γ, β, and α genes.

Analogous to developing B-cells, a variety of cellular antigens can be detected at different stages of T-cell development (Fig. 4). The earliest antigens expressed are TdT and CD7. The CD3 antigen, which is part of the protein complex associated with the T-cell receptor (Fig. 3B), is present early primarily in the cytoplasm and manifests on the cell surface at a later stage. The common thymocyte stage is defined by expression of CD1a, the common thymocyte antigen, and is frequently associated with coexpression of the CD4 (helper/inducer) and CD8 (cytotoxic/suppressor) antigens. As T-cells reach the mature stage, they express either CD4 or CD8, but not both. Similar to B-cell neoplasms, T-cell neoplasms occur owing to maturation arrest at various stages of T-cell development *(8)*. For example, lymphoblastic lymphoma frequently mimics normal common thymocytes showing expression of TdT, CD1a, cytoplasmic CD3, CD7, and coexpression of CD4 and CD8 (Fig. 4). Other examples of neoplastic counterparts to normal precursors include peripheral T-cell lymphoma, cutaneous T-cell lymphoma (mycosis fungoides), and the T-cell type of lymphoproliferative disorder of granular lymphocytes, which are all neoplasms of mature T-cells *(1)*.

2.3. B-Cell Immunoglobulin and T-Cell Receptor Gene Rearrangements

The B-cell immunoglobulin and T-cell receptors are involved in the process of antigen recognition by normal B- and T-lymphocytes. These receptors are structurally similar, being heterodimer proteins linked by disulfide bonds, and are composed of both variable (V) and constant (C) regions *(7)* (Fig. 3). The variable regions of these proteins are similarly involved in antigen recognition. The constant region of the immunoglobulin heavy-chain protein defines the nine immunoglobulin classes (IgG_1, IgG_2, IgG_3, IgG_4, IgA_1, IgA_2, IgM, IgD, and IgE) *(6)*. The genes which code for the B and T-cell receptors are also structurally similar and consist of a large number of exons, referred to as a supergene family, that undergo a similar process of DNA recombination leading eventually to the formation of functional receptor proteins *(3,6,7,10,11)*.

A general scheme of B-cell immunoglobulin and T-cell receptor gene rearrangements is shown in Fig. 5. The germline configuration refers to nonrearranged DNA. The exons that code for the variable regions of the immunoglobulin and T-cell receptors are referred to as V segments, diversity (D) segments, and junctional (J) segments, and those which code for the constant regions are referred to as C segments. The process of gene rearrangement first involves the selective apposition of one D segment with one J segment by deletion of the intervening coding and noncoding DNA sequences, resulting in a DJ rearrangement. By a similar process of rearrangement, a V segment, located in the 5' direction becomes apposed to D and J to form a VDJ rearrangement. Transcription to messenger RNA then occurs even though the VDJ segments are not yet directly apposed to C segments, which are remotely located in the 3'-direction. Subsequent splicing of the mRNA with deletion of noncoding sequences results in apposition of VDJ with C to form a VDJC mRNA, which can then be translated into an immunoglobulin or T-cell receptor protein. The genes coding for the immunoglobulin heavy chain protein and T-cell receptor β and δ proteins include V, D, J,

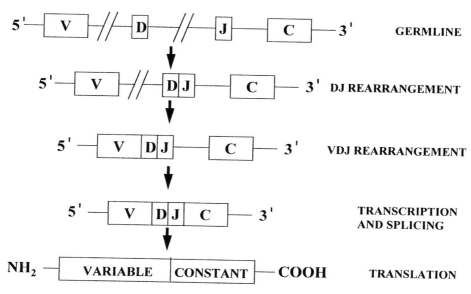

Fig. 5. Schematic diagram illustrating the sequential steps involved in immunoglobulin and T-cell receptor gene rearrangements. *See text* for discussion.

and C segments. The genes coding for the κ and λ light-chain proteins and the T-cell receptor α and γ proteins include only V, J, and C segments without D segments *(3,7,11)*.

The complex process of DNA recombination or rearrangement allows for tremendous diversity of both the humoral and cell-mediated immune systems, and the ability to detect a wide array of antigens *(3,6,7,10,11)*. The large number of V, D, J, and C segments results in many combinations that can be transcribed and translated to millions of different antigen receptors. A detailed diagram of the B-cell heavy-chain and the T-cell receptor β chain supergene families is shown in Fig. 6. The immunoglobulin heavy-chain gene consists of at least 100 V segments, approx 30 D segments, 6 J segments, and 9 C segments. The T-cell receptor β chain gene includes 75–100 V segments and two tandem DJC complexes, referred to as D1J1C1 and D2J2C2. Each DJC complex contains one D segment and one C segment. The first DJC complex contains six J segments (J_{B1} group) and the second DJC complex contains seven J segments (J_{B2} group) *(3,7,11)*.

2.4. Southern Blots and the Determination of B- and T-Cell Clonality

To establish a diagnosis of B- or T-cell malignancy, the ability to prove that a neoplastic population of B- or T-cells is monoclonal in origin is of central importance. A monoclonal, or simply, clonal cell population refers to a population of cells that share similar characteristics and are all derived from a single precursor cell. In lymphoid malignancies, clonality can be defined in several different ways. Clonality may be suggested based on traditional morphology if a monomorphous cell population is present, immunopathologically by showing the presence of monoclonal surface immunoglobulin (in the case of B-cell neoplasms), cytogenetically by demonstrating a recurrent chromosomal alteration, such as recurrent translocation, and by molecular genetics by demonstrating

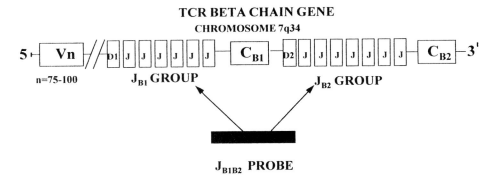

Fig. 6. Schematic diagram of the immunoglobulin heavy chain and the T-cell receptor β chain supergene families. To detect B-cell heavy-chain gene rearrangements by Southern blot analysis, a J_H probe, which recognizes heavy chain J segments is used. To detect T-cell receptor β chain gene rearrangements, a J_{B1B2} probe, which recognizes J segments in both the J_{B1} and J_{B2} groups, is used.

the presence of a clonal B- or T-cell gene rearrangement. In B- and T-cell neoplasms, the primary application of molecular genetics is to prove clonality in cases which are not morphologically malignant, and in which clonality cannot be proven immunopathologically. Southern blot analysis is a very sensitive and specific method for determining clonality, and may detect a monoclonal population that comprises as little as 1–5% of the total cell population *(3,7)*.

For Southern blot analysis, DNA is first extracted and purified from the cells that are to be analyzed. Fresh or frozen specimens are most suitable for Southern blot analysis of hematological disorders, and these include cell suspensions prepared from peripheral blood, bone marrow aspirates, and body fluids, and cell suspensions or cryostat sections prepared from tissues, such as lymph node or spleen. Separate samples of purified DNA are then digested with restriction enzymes *Eco*RI, *Hin*dIII, and *Bam*HI *(12)*. Restriction enzymes cleave DNA at specific sites by recognizing specific base pair sequences. The digested DNA fragments are then electrophoresed using agarose gels, which separate the DNA fragments according to molecular size. The DNA fragments are then transferred to a nylon membrane and hybridized with a specific DNA probe. DNA probe detection systems include radioactive labeling with ^{32}P, chemiluminescence, and colorimetric *(13)*.

DNA probes that are commonly used for detection of monoclonal B-cell populations are J_H, which recognizes the heavy-chain joining (J) segments, and J_K, which recognizes the κ light-chain joining (J) segments. DNA probes that are commonly used

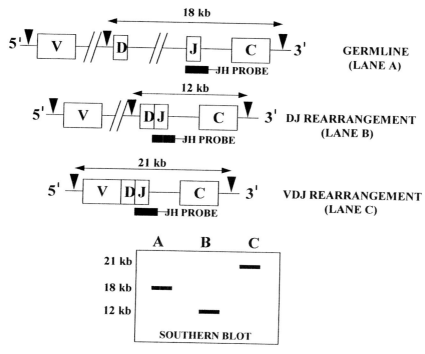

Fig. 7. Schematic diagram illustrating the Southern blot approach for detecting B-cell gene rearrangements. *See text* for discussion. Arrowheads identify restriction enzyme cleavage sites.

for detection of monoclonal T-cell populations are J_{B1B2} which recognizes the two groups of β chain joining (J) segments, and CT_B, which recognizes the two β chain constant (C) segments. The two DNA probes most commonly used in our laboratory are J_H and J_{B1B2}. Figure 6 shows their specific sites of recognition in the immunoglobulin heavy chain and T-cell receptor β chain genes in germline configuration.

The Southern blot approach for detecting B-cell gene rearrangements is shown schematically in Fig. 7. In reactive or polyclonal lymphocyte populations, the primary band identified with J_H probe is the germline band (Lane A). Thousands of different rearrangements are actually present in this lane, but individually, the rearrangements are too small to be detected. In a monoclonal B-cell population, all B-cells are derived from a single precursor cell and have identical gene rearrangements, which will be detected by Southern blots as a novel band. If the monoclonal B-cell population has a DJ rearrangement, numerous intervening coding and noncoding DNA sequences are deleted, resulting in a smaller fragment of DNA detected by the J_H probe (Lane B). If the monoclonal B-cell population has a VDJ rearrangement, a restriction enzyme cleavage site is also deleted, resulting in a larger fragment of DNA detected by the J_H probe (Lane C).

Southern blots using ^{32}P labeled DNA probes are shown in Figs. 8 and 9. Fig. 8 (Lanes 2, 5, and 8) shows the presence of clonal B-cell gene rearrangements which were detected with a J_H probe in a case of B-cell NHL. Figure 9 (Lanes 3, 6, and 9) shows the presence of clonal T-cell gene rearrangements, which were detected with

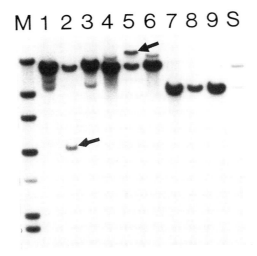

Fig. 8. Evaluation for B-cell clonality with Southern blots using J_H probe and restriction enzymes *Bam*HI (Lanes 1-3), *Eco*RI (Lanes 4–6), and *Hin*dIII (Lanes 7–9). Each restriction enzyme has a control lane identifying the germline configuration (Lanes 1, 4, and 7). Clonal B-cell gene rearrangements are identified in a case of B-cell NHL (Lanes 2, 5, and 8) with novel bands present in lanes 2 and 5 (arrowheads). Only the germline configuration is identified in a lymph node biopsy showing reactive hyperplasia (Lanes 3, 6, and 9). M, marker lane; S, sensitivity control lane with 5% DNA.

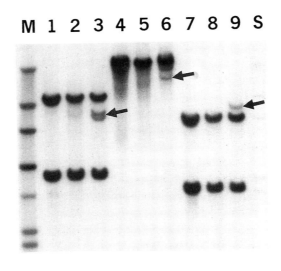

Fig. 9. Evaluation for T-cell clonality with Southern blots using J_{B1B2} probe and restriction enzymes *Eco*RI (Lanes 1–3), *Bam*HI (Lanes 4–6), and *Hin*dIII (Lanes 7–9). Each restriction enzyme has a control lane identifying the germline configuration (Lanes 1, 4, and 7). Clonal T-cell gene rearrangements are identified in a case of T-cell NHL (Lanes 3, 6, and 9) with novel bands present in each lane (arrowheads). Only the germline configuration is identified in a lymph node biopsy showing reactive hyperplasia (Lanes 2, 5, and 8). M, marker lane; S, sensitivity control lane with 5% DNA.

J_{B1B2} probe in a case of T-cell NHL. In each set of blots, a marker lane (Lane 1) consisting of predigested fragments of λ phage DNA is present to establish restriction fragment sizes. Separate DNA samples are digested with three restriction enzymes, *Eco*RI, *Hin*dIII, and *Bam*HI, for both B- and T-cell probes. With each enzyme digest, a control lane consisting of normal placental DNA is run to identify the germline configuration. A novel band refers to any band occurring in a lane other than:

1. A germline band;
2. A crosshybridization band, which occurs owing to hybridization of the probe to partially homologous DNA sequences in other areas of the genome; or
3. A partial digest band, which occurs owing to incomplete digestion of DNA by a restriction enzyme.

A diagnosis of a clonal B- or T-rearrangement is established according to the guidelines established by Cossman et al. *(12)*, which require the identification of at least two novel bands that may be present either in two separate enzyme digests or may both be present in the same enzyme digest.

2.5. The PCR and B- and T-Cell Clonality

The polymerase chain reaction (PCR) technique is becoming an increasingly popular method for evaluating the presence or absence of B- and T-cell clonality in lymphoid neoplasms *(14)*. This powerful method of DNA analysis allows for the evaluation of minute quantities of DNA by a process of DNA amplification. Analogous to Southern blot methods, the application of PCR to detect B- and T-cell clonality involves evaluation of gene rearrangements in those segments of DNA that code for the variable regions of the immunoglobulin and T-cell receptors. Each variable (V) segment of DNA has a unique DNA sequence that contributes to the great diversity of the immunoglobulin and T-cell receptor antigen recognition sites. In addition, short sequences of DNA are shared by nearly all of the V segments that can be recognized by a primer referred to as a consensus V region primer. In a similar fashion, short sequences of DNA shared by nearly all of the J segments can be recognized by a consensus J region primer *(14,15)*.

A diagram illustrating the application of PCR to detect B-cell heavy-chain gene rearrangements using V_H and J_H consensus primers is shown in Fig. 10, and an ethidium bromide-stained PCR gel is shown in Fig. 11. In order to amplify a segment of DNA by PCR successfully, the primers must recognize DNA sequences within a short segment of DNA. In the germline configuration, because V and J segments are widely separated, no significant DNA product is obtained following amplification by PCR (Fig. 10 Lane A and Fig. 11 Lanes 2 and 3). If a VDJ rearrangement occurs, the proximity of the V and J segments allows for the production of an amplified DNA product. A polyclonal B-cell population has a large number of VDJ rearrangements, which differ in size resulting in a smear pattern (Fig. 10, Lane B; Fig. 11, Lanes 4 and 5). In contrast, monoclonal B-cell populations contain identical VDJ rearrangement that results in the formation of a distinct band (Fig. 10, Lane C; Fig. 11, Lanes 6 and 7).

Although the Southern blot method has been the "gold standard" for demonstrating clonality in lymphoid neoplasms, PCR offers distinct advantages *(14,16)*. Whereas Southern blotting is costly and labor-intensive, requiring 7–10 d to obtain a result, PCR can be performed at a lower cost in just 1–2 d. In addition, Southern blotting requires a

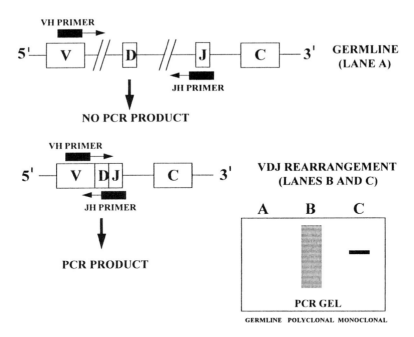

Fig. 10. Schematic diagram illustrating the PCR approach for detecting B-cell gene rearrangements. *See text* for discussion.

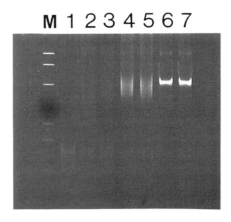

Fig. 11. B-cell gene rearrangement patterns shown in PCR gels after ethidium bromide staining using J_H and V_H consensus primers. In the germline configuration, no PCR product is obtained (Lanes 2 and 3). Polyclonal B-cell populations have a characteristic smear pattern (Lanes 4 and 5). Monoclonal B-cell populations are characterized by a single distinct band (Lanes 6 and 7). Lane M, molecular size marker; Lane 1, blank. (Courtesy of G. J. Tsongalis, Hartford Hospital.)

relatively large amount of high-quality intact DNA, and must be obtained from fresh or frozen tissue samples. In contrast, because the amplification of DNA by PCR requires only short segments of DNA, PCR analysis can be performed on small samples of

DNA and on DNA that is of low quality or only partially intact (such as DNA extracted from paraffin-embedded tissues). Finally, although Southern blotting may detect a 1–5% clonal lymphoid population, PCR may detect as small as a 0.1% clonal lymphoid population *(17)*.

Despite the many advantages of PCR in evaluating for B- and T-cell clonality, the technique is associated with a higher percentage of false-negative results than Southern blotting. This high false-negative rate likely occurs because of the inability of consensus V primers to recognize complementary DNA sequences in all of the V segments, and because of the inability of V and J primers to recognize genetic alternations, such as partial rearrangements (DJ rearrangements), and chromosomal translocations and somatic mutations involving the antigen receptor gene loci *(14,18)*.

2.6. Chromosomal Translocations in NHL

A number of specific, nonrandom chromosomal translocations have been described in association with different subtypes of NHL. These translocations can be demonstrated by traditional cytogenetic methods, as well as by molecular genetic methods which include Southern blotting, PCR, and fluorescence *in situ* hybridization (FISH). Because the demonstration of cytogenetic abnormalities in lymphoid neoplasms with traditional cytogenetic methods is technically difficult, especially in low-grade neoplasms that are associated with a low mitotic rate, molecular approaches currently are the methods of choice. The majority of cases of NHL can be accurately classified based primarily on morphological and immunopathological characteristics; however, in select cases, the demonstration of a specific chromosomal translocation may help confirm a diagnosis. For example, the demonstration of a t(8;14) in a lymphoma that is morphologically and immunopathologically suspicious for Burkitt's lymphoma would confirm this diagnosis *(5)*. More importantly, the ability to detect specific chromosomal translocations in lymphomas by highly sensitive methods, such as PCR, provides a means potentially to monitor patient therapy and to follow patients for evidence of minimal residual disease.

Chromosomal translocations in both leukemia and lymphoma often involve the transposition of a proto-oncogene from one chromosome to another. Proto-oncogenes are defined as normal cellular genes that are involved in the regulation of cellular processes, such as growth and proliferation, and have the potential to contribute to neoplastic transformation when they are structurally or functionally altered, as occurs with chromosomal translocations *(19)*. Proto-oncogenes can be categorized as promoters of cell growth and proliferation (category I), tumor suppressor genes, which normally inhibit cell growth and proliferation (category II), and genes that regulate programmed cell death or apoptosis (category III) *(20)*. Examples of proto-oncogenes that are involved in lymphomagenesis include:

1. c-*myc*, which is a category I proto-oncogene involved in the pathogenesis of Burkitt's lymphoma and is normally present on chromosome 8 *(5,19)*: In Burkitt's lymphoma, a t(8;14), t(2;8), or t(8;22) results in the juxtaposition of c-*myc* from chromosome 8 to the heavy- or light-chain loci on chromosomes 14, 2, or 22 with resultant deregulation of c-*myc*.
2. *bcl*-1 which is also a category I proto-oncogene and is involved in the pathogenesis of mantle cell lymphoma *(19,21,22)*. The *bcl*-1 locus includes the PRAD-1 cyclin gene, which is normally located on chromosome 11 and is involved in the regulation of cell-cycle

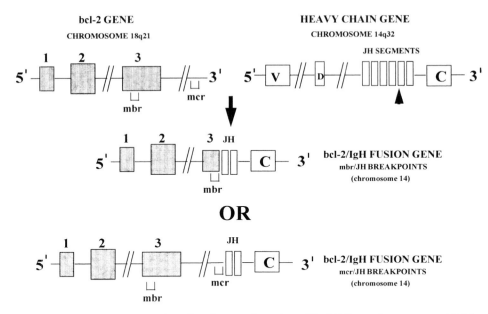

Fig. 12. Schematic diagram showing the translocation of *bcl*-2 from chromosome 18 (shaded boxes) to the heavy-chain gene (IgH) on chromosome 14 (open boxes) resulting in a *bcl*-2/IgH fusion gene. For *bcl*-2, most breaks occur in either the mbr or mcr regions. Breakpoints in the heavy-chain gene involve JH segments (arrowhead). The translocation may involve mbr and JH breakpoints (middle panel) or mcr and JH breakpoints (lower panel).

progression. In mantle cell lymphoma, a t(11;14) results in the juxtaposition of *bcl*-1 from chromosome 11 to the heavy-chain locus on chromosome 14 with resultant deregulation of PRAD-1.

3. *bcl*-2, which is unique, category III proto-oncogene involved in the pathogenesis of follicular lymphoma *(19–21)*.

The remainder of this section will focus on biological and molecular aspects of *bcl*-2. Apoptosis or programmed cell death is part of normal homeostasis, and is the body's way of maintaining a delicate balance between cell proliferation and cell death. The proto-oncogene *bcl*-2 normally resides on chromosome 18 and is involved in blocking apoptosis *(20)*. In healthy adults expression of *bcl*-2 is limited to long-lived cells, which include some subsets of normal T- and B-lymphocytes. In follicular lymphoma, *bcl*-2 becomes overexpressed after being translocated from chromosome 18 to the heavy-chain locus on chromosome 14. The overexpression of *bcl*-2 is likely one step in the process of lymphomagenesis, with elevated levels of *bcl*-2 extending the life-span of neoplastic cells *(20)*. The t(14;18) has been reported in up to 80–90% of cases of follicular lymphoma and less frequently in other types of hematopoietic and nonhematopoietic malignancies *(21)*.

Figure 12 schematically shows the reciprocal translocation involving the *bcl*-2 locus on chromosome 18q21 and the immunoglobulin heavy-chain locus (IgH) on chromosome 14q32. The *bcl*-2 gene contains three exons, including exon 1, which is a noncoding exon (upper panel, Fig. 12). The majority of chromosomal breaks occur in two regions referred to as the major breakpoint cluster region (mbr), where 50–75% of

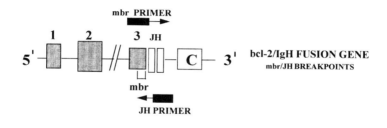

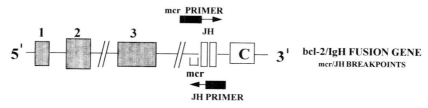

Fig. 13. Analysis for *bcl*-2/IgH gene rearrangements by PCR involves two separate primer combinations—mbr and J$_H$ primers **(top)** and mcr and JH primers **(bottom)**. *See text* for discussion.

the breaks occur, and the minor breakpoint cluster region (mcr), where 20–40% of the breaks occur *(20,21)*. The mbr is located in exon 3 and the mcr is located downstream in the 3'-direction from exon 3. The breakpoints in the heavy chain locus involve the J$_H$ segments. The t(14;18) results in a *bcl*-2/IgH fusion gene as depicted in the middle and lower panels of Fig. 12.

Analysis for the presence of *bcl*-2/IgH gene rearrangements can be performed by both Southern blotting and PCR. PCR is especially suited for analyzing for *bcl*-2/IgH rearrangements, because the *bcl*-2 and J$_H$ breakpoints are located within a short segment of DNA *(23)*. Analysis by PCR is performed using two separate primer combinations to analyze for breaks at both the major and minor breakpoint cluster regions—a combination of mbr and J$_H$ primers and a combination of mcr and J$_H$ primers (Fig. 13). If a t(14;18) and hence a *bcl*-2/IgH rearrangement has not occurred, no PCR product will be obtained following amplification.

3. HODGKIN'S DISEASE

Hodgkin's disease is the second major category of lymphoma and is generally considered to be more treatable and curable than NHL. The diagnosis is primarily a morphological diagnosis and is based on the identification of Reed-Sternberg (RS) cells and RS variants, which are considered to be the malignant cells, in association with a predominant background cell population that consists of benign inflammatory cells. In the majority of cases, RS cells and variants comprise <1% of the total cell population. The origin of the RS cell has remained an enigma, although a variety of cells have been implicated as the cell of origin, including B- and T-lymphocytes, granulocytes, histiocytes, dendritic reticulum cells and interdigitating reticulum cells. Current theories favor B- or T-lymphocytes as the cell of origin *(24)*.

Immunopathological studies often contribute to establishing a diagnosis of Hodgkin's disease, particularly in cases with atypical morphological features. RS cells and variants express the CD15 and CD30 antigens in the majority of cases of classical Hodgkin's disease (nodular sclerosis and mixed cellularity subtypes) *(1)*. In any subtype of Hodgkin's disease, RS cells and variants may also express B- or T-cell antigens, which is one piece of evidence suggesting their origin from B- or T-lymphocytes *(25)*. RS variants in the majority of cases of lymphocyte predominance Hodgkin's disease express the B-cell-associated antigen, CD20 (Fig. 1B).

Despite immunopathological evidence of B- or T-cell antigen expression on RS cells in some cases of Hodgkin's disease, the majority of cases fail to show evidence of clonal B- or T-cell gene rearrangements by Southern blot or PCR methods when performed on whole tissue sections. The inability to demonstrate clonal B or T-cell gene rearrangements may be related to the small percentage of RS cells present in most cases of Hodgkin's disease. However, rearrangements of the immunoglobulin heavy- and light-chain genes and T-cell receptor genes have been reported in some cases of Hodgkin's disease *(24)*, especially in cases with a relatively high percentage of RS cells and variants *(26)*. Recently, investigators have demonstrated that by isolating individual B-cell antigen-positive RS cells by micromanipulation of whole tissue sections and applying PCR to detect rearrangements of immunoglobulin V region genes, in some case of Hodgkin's disease RS cells are monoclonal, and in some cases they are polyclonal *(27)*. The demonstration of both monoclonal and polyclonal rearrangements in RS cells supports the concept that Hodgkin's disease is a heterogenous disorder and is strong evidence that in some cases RS cells are of B-cell origin *(27)*.

4. THE MYELOID MALIGNANCIES: ACUTE MYELOGENOUS LEUKEMIA (AML), MYELOPROLIFERATIVE DISORDERS, AND MYELODYSPLASTIC SYNDROMES

The myeloid malignancies are a diverse group of hematopoietic neoplasms that include as general categories of disease AML, the chronic myeloproliferative disorders, and the myelodysplastic syndromes. All of these diseases are clonal disorders that arise from the neoplastic transformation of a multipotent stem cell. AML and the chronic myeloproliferative disorders are disorders of cell proliferation and are usually associated with elevated peripheral blood counts. In contrast, the myelodysplastic syndromes are disorders of cell maturation and are usually associated with peripheral blood cytopenias and dysplastic morphology. A specific diagnosis can be established in most cases based on a combination of clinical features, morphology, cytochemical studies, and in some cases, immunopathological studies. In addition, traditional cytogenetic analysis has become a critical part of the clinical evaluation of these disorders, providing important information that may be useful in establishing both a correct diagnosis and assessing prognosis. For example, a variant of acute myelomonocytic leukemia associated with increased bone marrow eosinophils and cytogenetic abnormalities involving the long arm of chromosome 16 is recognized to be a favorable subtype of AML typically associated with long-term clinical remissions following induction chemotherapy *(28)*. Finally, the recent application of molecular genetic methods, including Southern blotting, PCR, and FISH, has further advanced our diagnostic capabilities. The following sections will focus on chronic myelogenous leukemia and the molecular genetics of the Philadelphia chromosome, briefly summarize applications of FISH, and expand on the concept of minimal residual disease.

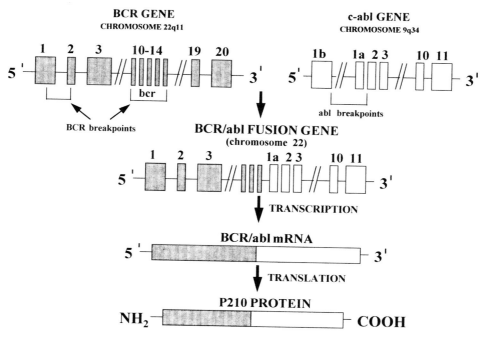

Fig. 14. Schematic diagram showing the translocation of the c-*abl* gene from chromosome 9 (open boxes) to the BCR gene on chromosome 22 (shaded boxes) resulting in a BCR/*abl* fusion gene. For c-*abl*, most breaks occur between exon 1b and exon 2. The majority of breaks in the BCR gene occur in the breakpoint cluster region (bcr), and a smaller number occur between exon 1 and exon 2. A t(9;22), which involves the bcr region, results in a BCR/*abl* fusion gene, which is transcribed to a chimeric BCR/*abl* mRNA and translated to a chimeric P210 protein.

4.1. Chronic Myelogenous Leukemia (CML) and the Philadelphia Chromosome

The myeloproliferative disorders include CML, polycythemia vera, essential thrombocythemia, and myelosclerosis with myeloid metaplasia. Although each of these disorders usually presents with distinct clinical and morphological features, it is common for cases to present with overlapping features, especially in the early stages of the diseases *(29)*. Clinically, CML is characterized by a triphasic clinical course with an initial chronic phase, followed by an accelerated phase, and terminating in a blast crisis *(30)*. In cases of suspected chronic-phase CML with overlapping clinical features, the identification of the presence of a Philadelphia (Ph[1]) chromosome by cytogenetic or molecular genetic methods confirms this diagnosis. Evolution of chronic-phase CML to accelerated phase and blast crisis is usually associated with the acquisition of additional chromosomal abnormalities *(29,30)*. The Ph[1] chromosome may also be observed in acute lymphocytic leukemia (ALL) in 30% of adult cases and 5% of childhood cases, and is associated with an unfavorable prognosis *(31)*.

The Ph[1] chromosome is a shortened chromosome 22 that arises from a reciprocal translocation involving the long arms of chromosomes 9 and 22 *(21,29,30)*. The translocation involves the c-*abl* proto-oncogene, which is normally present on chromosome 9q34, and the BCR gene on chromosome 22q11 (Fig. 14). The c-*abl* proto-oncogene

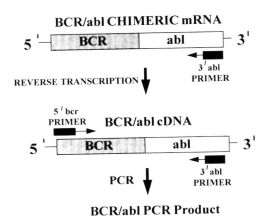

Fig. 15. Analysis for BCR/*abl* gene rearrangements by PCR using chimeric BCR/*abl* mRNA as a template. Using reverse transcriptase and a 3'-*abl* primer, a BCR/*abl* complementary DNA (cDNA) strand is produced. The cDNA can then be directly analyzed by PCR with 5'-*bcr* and 3'-*abl* primers, resulting in a BCR/*abl* PCR product.

consists of 11 exons that code for a protein product designated P145. This protein belongs to a family of tyrosine kinases, which are involved in the control of cellular growth. The majority of breakpoints in c-*abl* occur between exon 1b and exon 2. The BCR gene consists of 20 exons and includes a central breakpoint cluster region (bcr) where the majority of breakpoints in CML occur. The juxtaposition of *abl* with BCR results in the formation of a BCR/*abl* fusion gene, which is subsequently transcribed into a chimeric BCR/*abl* mRNA, and translated into a chimeric BCR/*abl* protein product referred to as P210 (Fig. 14). The chimeric P210 protein has enhanced tyrosine kinase activity compared to the normal P145 and is likely involved in the pathogenesis of CML. In Ph[1]-positive ALL, approx 50% of cases are associated with a chimeric P210 protein, and the remaining cases are associated with a chimeric P190 protein that also has increased tyrosine kinase activity *(31)*.

Molecular genetic methods for detecting BCR/*abl* gene rearrangements are recommended in any patient who has clinical features that are suspicious for CML, but absence of a detectable Ph[1] chromosome by routine cytogenetic analysis. Approximately 5–10% of patients will be Ph[1]-chromosome-negative by cytogenetic analysis, but a significant number of these patients will have BCR/*abl* gene rearrangements. Patients that are Ph[1]-chromosome-negative, but have BCR/*abl* gene rearrangements are clinically and morphologically indistinguishable from Ph[1]-chromosome-positive patients *(21)*.

To establish a diagnosis of CML in Ph[1]-chromosome-negative patients and for monitoring patients for response to therapy and evidence of minimal residual disease, detection of BCR/*abl* rearrangements by PCR is the method of choice (Fig. 15) *(32)*. In contrast to the *bcl*-2/IgH gene breakpoints, which occur within a short segment of DNA and allow for direct PCR analysis of DNA, the breakpoints for BCR/*abl* span a large segment of DNA, which prevents direct analysis. To circumvent this, the PCR approach for detecting BCR/*abl* rearrangements utilizes BCR/*abl* chimeric mRNA as a template (Fig. 15). Transcription of BCR/*abl* DNA to chimeric mRNA brings the primer annealing sites closer together, so that a region suitable for amplification, owing to its smaller size, is formed. Using reverse transcriptase and a 3'-*abl* primer, a complementary DNA strand is first produced. The cDNA can then be directly analyzed with 5'-*bcr* and 3'-*abl* primers with a resultant PCR product. If a t(9;22) and hence a BCR/*abl* rearrangement have not occurred, no PCR product will be obtained following amplification.

5. FISH

FISH can be used to diagnose and monitor hematological diseases. The technique utilizes fluorochrome labeled DNA probes to detect chromosomal abnormalities microscopically in cells prepared on peripheral blood smears, bone marrow aspirate smears, and formalin-fixed, paraffin-embedded histological sections. The major advantages of FISH over traditional cytogenetics are that FISH:

1. Does not require fresh, viable tissue;
2. Can be used to analyze interphase (nondividing) cells; and
3. Allows for the analysis of many more cells *(33)*.

FISH is most effectively used when screening a cell population in question for a specific chromosomal abnormality that was not detected by cytogenetic analysis. FISH can also be used to monitor therapy and to evaluate patients for evidence of minimal residual disease. Examples of chromosomal abnormalities in hematological neoplasms that can be readily identified using FISH include:

1. t(15;17), which is characteristic of acute promyelocytic leukemia (AML-M3) and when identified helps distinguish AML-M3 from other subtypes of AML;
2. t(9;22), which was discussed in detail in the preceding section; and
3. Trisomy 8, which is commonly observed in myelodysplastic syndromes and may help confirm a diagnosis of suspected myelodysplasia.

6. DETECTION OF MINIMAL RESIDUAL DISEASE

Minimal residual disease (MRD) refers to the presence of a residual clone of malignant cells in a patient that cannot be detected by standard pathological and radiological staging approaches and may eventually result in disease relapse *(34)*. For example, at presentation, patients with acute leukemia have a tumor burden consisting of 10^{12} leukemic cells, which is readily detectable by microscopic examination of the bone marrow. Following induction chemotherapy, the tumor burden is reduced by several orders of magnitude, resulting in clinical remission (defined as <5% bone marrow blasts); however, an undetectable residual tumor burden of 10^8 or 10^9 leukemic cells may still remain *(4)*. Traditional morphological assessment of the bone marrow cannot distinguish a patient with MRD of 10^9 leukemic cells from a patient with no leukemic cells.

The presence of MRD in patients with leukemia and lymphoma has been assessed by a variety of approaches, including traditional morphology, immunophenotypic analysis by flow cytometry, cell culture methods, conventional cytogenetics, and molecular methods, which include fluorescence *in situ* hybridization (FISH), Southern blotting, and PCR *(4)*. Each of these methods has advantages and disadvantages. With the exception of PCR, the approaches listed lack sensitivity and are capable of detecting approx a 1% malignant cell population. In contrast, PCR is significantly more sensitive and has the capability of detecting one malignant cell among 10^5–10^6 normal cells *(34,35)*. In order to evaluate for the presence of MRD by PCR, the malignant cell must have a unique set of DNA sequences that allow for distinction from normal cells. Evaluation for the presence of chromosomal translocations such as t(14;18)(q32;q21) in follicular, NHL and t(9;22)(q34;q11) in ALL and CML, are ideal for detecting MRD. An alternative approach in B- and T-cell malignancies involves detection of immuno-globulin and T-cell receptor gene rearrangements. A variety of PCR based strategies have been devised based on the premise that each clone of malignant B- or T-cells has a unique VDJ rearrangement that can be used as a molecular marker to probe for the presence of MRD *(4)*.

The ability to detect MRD more precisely would be expected to improve clinical management by optimizing therapy *(4,34,35)*. In some diseases, the presence of sig-nificant MRD may be a predictor of disease relapse, requiring more aggressive thera-peutic approaches, such as bone marrow transplantation. In contrast, patients with little or no residual MRD may require less intensive therapy, thus reducing patient exposure to potentially toxic drugs.

7. CONCLUSION

Molecular genetic techniques are powerful tools which have greatly enhanced our ability to diagnose and classify hematological diseases precisely. In lymphoid neo-plasms, the ability to prove or disprove the presence of B- or T-cell clonality by either immunopathological or molecular genetic approaches is often central to establishing a correct diagnosis. In both myeloid and lymphoid neoplasms, the identification of a specific chromosomal abnormality may be useful in confirming a diagnosis in cases that are otherwise inconclusive. This same chromosomal abnormality may subsequently be used as a marker to evaluate patients for response to therapy and for evidence of MRD. The field of molecular genetics is continually expanding our understanding of the basic molecular alterations involved in the pathogenesis of hematological diseases. By understanding basic disease mechanisms, it is likely that future therapies for hematological diseases will become more refined.

8. CASE EXAMPLE

A 68-yr-old woman presented with gastrointestinal bleeding. Endoscopic examina-tion of the stomach revealed thickened gastric folds with multiple small ulcers. Micro-scopic examination of endoscopic biopsies obtained adjacent to the gastric ulcers showed a dense lymphoid infiltrate, which had a varied histological appearance. The infiltrate was characterized by the presence of obvious benign, reactive germinal cen-ters and plasma cells in association with sheets of abnormal small lymphoid cells, which focally infiltrated normal gastric glands forming so-called lymphoepithelial lesions (Fig. 16). In areas, gastric glands were obliterated.

The microscopic findings suggested a differential diagnosis which included chronic gastritis and a type of NHL referred to as a low-grade, B-cell lymphoma of mucosal-associated lymphoid tissue (MALT). To distinguish chronic gastritis from an NHL, it was necessary to evaluate the biopsy for clonality, since chronic gastritis is a polyclonal process and NHL is a monoclonal process. Immunopathological studies performed on tissue sections clearly showed polyclonal surface immunoglobulin expression in benign reactive follicles, but were inconclusive in the sheets of abnormal small lymphocytes.

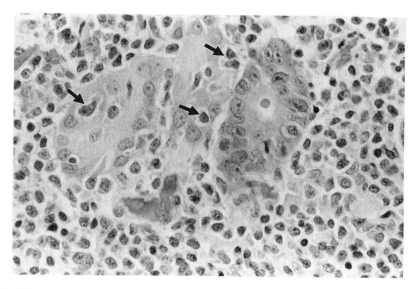

Fig. 16. Histological section of the gastric biopsy showing infiltration of normal gastric glands by abnormal small lymphoid cells (arrows) forming lymphoepithelial lesions. H & E stain ×500.

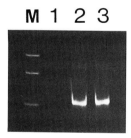

Fig. 17. PCR gel stained with ethidium bromide after amplification of DNA with J_H and V_H consensus primers. A single distinct band is present indicative of a monoclonal B-cell population. Studies performed in duplicate, Lanes 2 and 3. Lane M, molecular size marker; Lane 1, blank (courtesy of G. J. Tsongalis, Hartford Hospital).

Molecular genetic studies were then performed to evaluate the biopsy further for clonality. Because the quantity of DNA extracted from the small gastric biopsy was insufficient for Southern blot analysis, studies were performed by PCR. To evaluate for B-cell clonality, PCR studies were performed using J_H and V_H consensus primers and showed the presence of a single distinct band, which indicated the presence of a monoclonal B-cell population (Fig. 17).

A diagnosis of low-grade, B-cell lymphoma of MALT was established in this gastric biopsy based on the demonstration of a monoclonal B-cell population by PCR in association with the characteristic histologic features. These lymphomas typically arise in lymphoid tissue intimately associated with mucosal sites, such as the gastrointestinal tract, lung, and salivary gland and are often difficult to distinguish histologically from chronic inflammatory disorders, such as chronic gastritis, because the neoplastic lymphoid cells are usually associated with many benign, reactive lymphoid cells, including reactive germinal centers. This case illustrates a common diagnostic problem confronting the pathologist and demonstrates the contribution of molecular genetic methods to resolving these problems.

REFERENCES

1. Harris, N. L., Jaffe, E. S., Stein, H., Banks, P. M., Chan, J. K. C., Cleary, M. L., et al. A revised European-American classification of lymphoid neoplasms: a proposal from the International Lymphoma Study Group. *Blood* **84:**1361–1392, 1994.
2. Jaffe, E. S. The role of immunophenotypic markers in the classification of non-Hodgkin's lymphomas. *Semin. Oncol.* **17:**11–19, 1990.
3. Cossman, J., Uppenkamp, M., Sundeen, J., Coupland, R., and Raffeld, M. Molecular genetics and the diagnosis of lymphoma. *Arch. Pathol. Lab. Med.* **112:**117–127, 1988.
4. Campana, D. and Pui, C.-H. Detection of minimal residual disease in acute leukemia: methodologic advances and clinical significance. *Blood* **85:**1416–1434, 1995.
5. Medeiros, L. J., Bagg, A., and Cossman, J. Application of molecular genetics to the diagnosis of hematopoietic neoplasms, in *Neoplastic Hematopathology*, Knowles, D. M., ed., Williams and Wilkins, Baltimore, pp. 263–298, 1992.
6. Cooper, M. D. B lymphocytes: normal development and function. *New Engl. J. Med.* **317:**1452–1456, 1987.
7. Sklar, J. Antigen receptor genes: structure, function, and techniques for analysis of their rearrangements, in *Neoplastic Hematopathology*, Knowles, D. M., ed., Williams and Wilkins, Baltimore, pp. 215–244, 1992.
8. Foon, K. A. and Todd, R. F. Immunologic classification of leukemia and lymphoma. *Blood* **68:**1–31, 1986.
9. Spits, H., Lanier, L. L., and Phillips, J. H. Development of human T and natural killer cells. *Blood* **85:**2654–2670, 1995.
10. Royer, H. D. and Reinherz, E. L. T lymphocytes: ontogeny, function, and relevance to clinical disorders. *New Engl. J. Med.* **317:**1136–1142, 1987.
11. Gill, J. I. and Gulley, M. L. Immunoglobulin and T cell receptor gene rearrangement. *Hematol. Oncol. Clin. North Am.* **8:**751–770, 1994.
12. Cossman, J., Zehnbauer, B., Garrett, C. T., Smith, L. J., Williams, M., Jaffe, E. S., Hanson, L. O., and Love, J. Gene rearrangements in the diagnosis of lymphoma/leukemia. Guidelines for use based on a multiinstitutional study. *Am. J. Clin. Pathol.* **95:**347–354, 1991.
13. Hodges, K. A., Kosciol, C. M., Rezuke, W. N., Abernathy, E. C., Pastuszak, W. T., and Tsongalis, G. J. Chemiluminescent detection of gene rearrangements in hematologic malignancy. *Ann. Clin. Lab. Sci.*, in press.
14. Medeiros, L. J. and Weiss, L. M. The utility of the polymerase chain reaction as a screening method for the detection of antigen receptor gene rearrangements. *Hum. Pathol.* **25:**1261–1263, 1994.
15. Macintyre, E. A. The use of the polymerase chain reaction in hematology. *Blood Rev.* **3:**201–210, 1989.
16. Sioutos, N., Bagg, A., Michaud, G. Y., Irving, S. G., Hartmann, D. P., Siragy, H., Oliveri, D. R., Locker, J., and Cossman, J. Polymerase chain reaction versus Southern blot hybridization. Detection of immunoglobulin heavy-chain gene rearrangements. *Diagn. Mol. Pathol.* **4:**8–13, 1995.
17. Weiss, L. M. and Spagnolo, D. V. Assessment of clonality in lymphoid proliferations. *Am. J. Pathol.* **142:**1679–1682, 1993.

18. Segal, G. H., Jorgensen, T., Scott, M., and Braylan, R. C. Optimal primer selection for clonality assessment by polymerase chain reaction analysis: II. Follicular lymphomas. *Hum. Pathol.* **25**:1276–1282, 1994.

19. Gaidano, G. and Dalla-Favera, R. Protooncogenes and tumor suppressor genes, in *Neoplastic Hematopathology.* Knowles, D. M., ed., Williams and Wilkins, Baltimore, pp. 245–261, 1992.

20. Korsmeyer, S. J. Bcl-2 initiates a new category of oncogenes: regulators of cell death. *Blood* **80**:879–886, 1992.

21. Crisan, D., Chen, S-T., and Weil, S. C. Polymerase chain reaction in the diagnosis of chromosomal breakpoints. *Hematol. Oncol. Clin. North Am.* **8**:725–750, 1994.

22. Banks, P. M., Chan, J., Cleary, M. L., Delsol, G., De Wolf- Peeters, C., and Gatter, K. Mantle cell lymphoma. A proposal for unification of morphologic, immunologic, and molecular data. *Am. J. Surg. Pathol.* **16**:637–640, 1992.

23. Ngan, B.-Y., Nourse, J., and Cleary, M. L. Detection of chromosomal translocation t(14;18) within the minor cluster region of *bcl*-2 by polymerase chain reaction and direct genomic sequencing of the enzymatically amplified DNA in follicular lymphomas. *Blood* **73**:1759–1762, 1989.

24. Haluska, F. G., Brufsky, A. M., and Canellos, G. P. The cellular biology of the Reed-Sternberg cell. *Blood* **84**:1005–1019, 1994.

25. Agnarsson, B. A. and Kadin, M. E. The immunophenotype of Reed-Sternberg cells. A study of 50 cases of Hodgkin's disease using fixed frozen tissues. *Cancer* **63**:2083–2087, 1989.

26. Weiss, L. M., Strickler, J. G., Hu, E., Warnke, R. A., and Sklar, J. Immunoglobulin gene rearrangements in Hodgkin's disease. *Hum. Pathol.* **17**:1009–1014, 1986.

27. Hummel, M., Ziemann, K., Lammert, H., Pileri, S., Sabattini, E., and Stein, H. Hodgkin's disease with monoclonal and polyclonal populations of Reed-Sternberg cells. *New Engl. J. Med.* **333**:901–906, 1995.

28. Larson, R. A., Williams, S. F., Le Beau, M. M., Bitter, M. A., Vardiman, J. W., and Rowley, J. D. Acute myelomonocytic leukemia with abnormal eosinophils and inv (16) or t(16;16) has a favorable prognosis. *Blood* **68**:1242–1249, 1986.

29. Vardiman, J. W. Chronic myelogenous leukemia and the myeloproliferative disorders, in *Neoplastic Hematopathology*, Knowles, D. M., ed., Williams and Wilkins, Baltimore, pp. 1405–1438, 1992.

30. Kurzrock, R., Gutterman, J. U., and Talpaz, M. The molecular genetics of Philadelphia chromosome-positive leukemias. *New Engl. J. Med.* **319**:990–998, 1988.

31. Copelan, E. A. and McGuire, E. A. The biology and treatment of acute lymphoblastic leukemia in adults. *Blood* **85**:1151–1168, 1995.

32. Kawasaki, E. S., Clark, S. S., Coyne, M. Y., Smith, S. D., Champlin, R., Witte, O. N., and McCormick, F. P. Diagnosis of chronic myeloid and acute lymphocytic leukemias by detection of leukemia-specific mRNA sequences amplified in vitro. *Proc. Natl. Acad. Sci. USA* **85**:5698–5702, 1988.

33. Cowan, J. M. Fishing for chromosomes: the art and its applications. *Diagn. Mol. Pathol.* **3**:224–226, 1994.

34. Negrin, R. S. and Blume, K. G. The use of the polymerase chain reaction for the detection of minimal residual malignant disease. *Blood* **78**:255–258, 1991.

35. Sklar, J. Polymerase chain reaction: the molecular microscope of residual disease. *J. Clin. Oncol.* **9**:1521–1524, 1991.

Molecular Techniques in Laboratory Diagnosis
of Infectious Diseases

Jaber Aslanzadeh

1. INTRODUCTION

Accurate and timely diagnosis of infectious diseases is essential for proper medical management of patients. The prompt detection of the microbial pathogen also enables care providers to institute adequate measures to interrupt transmission to the susceptible population in the hospital or community. In the past, diagnoses of infectious diseases has usually been dependent on isolation of the infective agent by culture technique. Although this approach seemed adequate to identify the majority of common infections, the approach was not reliable for detection of organisms that were difficult or failed to grow in vitro or had a long incubation time. In fact, in many cases, the patient would recover long before the laboratory results became available. Because of these problems, there has been great demand for alternative techniques that would allow direct detection of infectious agents in clinical samples. Rapid antigen detection tests, such as latex agglutination, enzyme immunoassay (EIA), and direct and indirect fluorescent antibody tests, were developed and, although generally reliable, have a number of limitations. These include limited sensitivity when organisms are not prevalent or do not shed large amounts of antigen into infected tissue and necessity for antigen to react rapidly with the test antibody *(1)*. For these reasons there has been an interest and demand for newer methods for diagnosis of infectious diseases pathogens.

In the 1990s molecular techniques, including DNA probes and polymerase chain reaction (PCR), were introduced in clinical microbiology laboratories. Today molecular techniques are used routinely to detect an ever-increasing number of organisms. For example, DNA probes are now used routinely for culture confirmation of mycobacteria and have replaced laborious and time-consuming protocols, such as hyphea to yeast conversion or exoantigen extraction for diagnosis of dimorphic fungi *(2,3)*.

2. SPECIFIC MOLECULAR TECHNIQUES

2.1. DNA Probe Hybridization Assays

A nucleic acid probe is a defined fragment of DNA, radioactively or chemically labeled and used to locate specific nucleic acid sequences by hybridization. To develop a probe for a given organism, a unique "signature sequence" must be identified and

From: Molecular Diagnostics: For the Clinical Laboratorian
Edited by: W. B. Coleman and G. J. Tsongalis Humana Press Inc., Totowa, NJ

produced in sufficient quantity using either a DNA synthesizer or simple cloning protocols. The probes are labeled either during or after their production with a labeling agent. Depending on the type of label used, the sensitivity of detection may range from 10^4–10^6 organisms.

The two primary types of DNA probe hybridization assays are membrane and liquid hybridization. The membrane hybridization relies on lysing the target organism and fixing the liberated DNA onto a nylon membrane. Membrane is then probed with a radioactive or chemiluminescent labeled oligonucleotide probe that hybridizes to a unique sequence on the target DNA. In contrast, liquid hybridization does not rely on solid phase to immobilize the liberated DNA; following cell lysis, the liberated DNA directly hybridizes with the labeled probe.

The hybridization protection assay (Gen-probe) is the leading liquid hybridization test used routinely in clinical laboratories. The assay relies on use of an acridinium ester-labeled DNA probe that is homologous to the ribosomal RNA of the target organism. After ribosomal RNA is released from the organism, the labeled DNA probe combines with the target organism's ribosomal RNA to form a stable DNA:RNA hybrid. When the DNA–RNA hybrid is formed, the acridinium ester is oriented within the hybrid. The excess unbound probe is then hydrolyzed with selection reagent whereas the acridinium within the hybrid is protected from inactivation. Subsequent addition of an alkaline peroxide solution elicits chemiluminescence from protected acridinium ester. The amount of light emitted is proportional to the amount of hybridized probe *(2,3)*.

As of this writing, over 30 commercially developed probe assays (membrane or liquid hybridization) have been approved by FDA for use in clinical laboratories. Although the ultimate goal of these assays is to detect organisms directly from patient samples, the majority of these probes are intended for culture identification *(4–19)*. Table 1 shows the sensitivity and specificity of probe assays for an array of organisms.

2.2. Branched DNA (bDNA) Signal Amplification

The bDNA signal amplification system (Chiron, Emeryville, CA), which is quantitative as well as qualitative, utilizes multiple probes with each probe attached to multiple reporter molecules. As depicted in Fig. 1, the assay is performed in a 96-well ELISA plate *(20)*.

The bDNA reporter probes are synthesized to form a bristle-like structure. Hanging from each of the 15 bristles on the probe are one to three alkaline-phosphatase reporter molecules that are attached by complementary DNA tethers. This "ornaments-on-a-tree" approach allows the signal to be highly amplified at each target probe site. After introduction of a chemiluminescent substrate that is activated by alkaline-phosphatase probes, the signal is easily quantified through an ELISA-type plate reader *(20)*.

The bDNA signal amplification has been used effectively to quantitate hepatitis B virus DNA, human immunodeficiency virus (HIV)-RNA, Hepatitis C virus (HCV)-RNA, and cytomegalovirus (CMV) DNA *(20)*. These assays appear to be highly specific, do not react with genetically related viruses, and can detect as few as 10^3 viral particles. Perhaps the most promising aspect of this assay is the ability to monitor the effects of interferon therapy on hepatitis B virus and HCV, and the effects of such experimental drug therapy, such as protease inhibitors, on HIV *(21)*.

Table 1
List of Available Nucleic Acid Probes for Culture Confirmation or Direct Detection of Microorganisms from Clinical Specimens

Organism	Direct detection	Culture confirmation	Solid hybridization	Liquid hybridization	Sensitivity, %	Specificity, %	References
C. trachomatis	+			+	95.2 female / 77.2 male	98.2 female / 99.6 male	4
Neisseria gonorrhoeae	+			+	100	99.7	5
N. gonorrhoeae		+		+	100	100	5
Gardnerella vaginalis	+	+	+		95	96	7
Group A streptococcus	+			+	90	98	7
L. pheumonphila				+	~70	97	9
Campylobacter sp.		+		+	100	100	10
Streptococcus agalactiae		+		+	100	100	11
H. influenzae		+		+	98.4	100	12
Enterococus sp.		+		+	100	100	12
MSRA		+		+	95	92	12
M. tuberculosis complex		+		+	100	100	2
Micobacterium avium complex		+		+	97.2	100	13
Micobacterium kansasii		+		+	72.8	100	14
Micobacterium gordonae		+		+	98.7	100	15
S. pneumoniae		+		+	100	100	16
Listeria monocytogenes		+		+	100	100	17
Blastomyces dermatitidis		+		+	97.3	100	3
Coccidioides immitis		+		+	100	100	3
Cryptococcus neoformans,		+		+	100	100	3
H. capsulatum		+		+	100	100	3
Human papillomavirus	+		+		53	?	18
Trichomonas vaginalis	+		+		89	98	19

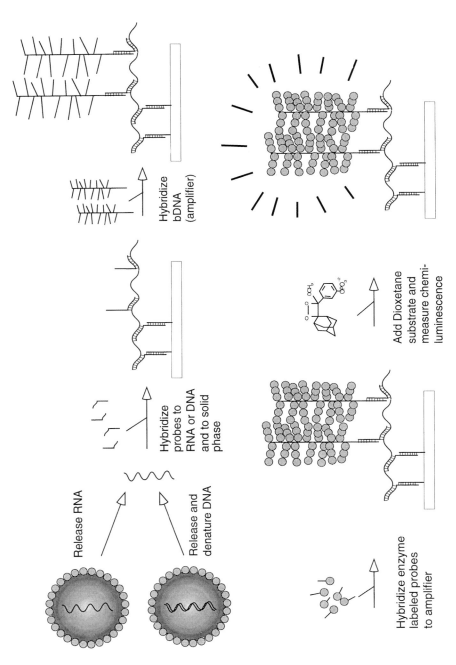

Fig. 1. Chiron bDNA signal amplification assay. Reproduced with permission from the Chiron Corporation (Emeryville, CA) (20).

Release RNA

Release and denature DNA

Hybridize probes to RNA or DNA and to solid phase

Hybridize bDNA (amplifier)

Hybridize enzyme labeled probes to amplifier

Add Dioxetane substrate and measure chemi-luminescence

2.3. PCR

The PCR is a widely used and powerful technique to detect the presence of an infectious agent in clinical specimens. The method involves repeated cycles of primer-mediated, enzymatic amplification of a specific DNA sequence. Because the number of pathogens in a clinical sample may vary significantly depending on the source, nature of infection, and time of collection, the clinical samples should be processed in a manner that will yield the highest possible number of target sequences. Moreover, to increase the assay sensitivity, it is recommended that the primers be directed to amplify sequences for which there are more than one copy per organism, such as insertion sequences, ribosomal DNA, or plasmid *(22)*.

2.4. Specimen Processing

Specimens submitted to the clinical laboratory with the exception of clear nonbloody spinal fluid should be subjected to a DNA extraction procedure. In our laboratory the Isoquick DNA extraction method, which uses chaotropic agent (guanidine thiocyanate), has proven to be a simple and effective for extraction of nucleic acid from most clinical samples. It is recommended that tissue be lysed with sodium dodecyl sulfate or other lysing agent and digested with enzyme (proteinase K) before sequential extraction with phenol chloroform and ethanol precipitation. The type of infecting organism should be a primary consideration in deciding whether to extract nucleic acid from the whole blood, plasma, or leukocyte suspension. For example, whole blood should be used for extracting DNA from intraerythrocytic organisms, such as babesia or malaria, whereas separated leukocytes are more appropriate for CMV. Plasma or serum should be used to extract nucleic acid when the target organism is found in the cell-free fraction. For urine specimens, DNA should be extracted from at least 1 mL of urine immediately after collection. If a prolonged delay is expected the urine should be mixed with an equal volume of ethanol and stored at 4°C. Several protocols have been recommended that are compatible for culture and DNA extraction from sputum. Extraction of DNA from sputum from patients suspected of mycobacterial infection has been most challenging in part because of low copy number present in the specimen and difficulty in lysing the organisms with simple enzymatic digestion of the bacterial cell wall. In addition, PCR has been used in specimens, such as bone, saliva, semen, and formalin-fixed paraffin-embedded tissues, with each specimen requiring specific extraction protocols.

Specimen processing must eliminate PCR inhibitors that may be present in a clinical specimen. The exact mechanisms by which PCR inhibitors interfere with amplification are not fully understood. It is believed that PCR inhibitors interact with nucleic acid or enzyme *Taq* polymerase. The single most important problem with the use of PCR in diagnostic laboratories is false-positive reaction owing to contaminating nucleic acid. The most common source of this contamination is the amplicons from previous PCR reactions. Such contamination can be minimized by meticulous laboratory technique, separation of the work areas, exposing the reaction mix to UV light, autoclaving, and treating the reaction mix with multiple enzymes or bleach. Longo et al. employed a two-step sterilization technique to control contamination *(23)*. Initially, dTTP was substituted with dUTP in all PCR products. All subsequent reactions were pretreated with uracil N glycosylase (UNG), followed by thermal inactivation of UNG. Isaacs et al. showed that the addition of psoralen to the reaction vessel followed by post-PCR activation of this compound, through exposure to long wave UV light, effectively modified PCR products and prevented their amplification in subsequent reactions *(24)*. Similarly, Aslanzadeh used hydroxylamine hydrochloride to sterilize PCR products. Hydroxylamine hydrochloride is a mutagenic agent that binds and chemically modifies nucleic acid *(25)*. It reacts preferentially with cytosine and prevents it from pairing with guanine. However, the modified cytosine is able to bind to adenine, which subsequently binds to thymine and disrupts normal nucleic acid pairing. Currently, isopsoralen and UNG are the two most common and reliable methods for sterilization of amplicons.

3. MOLECULAR TECHNIQUES
FOR DETECTION OF SPECIFIC DISEASE SYNDROMES

3.1. Respiratory Tract Infection

Molecular techniques have been developed to detect a large number of respiratory infections. Specific examples of how molecular techniques are used to make the diagnoses of respiratory tract infections are presented blow.

3.1.1. Legionella pneumophila

L. pneumophila is a gram-negative nutritionally fastidious organism that can cause pneumonia, especially in immunocompromised individuals. Because of its fastidious nature, the organism may require several days to grow and is detectable on culture in only 70–90% of cases *(26)*. Similarly, direct fluorescence antibody (DFA) performed on respiratory specimens suffers from lack of sensitivity and specificity *(27)*.

Several PCR assays have been evaluated for the diagnosis of legionella. Jaulhac et al. detected legionella from bronchoalveolar lavage (BAL) with a pair of primers that amplify a unique sequence of the gene coding for macrophage infectivity promoter (mip) *(28)*. In addition to *L. pneumophila*, these primers detected other legionella species, including *Legionella bozemanii* and *Legionella micdadei*. The assay was able to detect as few as 25 organisms/mL of BAL. Kessler et al. used a commercially developed PCR kit (EnviroAmp) in a prospective study to detect legionella in respiratory specimens *(29)*. The sensitivity of this assay was superior to that of DFA. Lindsay et al. demonstrated legionella-specific DNA (mip gene) in acute and convalescent sera from five patients with Legionnaires' disease, but not in sera from 100 control sera *(30)*. Jonas et al. developed a PCR assay with primers directed to amplify unique sequence from 16S rRNA and a nonradioactive EIA based detection system *(31)*. The assay can detect as few as 10 organisms/mL of BAL, and preliminary data suggest that the assay is highly sensitive and specific.

3.1.2. Chlamydia pneumoniae

C. pneumoniae is an obligate intracellular pathogen causing upper and lower respiratory tract infection responsible for approx 10% of cases of community acquired pneumonia. The organism is difficult to culture in vitro and has low sensitivity (50–75%). Although serologic tests, such as microimmunofluorescent (MIF) and complement fixation can provide useful information, they are often difficult to interpret.

PCR has been shown to be a rapid, sensitive, and specific test for laboratory diagnosis of this infection. Several investigators have developed PCR assays that amplify unique sequences from 16S rRNA gene and *Pst*I restriction fragments *(33)*. The assay can detect as few as 0.4–40 inclusion-forming units/sample. Similarly, a PCR assay that amplifies a 145-bp fragment of the chlamydial omp1 gene has been developed *(34)*. The chlamydial species were differentiated from each other by digestion of PCR product with restriction enzyme *Eco*RI and either *Hin*dIII or *Pst*I. Black et al. developed a nested PCR assay that detected a 16S rRNA gene of *C. pneumoniae* without need for extensive DNA purification steps *(35)*. The nested PCR was shown to be as sensitive as culture or serology for detection of infection with this organism. Gydons et al. assessed the utility of a PCR-EIA for detecting chlamydia in nasopharyngeal specimens from 56 patients with respiratory symptoms and 101 negative controls *(36)*. The assay amplified a fragment from a conserved region of 16S rRNA that was detected following hybridization with biotin labeled probe. In comparison to culture and/or DFA, this assay had a sensitivity of 76.5% and a specificity of 99.0%. Recently, Pruckl et al. showed the utility of PCR for detecting chlamydia in gargled-water specimens obtained from 193 children with acute or chronic respiratory infections *(37)*.

3.1.3. Mycoplasma pneumoniae

M. pneumoniae accounts for approx 20% of community-acquired pneumonias, especially in the younger population. Mycoplasma is the smallest free living organism that lacks a cell wall. Recovery of *M. pneumoniae* requires special media and may take 7–21 d. The complement fixation test is widely available with a sensitivity of 50–80%. A serum cold agglutination titer of 1:64 is present in about 50% of infected patients.

PCR provides the potential for early and reliable diagnosis of this infection. Garret and Bonnet developed an assay that amplified a 144-bp segment of the *M. pneumoniae* genome *(38)*. Others have used primers that amplify unique sequences from 16S rRNA and P1 adhesion protein *(39–41)*. Luneberg et al. developed a PCR assay that detected 950 bp from the gene encoding elongation factor Tu (tuf) *(42)*. Using nonradioactive hybridization (biotin) in a microtiter plate, this assay was then used to detect mycoplasma in throat swabs and had a sensitivity and specificity of 90 and 97%, respectively.

3.1.4. Mycobacterium tuberculosis

M. tuberculosis (MTB) remains an important public health problem, in part because of an increasing number of susceptible individuals who are poorly nourished and live in crowded conditions, such as AIDS patients and homeless people. The organism is transmitted from person to person, making early diagnosis and effective treatment an important step in preventing further spread of the disease. Currently, the diagnosis of MTB depends on visualizing acid fast bacilli (AFB) in clinical specimens and culturing the organism. The AFB stain has a sensitivity of 22–80%. Although culture is the "gold standard," it may take 6–8 wk before a positive culture is detected. While the use of DNA probes has significantly reduced the time from which a visible colony is detected and culture is confirmed, direct detection of the organism from a clinical sample is not yet available.

Several PCR, commercial and in house developed, assays have been evaluated for rapid diagnosis of MTB. These assays differ in primer, sample preparation and PCR product detection techniques. Hance et al. demonstrated the use of PCR with a primer set that amplified a segment of a gene coding for a 65-kDa antigen that is common to all mycobacteria *(43)*. Within these gene segments are variable regions that are specific for different mycobacterial species. A PCR developed by Cousins et al. relied on amplifying a unique segment within the gene coding for MPB64 or MPB70 antigens *(44)*. This PCR had a sensitivity of 97%. Similarly, PCR has been developed using primers that amplify conserved areas of insertion sequence IS6610/IS986 *(45)*. The advantage of these PCR protocols is that they may be more sensitive, since multiple copies of these target sequences are present per organism. The overall sensitivity of these assays when applied to clinical samples is reported to range from 60 to 100%. The reported sensitivity of the commercially developed PCR kits range from 50% for smear negative samples to 93% for smear positive samples. Commercial assays other than PCR, such as the ligase chain reaction (LCR), strand displacement amplification reaction, transcription-based amplification, and Q β replicase reactions, are under development and appear promising *(46)*.

4. CNS INFECTIONS

The major CNS infection syndromes are meningitis, encephalitis, myelitis, and brain abscess. A large variety of organisms can cause CNS infections. Molecular techniques have been successful in diagnosing some of these infections.

4.1. Herpes Simplex Virus Encephalitis (HSVE)

HSVE is the most common sporadic cause of encephalitis and can result in severe morbidity or mortality. The successful use of acyclovir in reducing morbidity and mortality when administered early in the course of infection has made rapid diagnosis of HSVE of great importance *(47)*. Unfortunately, the clinical diagnosis of HSVE is not highly specific, since HSVE can mimic other CNS disorders. Laboratory diagnosis of HSVE has been difficult. Culture of cerebrospinal fluid (CSF) is usually negative. Serologic analysis of simultaneously drawn CSF and serum samples as well as demonstration of intrathecally synthesized IgM may be diagnostic, but not until after 3–10 d following the onset of neurological symptoms *(48)*.

The efficacy of PCR in detecting HSV in CSF specimens from patients with documented HSVE has been reported *(49)*. In a recent study, Lakeman and Whitley used PCR to detect HSV DNA in CSF from 53 (98%) of 54 patients with biopsy-proven HSVE and proposed the technique be used as the standard test for diagnosis of HSVE *(50)*. In each case, PCR was performed with two sets of primers that amplified unique sequences from DNA polymerase and glycoprotein B genes. Both primer sets detect HSV-1 and HSV-2, and do not crossreact with other herpes viruses. There was no effect of antiviral therapy during the first week of treatment on detection of HSV DNA in CSF. However, the effect of antiviral therapy on detection of HSV DNA became evident during the second week of treatment, when only 47% of the specimens remained PCR-positive. Only 4 (21%) of the 19 specimens obtained from 18 patients 2 wk after therapy were PCR-positive.

4.2. Lyme Disease

Lyme disease is a multisystem disorder that is characterized by dermatologic, neurologic, cardiac, and rheumatic manifestations. It is caused by the spirochete *Borrelia burgdorferi*, which is transmitted to humans through the bite of the tick, *Ixodes dammini*, or related ixodid tick. Lyme disease is the most commonly reported vector-borne disease in the United States *(51)*.

Lyme disease typically occurs in three stages. The first stage is characterized by erythema migrans or nonspecific influenza-like symptoms. The second stage usually begins weeks to months after the onset of illness. In approx 15% of untreated patients, it includes disease of the CNS and/or peripheral nervous system (e.g., meningitis, cranial neuritis, particularly Bell's palsy, radiculopathies, plexopathies, or peripheral neuropathies). The third stage, which begins weeks to years after the first, occurs in approx 60% of untreated patients and consists of arthritis and late neurologic complications. The neurologic complications include neuropsychiatric symptoms, focal CNS disease, severe incapacitating fatigue, or a multiple sclerosis-like demyelinating disease.

Lyme disease is diagnosed serologically either by indirect immunofluorescence staining or by the more sensitive and specific enzyme-linked immunosorbent assay (ELISA) followed by Western blot analysis. Since these tests and their reagents are not yet standardized, variations in results are common. False negative results may be obtained during the first weeks of infection, since antibody is usually not detectable until 4–6 wk after the onset of illness. False-positive findings may occur in patients with other spirochetal disease, such as syphilis and relapsing fever.

Persing et al. developed PCR assays that detected unique sequences from borrelia outer surface protein (OspA) and flagellin (fla) genes *(52)*. Initially, they employed these assays to examine museum specimens of *I. dammini* for the presence of borrelia DNA. The assay was subsequently shown to be effective in detecting borrelia in synovial fluid. Kruger and Pulz employed a similar PCR assay that detected borrelia-specific DNA in CSF from two patients with neuroborreliosis *(53)*. These initial studies demonstrate that PCR could be useful for laboratory diagnosis of neuroborreliosis. PCR has also been useful to diagnose other CNS infections including *Toxoplasma gondii* encephalitis, neurosyphilis, and tuberculosis meningitis.

5. SEXUALLY TRANSMITTED DISEASES

In the last two decades, the number of sexually transmitted diseases has expanded greatly and now includes over 25 known pathogens. Significant efforts have been made to develop molecular techniques for rapid and reliable diagnosis of these infections.

5.1. Chlamydia trachomatis

C. trachomatis is an obligate intracellular pathogen. It is the major cause of nongonococcal urethritis and epididimitis in men and cervicitis, uritheritis, endomitritis, and salpangitis in women. The agent may cause inclusion conjunctivitis in neonates that acquire the agent during passage through an infected birth canal. The "gold standard" for diagnosis of chlamydial infections is culture in McCoy followed by fluorescent antibody staining. Because cell culture is relatively demanding, nonculture detection methods, such as the ELISA and DNA probe-based assays, have been developed. The DNA probe assay has been shown to have sensitivity similar to that of antigen detection *(54)*.

C. trachomatis possesses a cryptic plasmid of which there are 7–10 copies in each elementary body. This plasmid is the target of most amplification reactions. Loeffelholz et al. developed a rapid PCR (amplicor) for detecting a conserved region within the plasmid that required minimal specimen preparation *(55)*. They compared PCR with culture using 503 cervical specimens. After resolution of discrepant specimens with a confirmatory PCR assay directed against the chlamydial outer membrane, PCR had a sensitivity of 97% and specificity of 99.7%, whereas culture had a sensitivity of 85.7% and specificity of 100%. Similarly, they compared PCR with Chlamydiazyme (Abbott Diagnostics) in 375 cervical specimens. PCR had a sensitivity and specificity of 100%, whereas EIA had a sensitivity of 58.8% and specificity of 100%.

LCR is an alternative amplification technique for diagnosis of chlamydia that is under development. Preliminary data show that the test has a sensitivity and specificity of 85 and 99.5%, respectively *(56)*.

5.2. HIV

HIV-1 and HIV-2 are the etiologic agents of AIDS. The virus by itself does not produce most of the illness and death associated with the infection. The virus infects lymphocytes causing progressive loss of T-helper cells. The loss of lymphocytes, cause generalized immunosuppression and the patient is at risk from opportunistic infections with such organisms as *Pneumocystis carinii*, HSV, *Toxoplasma*, *Cryptococous*, CMV, and *Mycobacteria*.

Methods for detection of individuals infected with HIV provide a vital key in attempts to curtail the spread of the virus. Although the virus can be cultivated in vitro, it is time-consuming, laborious, and expensive. Most laboratories use enzyme immunoassay EIA for initial diagnosis and Western blot for conformation of positive samples. A rapid latex agglutination test that can be performed in about 5 min is available and requires minimal laboratory facilities *(57)*. The sensitivity of this test ranges from 71–91% and specificity of 93–99%. Similarly, a p24 antigen detection kit can detect picograms of this antigen in patient's sera *(58)*. This test is most useful in the early stage of illness, when the patient may be negative by other tests.

Several PCR-based amplification assays have been developed for detecting HIV infections using primers directed to amplify unique sequences from the conserved regions of *gag, pol, env, vpr, nef,* and *ras* genes *(59)*. He et al. developed a PCR assay that was coupled with solution hybridization for detecting the PCR products *(60)*. The assay detected as few as five copies of HIV-1 DNA in lysate of 100,000 peripheral blood mononuclear cells (PBMCs) from a seronegative control individual. Currently, PCR is the most sensitive method of detecting HIV infections. The procedure is most useful for resolving indeterminate serologic results and evaluating the HIV status of neonates born to infected mothers. Similarly, PCR has been used to evaluate AZT resistance as well as quantitate virion number and response to treatment *(61)*. Bush et al. developed a self-sustained sequence replication (3SR) that detected as few as 12 HIV-1 RNA copies *(62)*. Similarly, bDNA signal amplification has been shown to be reliable for detecting and quantifying viral particles in the infected individuals *(63)*.

6. GASTROINTESTINAL TRACT AND LIVER DISEASE

6.1. Hepatitis C Virus

HCV is believed to be the etiologic agent of most cases of nonA, nonB (NANB) hepatitis. The virus is a 9.4-kb positive stranded RNA virus, whose genome structure closely resembles the flaviviruses. The virus is thought to code a polyprotein of 3010 amino acids, which are then posttranslationally modified into the viral products. Antibody generated to a number of these proteins is the base of the current serodiagnosis of

HCV infection. Patients who acquire HCV infections through blood transfusion seroconvert within 6 mo after transfusion, with a mean time of seroconversion of about 5 mo. Although individuals who are chronic carriers of HCV usually have antibody to viral antigens in their serum, most acutely infected patients do not. It is also not possible to know whether an anti-HCV-positive patient is a virus carrier or has simply recovered from a past infection.

Because HCV RNA is present in the sera soon after infection, PCR has been used to diagnose HCV infections and monitor the progress of patients who are undergoing systemic interferon therapy *(64)*. The detection of HCV RNA begins with initial reverse transcription to create a cDNA copy of the extracted viral RNA sequences. HCV RNA has been detected in the sera of 96% of HCV positive patients. The assay can be used as early as 1 wk after onset of symptoms. Because the 5' untranslated region of the virus is 98% conserved among different strains, primers that amplify this region have been used by a majority of the investigators *(65)*. In addition, a nested approach can be used to increase assay sensitivity by which first-round amplification products (usually 30–40 cycles) are subjected to a second round of PCR (30–40 cycles) with an internal set of primers. PCR products are then electrophoresed in an agarose gel to enable detection by ethidium bromide staining. An alternative approach to the nested PCR is the use of a single-step PCR combined with a sensitive detection method, such as Southern blot hybridization.

6.2. Clostridium difficile

C. difficile is the primary cause of antibiotic associated-colitis, a diarrheal illness that may be severe and associated with the development of pseudomembranous colitis. The organism is part of the normal flora in >50% of neonates. The number decreases to <4% by the age 2 yr. Hospitalized patients frequently become colonized with this organism with subsequent disturbance of the normal flora as a result of the use of antibiotics, such as clindamycin, ampicillin, and cephalosorins. The organism produces at least two toxins: an enterotoxin (toxin A) and a cytotoxin (toxin B). Most strains produce either both toxins or none at all. Toxin A induces a positive fluid response in the rabbit ligated illeal loop assay and probably is the main virulence factor. Nontoxinogenic strains are probably avirulent *(66)*.

Currently, *C. difficile* is diagnosed by detection of toxins A and B by EIA, latex agglutination, or cell-culture cytotoxicity assay. Detection of organism by culture is not reliable. The cytotoxicity assay in conjunction with neutralization of the toxin cytopatheic effects using antitoxin B is considered the "gold standard." Degradation of toxin proteins by proteases that are present in stool are a source of false negative results *(66)*. Several PCR assays have been developed that detect the 16S rRNA gene and the gene coding for toxins A and B of *C. difficile*. Initial findings of these tests show that PCR has a greater sensitivity than that of culture or the toxin assays. Kato et al. used a PCR assay that detected a unique segment of the toxin A gene directly from stool specimens *(67)*. The inhibitory substances present in the stool were removed by an ion-exchange column after phenol-chloroform extraction. A total of 39 stool specimens were evaluated by PCR, and the results were in complete agreement with the cell culture assay. Gumerlock et al. used a PCR assay that detected a specific region within the gene coding for toxin B *(70)*. They examined 28 known toxigenic strains, and all were positive by this assay. Nontoxigenic strains did not produce PCR products. Kuhl et al. developed a PCR assay that detected a conserved region within the 16S rRNA gene *(69)*. The toxigenic strains were distinguished from nontoxigenic strains by PCR amplification of the toxin A and/or B gene sequences.

6.3. Escherichia coli O157, H7

Enterohemorrhagic *E. coli* (EHEC) are acquired through consumption of contaminated undercooked beef or contaminated milk. Like diphtheria, the organism is lysogenized by a bacteriphage that codes for two protein Shiga-like toxins 1 and 2 (verotoxin 1 and *2)*. These proteins inhibit protein synthesis and are active against Vero cells and HeLa cells. There are over 50 serotypes of EHEC. However, *E. coli* O157, H7 is the only serotype that is a threat to public health. Three to 5 d following ingestion, the organism may cause mild diarrhea or progressive bloody diarrhea with abdominal cramps (hemorrhage colitis). Patients are typically young. Serious systemic complications are thrombotic thrombocytopenic purpura and hemolytic uremic syndrome. Currently, the detection of the *E. coli* O157, H7 is extremely time-consuming. Isolation is based on the fact that *E. coli* O157, H7 does not ferment sorbitol and can be detected on a sorbitol-MacConkey agar medium. All sorbitol negative organisms are checked for the presence of O157 and H7 antigens. PCR offers a rapid and reliable detection of this organism in fecal samples. Pollard et al. developed a PCR assay that detected VT1 and VT2 gene sequences from 40 laboratory strains of *E. coli* O157, H7 *(70)*.

7. MOLECULAR METHODS FOR DETECTING ANTIMICROBIOL RESISTANCE

The resistance of microorganisms to antibiotics remains a major obstacle to the successful treatment of infected individuals. The major mechanisms of bacterial resistance include enzymatic inactivation of antibiotic, such as β-lactamase, decreased cell membrane permeability, such as bacterial resistance to tetracycline, altered target sites, such as low-affinity target for penicillin binding proteins, and altered metabolic pathway or bypass, as is in sulfonamide resistance. Several reliable culture-dependent approaches have been developed for detecting resistant organisms in clinical laboratories. All these tests rely on culturing the organism from the site of infection, propagating them in pure culture, and performing susceptibility tests using broth or agar dilution methods. Molecular techniques provide the opportunity for more rapid detection of resistant organisms in clinical samples. For example, PCR-based detection of mutations in the *rpo*B gene of MTB indicates resistance of the organism to rifampin, which, in turn, suggests the possibility of multidrug-resistant MTB *(71)*. Similarly the molecular technique can be used to determine resistance in cases in which the conventional minimum inhibitory concentration (MIC) is at or near breakpoint.

7.1. Resistance to β-Lactam Antibiotics

Methacillin-resistant *Staphylococcus aureus* (MRSA) is a common cause of nosocomial infections. Resistance is mediated by a production of low-affinity PBP2a or PBP2' encoded by the mecA gene *(72)*. Similarly, coagulase-negative staphylococci have become resistant by acquisition of this gene. Methacillin-resistant organisms are detected using traditional susceptibility tests, including disk diffusion, and broth and agar dilution tests. The expression of resistance in some strains is heterogeneous, complicating the detection of the resistant organisms with traditional techniques. In addition, some strains of *S. aureus* may be borderline resistant owing to production of large amount of β-lactamase *(72)*. PCR or DNA probe assays circumvent these problems. Several investigators have developed PCR assays to detect the mecA gene either directly or following the laboratory propagation of the organisms. In one study, a minimum of 500 CFU of *S. aureus* were required to detect the mecA gene *(73)*.

In recent years β-lactamase resistant *Streptococcus pneumoniae* have become a major global problem. Resistant strains are developed through acquisition of segments of streptococcal species chromosomal genes that result in altered forms of *S. pneumoniae* penicillin-binding proteins (PBPs). Because of the random nature of these transformations, DNA probes that would identify these insertions are not available. PCR-based assays that analyze the PBP 2B and 2X genes of 3F isolated appear to be promising *(74)*.

β-lactamase resistance among gram-negative bacteria is usually plasmid-mediated. Several plasmids, such as TEM, SHV, OXA, CARB, ROB, and β-lactamase, have been characterized in these organisms. Currently, it appears unrealistic to try to identify all these enzyme types among clinical isolates other than for epidemiological studies.

7.2. Aminoglycoside Resistance

The bacterial resistance to aminoglycosides is the result of production of aminoglycoside-modifying enzymes, such as phosphoryltransferase, nucleotidyltransferase, and acetyltransferase. Lack of unique sequence among the gene coding for the modifying enzymes, especially in gram-negative organisms, makes it difficult to use PCR and DNA probes for routine use in clinical laboratories *(75)*. Aminoglycoside resistance in gram positive organisms is more uniform, and PCR assays have been used to detect genes responsible for streptomycin resistance and high level gentamicin resistance.

7.3. Rifampin Resistance

Rifampin is a potent antituberculosis drug that has antibiotic activity against many bacteria. The compound is a large fat-soluble molecule that acts by inhibiting bacterial DNA-dependent RNA polymerase. Mutation in the *rpo*B gene, which encodes the β subunit of this enzyme, results in high-level resistance to rifampin in MTB and *Mycobacterium leprae*. Telenti et al. developed a PCR assay that amplifies a region of *rpo*B. They identified the mutations by single-stranded conformational polymorphism analysis of the amplification products *(71)*. Similarly, a PCR assay for detecting rifampin resistance in *M. leprae* has been developed *(76)*. Rifampin resistance also serves as an indicator for multidrug resistance in *M. tuberculosis*.

7.4. Vancomycin Resistance

Vancomycin was introduced in 1956 and marketed for its efficacy against penicillinase producing staphylococci. Following the introduction of antistaphylococccal penicillins and cephalosporins, vancomycin was used as alternative therapy for methacillin-resistant staphylococci and in patients allergic to penicillin or cephalosporins. Vancomycin exerts its antibacterial activity by inhibiting biosynthesis of a major structural polymer of the bacterial cell wall, peptidoglycan. The spectrum of vancomycin activity is limited to aerobic and anaerobic gram-positive organisms. Vancomycin is bactericidal against most gram-positive organisms except enterococci. The combination of gentamicin and vanomycin is synergistic against most strains of enterococci. The mechanism of enterococcal vancomycin resistance has been extensively studied. Two distinct phenotypes of acquired resistance, VanA and VanB, have been identified on the basis of their antibacterial activity against vancomycin and teicoplanin. VanA includes strains with inducible high-level resistance to vancomycin and teicoplanin. The resistance is transferred via conjugative transfer of an 11-kb transposon (Tn1546). The VanB phenotype includes strains of enterococci with high-level resistance to vancomycin, but susceptibility to teicoplanin. The vanB gene cluster is located on the chromosome as part of very large conjugative elements that can be transferred to a susceptible organism. Dutka-Malen et al. developed a PCR assay that simultaneously detects glycopeptide resistance and species identification of enterococci *(77)*. The assay is based on specific amplification of internal fragments of genes coding D-alanine:D-alanine ligases and related glycopeptide resistance proteins. The specificity of the assay was tested on five glycopeptide-resistant and 15 susceptible strains. The assay offers a specific and rapid alternative to the antibiotic susceptibility testing.

8. MOLECULAR EPIDEMIOLOGY

8.1. Plasmid Analysis

In recent years, several DNA based methods have been developed to type those organisms that were not distinguishable or difficult to discriminate by phenotypic typing techniques. Plasmid analysis is one of the earliest molecular-based techniques applied to epidemiological investigation. Plasmids are autonomous extrachromosomal DNA often carrying genes for antibiotic resistance. An organism may harbor several distinct plasmids. Plasmids have become valuable markers for comparing closely related strains of bacteria in epidemiologic studies, as well as studying the outbreaks of nosocomial infection *(78)*. The plasmid comparison can be carried one step further in specificity by cutting the plasmid DNA with specific restriction enzymes and examining the resulting fragments by agarose gel electrophoresis. The technique is highly reproducible, with good discriminatory power, and is easy to perform and interpret *(78)*.

8.2. Chromosomal DNA Analysis

This technique relies on the restriction endonuclease digestion of chromosomal DNA followed by electrophoresis of the resultant fragment in an ethidium bromide-stained agarose gel. The enzyme recognizes specific nucleotide sequences in DNA and digests them at all sites at which the sequence appears. Although the technique has been useful in the study of many organisms, such as *C. difficile*, it is difficult to interpret in part owing to the large number of restriction fragments that must be compared.

8.3. Southern Blot Analysis of Restriction Fragment Polymorphisms (RFLPs)

To improve on the specificity of chromosomal analysis, restriction fragments are blotted onto a nylon membrane followed by detection of particular restriction fragment with a labeled probe. Any variation in their number or migration is referred to as an RFLP. The discriminatory power of this technique is directly related to the size and number of fragment detected by the probe. For example, DNA probe directed to conserved regions of *E. coli* rRNA gene (ribotyping) will detect a wide range of organisms *(79)*. In general, ribotyping will produce an average of 10–15 RFLPs for organisms, such as *E. coli*, *Klebsiella*, *Hemophilus*, and *Staph spp*. In contrast, ribotyping of mycobacteria will produce one or two RFLPs, with limited epidemiological utility. *M. tuberculosis*, however, has insertion sequences (IS), such as IS6110, that are present in multiple repeats within the bacterial chromosome. DNA probe directed to the conserved regions of these insertion sequences are highly discriminatory among the species *(80)*.

8.4. Pulsed-Field Gel Electrophoresis

PFGE is a variation of agarose gel electrophoresis that can separate extremely long DNA molecules. Ordinary gel electrophoresis fails to separate such molecules, because steady electric field stretches them out so they travel end first through the gel in a snakelike configuration at a rate that is independent of their length. In PFGE, by contrast, the direction of the electric field is charged periodically, which forces the molecule to reorient before continuing to move snakelike through the gel. The reorientation takes more time for larger molecules, so they move more slowly. To obtain suitable unsheared DNA, the organism is embedded in agarose plugs followed by enzymatic lysing of the cell wall and digestion of the cellular proteins. The intact DNA is digested *in situ* with appropriate restriction enzymes. The PFGE of the digested chromosome will provide a 5–20 distinct fragment pattern ranging from 10–800 kb. The technique has been used successfully to discriminate strains of pathogens, such as *E. coli*, *Enterococci*, *Staphylococci*, and *Pseudomonas aeruginosa*.

8.5. PCR

The introduction of PCR has also provided a means for rapid and reliable typing of clinical isolates. These include restriction digestion of PCR products and analysis of the resulting fragments for polymorphisms. Rep-PCR is based on the use of primers directed to hybridize to short extragenetic repetitive sequences within the bacterial chromosome. When two sequences are located near each other, the DNA fragments between those sites are amplified. Finally, arbitrary primed PCR is based on the use of short primers (10 bases) that are not directed to amplify specific region. These primers hybridize randomly, and if two such sites are within a kilobase of each other, the amplification of these random targets occur. Although the technique is rapid, it has not been completely problem-free.

9. CONCLUSIONS

The introduction of molecular techniques, especially PCR, to clinical laboratories has provided powerful sets of new tools that have facilitated the detection and diagnosis of infectious diseases. Despite its initial promise, there has been limited success in the routine use of these techniques in clinical laboratory. In-house developed PCRs and similar assays are complex and cumbersome, and there is no complete agreement among investigators on the ideal set of primers, extraction protocol, or PCR product detection techniques. The laboratory technologist must therefore have special training and extensive understanding of the principles of molecular biology. In addition, false-negative results occur as a result of interfering substances and false positive results from amplicon contaminations of previous amplification reactions. Commercially developed PCR and similar amplification techniques have addressed some of these issues. Assays have been developed that are user-friendly and more compatible with average laboratory work flow, including fewer steps and minimal specimen preparation time. As these improvements are brought to the clinical laboratories and further improvements are made, molecular techniques will become an integral part of clinical microbiology laboratories.

REFERENCES

1. Yolken, R. H. Enzyme immunoassay for detection of infectious diseases antigens in body fluids: current limitation and future prospects. *Rev. Infect. Dis.* **4:**35, 1992.
2. Goto, M., Oka, S., Okuzumi, K., Kimura, S., and Shimada, K. Evaluation of acridinium-ester-labeled DNA probes for identification of *Mycobacterium tuberculosis* and *Mycobacterium avium-Mycobacterium intracellulare complex* in culture. *J. Clin. Microbiol.* **29:**2473–2476, 1991.
3. Stockman, L., Clark, K. A., Hunt, J. M., and Roberts, G. D. Evaluation of commercially available acridinium ester-labeled chemiluminescent DNA probes for culture identification of Blastomyces dermatitidis, *Coccidioides immitis, Cryptococcus neoformans*, and *Histoplasma capsulatum. J. Clin. Microbiol.* **31:**845–850, 1993.
4. Kluytmans, J. A. J., Niesters, H. G.M., Mouton, J. W., Quint, W. G. V., Ijpelaar, J. A. J., Van Rijsoort-Vos, J. H., et al. Performance of a nonisotopic DNA probe for detection of *Chlamydia trachomatis* in urogenital specimens. *J. Clin. Microbiol.* **29:**2685–2689, 1991.
5. Chapin-Robertson, K. C., Reece, E. A., and Edberg, S. C. Evaluation of the Gen Probe PACE II assay for the direct detection of *Neisseria gonorrhoeae* endocervical specimens. *Diagn. Microbiol. Infect. Dis.* **15:**212,213, 1992.
6. Lewis, J. S., Kranig-Brown, D., and Trainor, D. DNA probe confirmatory test for *Neisseria gonorrhoae. J. Clin. Microbiol.* **28:**2349–2350, 1990.
7. Briselden, A. M. and Hillier, S. L. Evaluation of affirm VP microbial identification test for *Gardnerella vaginalis* and *Trichomonas vaginalis. J. Clin. Microbiol.* **32:**148–152, 1994.
8. Steed, L. L., Korgenski, E. K., and Daly, J. A. Rapid detection of *Streptococcus pyogenes* in pediatric patient specimens by DNA probe. *J. Clin. Microbiol.* **31:**2996–3000, 1993.
9. Doebbeling, B. N., Bale, M. J., Koontz, F. P., Helms, C. M., Wenzel, R. P., and Pfaller, M. A. Prospective evaluation of the Gen Probe assay for detection of *Legionellae* in respiratory specimens. *Eur. J. Clin. Microbiol. Infect. Dis.* **7:**748–752, 1988.
10. Tenover, F. C., Carlson, L., Barbagallo, S., and Nachamkin, I. DNA probe culture confirmation assay for identification of thermophilic *Campylobacter* species. *J. Clin. Micrbiol.* **28:**1284–1287, 1990.
11. Daly, J. A., Clifton, N. L., Seskin, K. C., and Gooch, WM., III Use of rapid, nonradioactive DNA probes in culture confirmation tests to detect Streptococcus agalactiae, *Haemophilus influenzae*, and *Enterococcus* spp. from pediatric patients with significant infections. *J. Clin. Microbiol.* **29:**80–82, 1991.
12. Youmans, G. R., Davis, T. E., and Fuller, D. D. Use of chemiluminescent DNA probes in the rapid detection of oxacillin resistance in clinically isolated strains of *Staphylococcus aureus . Diagn. Microbiol. Infect. Dis.* **16:**99–104, 1993.
13. Drake, T. A., Hindler, J. A., Berlin, O. G. W., and Bruckner, D. Rapid identification of Mycobacterium avium complex in culture using DNA probers. *J. Clin. Microbiol.* **25:**1442–1445, 1987.
14. Tortoli, E., Simonetti, M. T., Lacchini, C., Penati, V., Piersimoni, C., and Morbiducci, V. Evaluation of a commercial DNA probe assay for the identification of *Mycobacterium* kansasii *Eur. J. Clin. Microbial. Infect. Dis.* **13:**264–267, 1994.

15. Walton, D. T. and Valesco, M. Identification of *Mycobacterium gordonae* from culture by the Gen Probe rapid diagnostic system: evaluation of 218 isolates and potential sources of false-negative results. *J. Clin. Microbiol.* **29:**1850–1854, 1991.

16. Denys, G. A. and Carey, R. B. Identification of *Streptococcus pneumoniae* with a DNA probe. *J. Clin. Microbiol.* **30:**2725–2727, 1992.

17. Okwumabua, O., Swaminathan, B., Edmonds, P., Wenger, J., Hogan, J., and Alden, M. Evaluation of a chemiluminescent DNA probe assay for the rapid confirmation of Listeria monocytogenes. *Res. Microbiol.* **143:**183–189,1992.

18. Delvenne, P., Fontaine, M. A., Delvenne, C., Nikkels, A., and Boniver, J. Detection of human papillomavirus in paraffin-embedded biopsies of cervical intraepithelial lesions: analysis by immunohistochemistry, in situ hybridization, and the polymerase chain reaction. *Mod. Pathol.* **7:**113–119, 1994.

19. Briselden, A. M. and Hillier, S. L. Evaluation of the affirm VP microbial identification test for *Gardnerella vaginalis* and *Trichomonas vaginalis*. *J. Clin. Microbiol.* **32:**148–152, 1994.

20. Urdea, M. S. synthesis and characterization of branched DNA (bDNA) for the direct and quantitative detection of CMV., HBV., HCV and HIV. *Clin. Chem.* **39:**725,726, 1993.

21. Lau, J. Y., Davis, G. L., Kniffen, J., Qian, K. P., Urdea, M. S., Chan, C. S., Mizokami, M., Neuwald, P. D., and Wilber, J. C. Significance of serum hepatitis C virus RNA levels in chronic hepatitis C. *Lancet* **341:**1501–1504, 1993.

22. Persing, D. H. In vitro nucleic acid amplification techniques, in *Diagnostic Molecular Microbiology Principles and Applications*, Persing, D. H., Smith, T. F., Tenover, F. C., and White, T. J., eds., American Society of Microbiology, Washington, DC, pp. 51–87, 1994.

23. Longo, M. C., Berninger, M. S., and Hartley, J. L. Use of uracil DNA glycosylase of control carry-over contamination in polymerase chain reaction. *Gene* **93:**25–128, 1990.

24. Isaacs, S. T., Tessman, J. W., Metchette, K. C., Hersat, J. E., and Cimino, G. D. Post-PCR sterilization: development and application to an HIV-1 diagnostic assay. *Nucleic Acid Res.* **19:**109–116, 1991.

25. Aslanzadeh, J. Application of hydroxylamine hydrocholoride for post-PCR sterilization. *Mol. Cell. Probes* **7:**145–150,1993.

26. Zuravleff, J. J., Yu, V. L., Shonnard, J. W., Davis, B. K., and Rihs, J. D. Diagnosis of Legionnaires' disease. An update of laboratory methods with new emphasis on isolation by culture. *JAMA* **250:**1981–1985, 1983.

27. Tenover, F. C., Edelstein, P. H., Goldstein, L. C., Sturge, J. C., and Plorde, J. J. Comparison of cross-staining reactions by *Pseudomonas spp.* and fluorescein-labeled polycolonal antibodies directed against *Legionella pneumophila*. *J. Clin. Microbiol.* **23:**647–649, 1986.

28. Jaulhac, B., Nowicki, M., Bornstein, N., Meunier, O., Prevost, G., Piemont, Y., Fleurette, J., and Monteil, H. Detection of *Legionella spp.* in bronchoalveolar lavage fluid by DNA amplification. *J. Clin. Microbiol.* **30:**920–924, 1992.

29. Kessler, H. H., Reinthaler, F. F., Pschaid, A., Pierer, K., Kleinhappl, B., Eber, E., and Marth, E. Rapid detection of Legionella species in bronchoalveolar lavage fluid with EnviroAmp Legionella PCR amplification and detection kit. *J. Clin. Microbiol.* **31:**3325–3328, 1993.

30. Lindsay, D. S., Abraham, W. H., and Fallon, R. J. Detection of mip gene by PCR for diagnosis of Legionnaires' disease. *J. Clin. Microbiol.* **32:**3068,3069, 1994.

31. Jonas, D., Rosenbaum, A., Weyrich, S., and Bhakdi, S. Enzyme- linked immunoassay for detection of PCR amplified DNA of legionella in bronchoalveolar fluid. *J. Clin. Microbiol.* **33:**1247–1252, 1995.

32. Gaydos, C. A., Quinn, T. C., and Eiden, J. J. Identification of *Chlamydia pneumoniae* by DNA amplification of the 16S rRNA gene. *J. Clin. Microbiol.* **30:**796–800, 1992.

33. Campbell, L. E., Melagosa, M. P., Hamilton, D. J., Kuo, C.-C., and Graystone, J. T. Detection of *Chlamydia pneumoniae* by polymerase chain reaction. *J. Clin. Microbiol.* **30:**434–439, 1992.

34. Rasmussen, S. J., Douglas, F. P., and Timms, P. PCR detection and differentiation of *Chlamydia pneumoniae*, *Chlamydia psittaci*, and *Chlamydia trachomatis*. *Mol. Cell. Probes* **6**:389–394, 1992.

35. Black, C. M., Fields, P. I., Messer, T. O., and Berdal, B. P. Detection of *Chlamydia pneumoniae* in clinical specimens by polymerase chain reaction using nested primers. *Eur. J. Clin. Microbiol. Infect. Dis.* **13**:752–756, 1994.

36. Gaydos, C. A., Eiden, J. J., Oldach, D., Mundy, L. M., Auwaerter, P., Warner, M. L., Vance, E., Burton, A. A., and Quinn, T. C. diagnosis of *Chlamydia pneumoniae* infection in patients with community acquired pneumonia by polymerase chain reaction enzyme immunoassay. *Clin. Infect. Dis.* **19**:157–160, 1993.

37. Pruckl, P. M., Aspock, C., Makristathis, A., Rotter, M. L., Wank, H., Willinger, B., and Hirschl, A. M. Polymerase chain reaction for detection of Chlamydia pneumoniae in gargled-water specimens of children. *Eur. J. Clin. Microbiol. Infect. Dis.* **14**:141–144, 1995.

38. Garret, M. and Bonnet, J. PCR detection of *Mycoplasma pneumoniae*, in *Diagnostic Molecular Microbiology Principles and Applications*, Persing, D. H., Smith, T. F., Tenover, F. C., and White, T. J, eds. American Society of Microbiology, Washington, DC, pp. 253–260, 1993.

39. vanKuppeveld, F. J., Johansson, K.-E., Galama, J. M., Kissing, J., Bolske, G., Hjelm, E., van der Logt, J. T., and Melchers, W. J. 16S rRNA based polymerase chain reaction compared with culture and serological methods for diagnosis of Mycoplasma pneumoniae infection. *Eur. J. Clin. Microbiol. Infect. Dis.* **13**:401–405, 1994.

40. Tjhie, J. H., vanKuppeveld, F. J., Roosendaal, R., Melchers, W. J. G., Gordijn, R., MacLaren, D. M., Walboomers, J. M. M., Meijer, C. J. L. M., and Van Den Brule, A. J. C. Direct PCR enables detection of *Mycoplasma pneumoniae* in patients with respiratory tract infections. *J. Clin. Microbiol.* **32**:11–16, 1994.

41. Leng, Z., Kenny, G. E., and Roberts, M. C. Evaluation of the detection limits of PCR identification of *Mycoplasma pneumoniae* in clinical samples. *Mol. Cell. Probes* **8**:125–130, 1994.

42. Luneberg, E., Jensen, J. S., and Frosch, M. Detection of *Mycoplasma pneumoniae* by polymerase chain reaction and nonradioactive hybridization in microtiter plates. *J. Clin. Microbiol.* **31**:1088–1094, 1993.

43. Hance, A. J., Grandchamp, B., Levy-Frebault, V., et al. Detection of and identification of mycobacteria by amplification of mycobacterial DNA. *Mol. Microbiol.* **3**:843–849, 1989.

44. Cousins, D. V., Wilton, S. D., Francis, B. R., and Gow, B. L. Use of polymerase chain reaction for rapid diagnosis of tuberculosis. *J. Clin. Microbiol.* **30**:255–258, 1992.

45. Anderson, A. B., Thybo, S., Godfery-Faussett, P., and Stoker, N. G. Polymerase chain reaction for detection of Mycobacterium tuberculosis in sputum. *Eur. J. Clin. Microbiol. Infect. Dis.* **12**:922–927, 1993.

46. Buxton, Q. A. D., Hendricks, A., Robinson, L., Shah, J., Lu, L., Vera-Garcia, M., King, W., and Olive, D. M. Comparison of amplified Q beta replicase and PCR assays for detection of *Mycobacterium tuberculosis*. *J. Clin. Microbiol.* **33**:860–867, 1995.

47. Whitely, R., Arvin, A., Prober, C., Burchett, S., Corey, L., Powell, D., Plotkin, S., Starr, S., Alford, C., Conner, J., Jacobs, R., Nahmias, A., and Soong, S. A controlled trial comparing vidarabine with acyclovir in neonatal herpes simplex virus infection. *New Engl. J. Med.* **324**:444–449, 1991.

48. Elitsur, Y., Carmi, R., and Sarov, I. HSV-specific serum/CSF antibody ratio in association with HSV serum IgM antibodies in diagnosis of herpes encephalitis in infants. *Isr. J. Med. Sci.* **19**:943–945, 1983.

49. Aslanzadeh, J., Osmon, D. R., Wilhelm, M. P., Espy, M. J., and Smith, T. F. A prospective study of the polymerase chain reaction for detection of herpes simplex virus in cerebrospinal fluid submitted to the clinical virology laboratory. *Mol. Cell. Probes* **6**:367–373, 1992.

50. Lakeman, F. D. and Whitley, R. J. Diagnosis of herpes simplex encephalitis: application of polymerase chain reaction to cerebrospinal fluid from brain-biopsied patients and correlation with disease. *J. Infect. Dis.* **171**:857–863, 1995.
51. Centers for Disease Control. Lyme disease United States, 1987 and 1988 *Morbid. Mortal. Wkly. Rept.* **38**:668–672, 1989.
52. Persing, D. H., Telford, S. R., Rys, P. N., Dodge, D. E., White, T. J., Malawista, S. E., and Spielman, A. Detection of Borrelia burgdorferi DNA in museum specimens of Ixodes dammini ticks. *Science* **249**:1420–1423, 1990.
53. Kruger, W. H. and Pulz, M. Detection of *Borrelia burgdorferi* in cerebrospinal fluid by the polymerase chain reaction. *J. Med. Microbiol.* **35**:98–102, 1991.
54. Clarke, L. M., Sierra, M. F., Lopez, D. N., Covino J. M., and McCormack, W. M. Comparison of the Syva Micro Track enzyme immunoassay and Gen-Probe PACE 2 with cell culture for diagnosis of cervical *Chlamydia trachomatis* infection in a high-prevalence female population. *J. Clin. Microbiol.* **31**:968–971, 1993.
55. Loeffelholz, M. J., Lewinski, C. A., Silver, S. R., Purohit, A. P., Herman, S. A., Buonagurio, D. A., and Dragon, E. A. Detection of *Chlamydia trachomatis* in endocervical specimens by polymerase chain reaction. *J. Clin. Microbiol.* **30**:2847–2851, 1992.
56. Schachter, J. and Stamm, W. E. Chlamydia, in *Manual of Clinical Microbiology*, Murry, P. R., Baron, E. J., Pfaller, M. A., Tenover, F. C., and Yolken, R. H., ed., American Society of Microbiology, Washington, DC, 1995.
57. Riggin, C. H. HIV-1 testing by latex agglutination. *Clin. Microbiol. News Lett.* **12**:35–38, 1990.
58. McDoneel, K. B., Chimel, J. S., Poggensee, L., Wu, S., and Phair, J. P. Predicting progression to AIDS: combined usefulness of CD4 lymphocyte counts and p24 antigenimia. *Am. J. Med.* **89**:706–712, 1990.
59. Mallet, F., Herbard, C., Brand, D., Chapuis, E., Cros, P., Allibert, P., Besnier, J. M., Barin, F., and Mandrand, B. Enzyme-linked oligosorbant assay for detection of polymerase chain reaction-amplified human immunodeficiency virus type 1. *J. Clin. Microbiol.* **31**:1444–1449, 1993.
60. He, Y., Coutlee, F., Saint-Antoine, P., Olivier, C., Voyer, H., and Kessous-Elbaz, A. Detection of polymerase chain reaction-amplified human immunodeficiency virus type 1 DNA with a digoxigenin-labeled RNA probe and an enzyme linked immunoassay. *J. Clin. Microbiol.* **31**:1040–1047, 1993.
61. Arens, M. Use of probes and amplification techniques for the diagnosis of human immunodeficiency virus (HIV-1) infections. *Diag. Microbiol. Infect. Dis.* **16**:165–172, 1993.
62. Bush, C. E., Donovan, R. M., Peterson, W. R. et al. Detection of human immunodeficiency virus type 1 RNA in plasma samples from high-risk pediatric patients by using the self-sustained sequence replication reaction. *J. Clin. Microbiol.* **30**:281–286, 1992.
63. Urdea, M. S., Wilber, J. C., and Yeghiazarian, T., et al. Direct and quantitative detection of HIV-1 RNA in human plasma with a branched DNA signal amplification assay. *AIDS* **7**:S11–S14, 1993.
64. Yoshioka, K., Kakuma, S., Wakita, T., Ishikawa, T., Itoh, Y., and Takayanagi, M. Detection of hepatitis C virus by polymerase chain reaction and response to interferon alpha therapy: relationship to genotypes of hepatitis C virus. *Hepatology* **16**:293–299, 1991.
65. Bukh, J. et. al. Importance of primer selection for the detection of hepatitis C virus RNA with polymerase chain reaction assay. *Proc. Natl. Acad. Sci. USA* **89**:187–191, 1992.
66. Onderdonk, A. B. and Allen, S. D. Clostridium, in *Manual of Clinical Microbiology*, Murry, P. R., Baron, E. J., Pfaller, M. A., Tenover, F. C., and Yolken, R. H., eds., American Society of Microbiology, Washington, DC, pp. 574–586, 1995.
67. Kato, N., Ou, C. Y., Kato, H., Bartley, S. L., Luo, C. C., Killgore, G. E., and Ueno, K. Detection of toxigenic Clostridium difficile in stool specimens by polymerase chain reaction. *J. Infect. Dis.* **167**:455–488, 1993.

68. Gumerlock, P. H., Tang, Y. J., Weiss, J. B., and Silva, J., Jr. Specific detection of toxigenic strains of Clostridium difficile in stool specimens. *J. Clin. Microbiol.* **31**:507–511, 1993.

69. Kuhl, S. J., Tang, Y. J., Navarro, L., Gumerlock, P. H., and Silva, J., Jr. Diagnosis and monitoring of Clostridium difficile infections with the polymerase chain reaction. *Clin. Infect. Dis.* **4**:S234–S238, 1993.

70. Pollard, D. R., Johnson, D. M., Lior, H., Tyler, S. D., and Rozee, K. R. Rapid and specific detection of verotoxin genes in *E. coli* by the polymerase chain reaction. *J. Clin. Microbiol.* **28**:540–545, 1990.

71. Telenti, A., Imboden, P., Marchesi, F., Schmidheini, T., and Bodmer, T. Direct automated detection of rifampicin resistant *Mycobacterium tuberculosis* by polymerase chain reaction and single strand confirmation polymorphism analysis. *Antimicrob. Agents Chemother.* **37**:2054–2058, 1993.

72. Chambers, H. F. Methicillin-resistant staphylococci. *Clin. Microbiol. Rev.* **1**:173-86, 1988.

73. Ubukata, K., Nakagami, S., Nitta, A., Yamane, A., Kawakami, S., Sugiura, M., and Konno, A. Rapid detection of the mecA gene in methicillin-resistant staphylococci by enzymatic detection of polymerase chain reaction products. *J. Clin. Microbiol.* **30**:1728–1733, 1992.

74. Munoz, R., Coffey, T. J., Daniels, M., et al. Intercontinental spread of a multiresistant clone of serotype 23F *Streptococcus pneumoniae*. *J. Infect. Dis.* **164**:302–306, 1991.

75. Shaw, K. J., Rather, P. N., Hare, R. S., and Miller, G. H. Molecular genetics of aminoglycoside resistance genes and familial relationships of aminoglycoside-modifying enzymes. *Microbiol. Rev.* **57**:138–163, 1993.

76. Honore, N. and Cole, S. The molecular basis of rifampin resistance in *Mycobacterium leprae*. *Antimicrob. Agents Chemother.* **37**:414–418, 1993.

77. Dutka-Malen, S., Evers, S., and Courvalin, P. Detection of glycopeptide resistance genotypes and identfication to the species level of clinically relevant enterococci by PCR. *J. Clin. Microbiol.* **33**:24–27, 1995.

78. Mayer, L. W. Use of plasmid profiles in epidemiologic surveillance of disease outbreaks and in tracing the transmission of antibiotic resistance. *Clin. Microbiol. Rev.* **1**:228–243, 1988.

79. Stull, T. L., LiPuma, J. J., and Edlind, T. D. A broad-spectrum probe for molecular epidemiology of bacteria:ribosomal RNA. *J. Infect. Dis.* **157**:280–286, 1988.

80. vanEmbden, J. D., Cave, M. D., Crawford, J. T., et al. Strain identification of *Mycobacterium tuberculosis* by DNA fingerprinting: recommendation for a standardized methodology. *J. Clin. Microbiol.* **31**:406–409, 1993.

Part IV
Issues for the Clinical Molecular Pathology Laboratory

Quality Control Issues
for the Clinical Molecular Pathologist

Daniel H. Farkas

1. INTRODUCTION

By the time you get to this chapter in this book, assuming you are reading the book in sequence, it should be clear that the tools of molecular biology have broad diagnostic applications within the clinical pathology laboratory. Furthermore, the methodology of molecular biology is also of paramount importance in the decidedly nondiagnostic field of gene therapy. This chapter describes some of the practical issues of quality control (QC) associated with generating accurate laboratory results.

2. QUALITY CONTROL

QC, as it relates to the clinical laboratory, is a set of principles and tasks implemented to provide the most accurate possible laboratory results via efforts to anticipate and avoid problems within a laboratory procedure before they occur. Appropriate QC reigns in every possible step that may cause a test or procedure to fail, or that would require its repetition and at the same time dramatically reduces troubleshooting. Superior QC guarantees that there will be no concerns about why a test failed; it should not. Of course, this is a naive view since we do not work in a perfect world and furthermore, some of the techniques in molecular biology are a bit temperamental. Despite this naiveté, usually our laboratory results do turn out accurately, which is owing, in no small part, to proper QC. Finally, the variable of human performance and human error, although minimized by properly trained and certified medical technologists, emphasizes the importance of absolute vigilance about the control of molecular pathology.

2.1. Instrumentation

The molecular pathology laboratory is no different from any other section of a hospital-based pathology laboratory with respect to the need for appropriate equipment maintenance, calibration, and documentation of same. The goal of course is safe, reliable, and accurate patient testing. Use of equipment should be documented either daily or at least with each use. Critical operating characteristics must be reviewed by performing and documenting key function checks. Routine preventative maintenance and instrument repair must also be documented. Review by the laboratory supervisor or

From: Molecular Diagnostics: For the Clinical Laboratorian
Edited by: W. B. Coleman and G. J. Tsongalis Humana Press Inc., Totowa, NJ

director must be done periodically. In our laboratory, I indirectly monitor instrument performance every time I review (and enter into the laboratory information system) test results. I formally check instrument performance logs at the beginning of each month. None of the above is unique to the molecular pathology laboratory.

The Commission on Laboratory Accreditation of the College of American Pathologists (CAP; 325 Waukegan Road, Northfield, IL 60093-2750; 847-446-8800) publishes inspection checklists for pathology laboratory sections; Section 12 is for molecular pathology. Not only is CAP certification necessary for laboratory accreditation, but the CAP has also been granted "deemed status" by the US federal government such that laboratories successfully completing a CAP inspection may consider themselves CLIA '88 certified (CLIA '88 is a federal law—Clinical Laboratory Improvement Amendments of 1988—enacted, among other things, to improve laboratory quality).

Among the instrumentation specifically mentioned in the CAP molecular pathology inspection checklist are spectrophotometers, signal detection instruments, film processing and photographic equipment, fume hoods, biological safety cabinets, electrophoresis equipment (including power supplies), pH meters, centrifuges, timers, balances, volumetric glassware, automatic pipets, and thermometers and temperature-dependent equipment, including, importantly, thermal cyclers. With the exception of thermal cyclers, none of the above items is unique to a molecular diagnostics laboratory. Instrument calibration must be done to confirm that an instrument is performing within established tolerance limits. Calibration periodicity may be established by the manufacturer or changed by the laboratory if it is deemed appropriate, e.g., if an instrument gets heavy or light use.

Spectrophotometers are important for accurate quantitation of extracted nucleic acids and are a mainstay of many molecular pathology laboratories, although alternative quantitation methods exist. With respect to QC, care should be taken to avoid specimen mix-up during DNA quantitation. One DNA solution looks identical to the next and quantitation in unmarked cuvets is an invitation to mix-up. Devise some protocol for avoiding this problem *(1)*. Equally important with respect to QC is taking absorbance readings of nucleic acid solutions within the linear range of the instrument. My lab determines this linear range (absorbance vs DNA concentration) quarterly using a standard DNA solution obtained commercially. The range is posted and all patient DNA solutions that absorb outside this range are appropriately diluted with buffer until absorbance falls within the linear range. Beyond this last point, the CAP inspection checklist asks specific questions about the calibration and maintenance of spectrophotometers.

Electrophoretic power supplies must be calibrated periodically with a voltmeter to confirm that the voltage displayed by the unit is actually the voltage being supplied to the circuit (created by the power supply, electrical leads, gel, and buffer). Clearly, such calibration must be documented. Thermal cyclers for performance of in vitro nucleic acid amplification, e.g. polymerase chain reaction (PCR) and ligase chain reaction (LCR), are key pieces of equipment in the molecular pathology laboratory and will become increasingly prevalent in other department sections, e.g., microbiology, histocompatibility, virology, and so forth. Before being placed into service and periodically thereafter (the interval is defined by the use the machine gets—the thermal cyclers in my lab are calibrated quarterly), temperature accuracy of individual wells of cyclers should be checked. Thermal cyclers are used at two to three different temperatures to achieve in vitro nucleic acid amplification, and each should be monitored during accuracy checks. The organization of the heating/cooling circuitry of the blocks of some thermal cyclers is such that it is redundant to check each well; only a fraction of them need be checked to assess the accuracy of the entire block. This issue should be investigated with the manufacturer of your particular instrument.

2.2. Results Reporting

Because molecular tests are multistep and largely unlike others performed in hospital laboratories, each component of a test used to generate results must be reviewed before interpretation and results are entered on the hospital computer system for pathologist verification. Even those molecular tests that are kit-based and similar to enzyme immunoassay tests are prone to a hazard unlike others in the clinical laboratory, namely amplicon carryover contamination associated with PCR-based tests (*see* Section 2.5.). Procedure worksheets, initialed and dated by the technologist performing the work, are used to document and monitor the progress of every specimen in the lab through the parts of the test being done. Review by the laboratory director, lead technologist, or medical director precedes results reporting. Clerical or computational errors that may contribute to poor or unusual results are detected at this stage.

Whether results are normal or abnormal should be periodically tabulated. Percent normal vs abnormal data should be available for all tests performed in accordance with a specific question on the CAP molecular pathology inspection checklist. With the checklist in hand, proper decisions can be made about how to organize the lab for appropriate quality assurance and quality control. National Committee for Clinical Laboratory Standards (NCCLS; Villanova, PA, 610-525-2435) guidelines are also available to guide new labs. NCCLS subcommittees have developed testing guidelines for molecular hematology-oncology, molecular microbiology, and molecular genetics.

2.3. Test Controls

Obviously, all test results must be controlled. There are multiple facets of molecular tests for which a positive and negative control must be included. The Southern blot-based B/T cell gene rearrangement test for lymphoproliferative disease genotyping should include a negative control for rearrangement (usually placental DNA), a positive control for hybridization (usually placental DNA), a positive control for rearrangement (DNA from a leukemic or lymphomatous patient or an appropriate cell line), a sensitivity control, and mol-wt markers (2). The aforementioned controls are for the detection portion of this test only. Multiple steps are involved in Southern blotting before one even reaches the detection portion of the test. Suitable controls and checkpoints must be and are "built in" to the DNA extraction, quantitation, restriction, electrophoresis, and transfer portions of this test (2,3).

PCR-based tests demand their own set of test controls. These include, but are not limited to, nucleic acid extraction controls, external (amplification of DNA known to contain and generate the amplicon of interest) and internal (amplification of a second target within the extracted DNA to control for the actual existence of amplifiable DNA in the sample) controls for the amplification reaction itself, restriction enzyme controls (if such analysis is part of the test), positive and negative controls for detection (regardless of the end point), and controls against contamination with extraneous amplicons from previously performed reactions *(4,5)*. When this many controls (and associated expenses) seem to become excessive and burdensome, always remember that the benchmark one is striving to achieve is the most accurate and reliable patient test result possible. Consider the financial and nonfinancial costs associated with an incorrect laboratory diagnosis.

For example, the completeness of restriction enzyme digestion must always be checked. Southern blot-based detection of the mutation that causes Fragile X syndrome has become the gold standard for this diagnosis *(6)*. Detection of the mutation responsible for Factor V_{Leiden} is a popular and useful new molecular diagnostic test for assessment of thrombotic risk *(7)*. Both of these tests depend on complete restriction enzyme digestion for an accurate result.

The genetic lesion responsible for Fragile X syndrome is detected by Southern blotting and probing the patient's DNA with a probe specific for the region of interest. Incomplete digestion with a restriction enzyme results in different sized fragments, all of which will be larger than the normal fragment. On completion of electrophoresis, these fragments will not have migrated as far as the completely digested DNA, because they are larger in mass. Without the proper control for completeness of restriction enzyme digestion, these artifactually large DNA fragments may lead to the incorrect interpretation that the patient is mosaic for the presence of Fragile X syndrome, i.e., possessing heterogeneous populations of cells all with varying degrees of the CGG amplification responsible for the disorder.

A molecularly based test for the detection of Factor V_{Leiden} depends on PCR amplification of a 267-bp region of interest in the gene for Factor V. This is the region that contains the specific missense mutation responsible for functional resistance to activated protein C (APC) leading to familial or recurring venous thrombosis. The missense mutation destroys one of two *Mnl*I restriction enzyme recognition sites in the amplicon. PCR is followed by digestion of the amplicon with the restriction enzyme, *Mnl*I. The 267-bp amplicon of normal individuals is converted by *Mnl*I digestion to 163-, 67-, and 37-bp bands (usually only the 163-bp band is used in the interpretation, although visualization of the smaller bands is relevant). Homozygous mutants have one site resistant to *Mnl*I digestion and display bands of 200 and 67 bp after gel electrophoresis. Heterozygotes show both the 200- and the 163-bp bands (and the smaller bands). The interpretation is straightforward, since one need only observe what combination of 163- and 200-bp bands is visible to determine if the patient is homozygous wild-type, heterozygous, or homozygous mutant. It is imperative to include a known heterozygote and a known normal DNA as controls for complete *Mnl*I digestion. It could also be argued that inclusion of a known homozygous mutant is prudent. If *Mnl*I digestion is incomplete, a homozygous wild-type individual could be misdiagnosed as heterozygous or homozygous mutant. Proper controls for complete *Mnl*I digestion guard against misinterpretation of a result in this test.

Prior to Southern blot-based testing, several hundred nanograms of restricted DNA should be electrophoresed in a so-called test gel to check for complete restriction. Larger-scale electrophoresis for Southern blotting may proceed if inspection of the test gel shows the familiar broad smear of restricted DNA indicative of complete digestion. Sometimes the test gel shows that continued digestion is necessary. When DNA yield is low or when a sample is precious, as is the case with most patient DNAs, the test gel pays important dividends. Time invested in a test gel for complete restriction enzyme digestion eliminates the need to set up a new test because the DNA did not digest properly. If the test gel shows that digestion was incomplete, only 500 ng have been used. Not using a test gel means one is gambling all the DNA one has committed to restriction has been completely cut. If the DNA was not cut, this would only be known after the DNA was electrophoresed in the analytical gel that is to be used for Southern transfer. One would then be faced with the difficult choice of aborting the test or attempting to purify the uncut DNA from the agarose gel. Test gel controls include an abundant DNA that has repeatedly been cut successfully by the relevant enzyme(s). Molecular-weight markers should also be included as a size reference in determining that a full array of DNA fragments has been generated *(3)*.

Reasons why DNA restriction may have failed or be only partially successful include omission of enzyme or buffer, or incorrect assembly of the reaction. The reaction may have been incubated at the wrong temperature (this shows the importance of periodic calibration of all temperature-dependent devices with an appropriate thermometer). Inhibitors may be present in the DNA that were not eliminated by the DNA extraction procedure being used. Finally, lack of restriction enzyme digestion of DNA may show that an older or often-used batch of enzyme may have finally lost its effectiveness *(3)*.

Even before DNA restriction is begun, DNA quality must be assessed. If DNA is not of good purity and high molecular weight, it may not yield satisfactory Southern blot results. Extracted DNAs should first be subjected to a "QC mini-gel" used to assess DNA quality. DNAs not meeting defined criteria are not subjected to further analysis, the test is aborted, and the appropriate actions taken, e.g., investigation into reasons why this may have happened and notification of the relevant physician(s) to offer the option of recollecting the specimens. Degraded DNA samples lack high-mol-wt components and appear as smears on ethidium bromide staining of agarose gels that have undergone electrophoresis. Some subjectivity is unavoidable in deciding if a particular DNA specimen has suffered too much degradation and is inappropriate for Southern blot-based testing. PCR-based tests are more forgiving of partially degraded DNAs, because there still may be enough target DNA of sufficient length for successful PCR.

Corroboration of the ability of PCR to amplify target DNA in a given patient specimen verifies that a negative result is a true negative and not a false negative resulting from the presence of a PCR inhibitor in that specimen. Options to perform this kind of quality control include coamplifying a constitutively expressed gene or coamplifying exogenously added nucleic acid, i.e., "spiking," along with the target of interest. This is a point specifically addressed in the CAP molecular pathology inspection checklist.

2.4. Using Biology for Quality Control

The *bcl*-2 (B cell leukemia and lymphoma-2) proto-oncogene becomes juxtaposed to the immunoglobulin heavy-chain (IgH) locus on chromosome 14 during the chromosomal translocation, t(14;18)(q32;q21). *bcl*-2 gene rearrangement is a hallmark of follicular lymphomas, since it is present in over 80% of them. This rearrangement is also associated with other lymphoid malignancies *(8)*.

For purposes of QC, one can exploit the fact that *bcl*-2 is juxtaposed to the IgH gene as a result of the translocation described. Often, *bcl*-2 and B/T cell gene rearrangement analysis are ordered simultaneously. Use of a *bcl*-2 gene probe and a probe directed against the immunoglobulin heavy-chain gene locus usually, but not always, detects identically sized fragments, when DNA is digested with the same enzyme *(8)*. Questions about band size and identity of true rearrangement bands may be resolvable by using this convenient "built-in" checkpoint.

Indirect linkage analysis for detection of mutations that may result in genetic disease is a powerful, technique. The accuracy of results is dependent on many factors, some of which are outside the control of the laboratory. It is important to note that nonpaternity within a family pedigree can adversely affect accuracy of results. Paternity testing may be considered as an important adjunct to linkage analysis for genetic disease.

Fragile X syndrome is caused by abnormal amplification of a CGG trinucleotide on the X chromosome such that affected individuals have many more than the up to 52 repeats of this trinucleotide than normal individuals have. There is a zone between normal and affected, and there is some overlap in this zone on the high end, i.e., between affected and transmitter. Ordinarily individuals in this zone are said to be transmitters or carriers of the mutation that can then be passed on to subsequent generations and manifested as the syndrome. However, the number of CGG repeats in carriers may extend into the low end of the number considered to be affected. Also, the number of repeats in an affected individual may be low enough to consider that individual as a carrier. Methylation status is used to differentiate between these possibilities. Thus, those affected with Fragile X syndrome have their affected *FMR*-1 gene hypermethylated, such that it is not expressed. The *FMR*-1 gene in those who are truly carriers is hypomethylated and is expressed. One can use methylation-sensitive restriction enzymes in Southern blot-based analysis for fragile X syndrome to determine the methylation status of *FMR*-1. One indirect benefit of this analysis is that it is gender-specific. Females have an inactivated X chromosome in their cells, and the genes on this inactive chromosome are unexpressed and hypermethylated; males have no inactive X chromosome. A distinctive male or female pattern is observed on performing this kind of analysis and can be used to check specimens against patients to help guard against specimen mix-up. For example, if during Southern blot-based Fragile X syndrome analysis, John's DNA shows the typical female pattern (on digestion with the appropriate methylation-sensitive restriction enzyme) and/or Mary shows the typical male pattern, one should consider that a specimen mix-up may have taken place. Similarly, for Fragile X syndrome analysis and for other genetic disease analysis, when gender is relevant to the information that is being gleaned from the test and passed on to patients, parents, physicians, and genetics counselors, laboratorians may appropriately consider the use of a Y chromosome-specific probe as an adjunct to determine accurately the sex of the patient who contributed the DNA for the test.

Inherited X-linked disorders can have dramatic effects in male offspring. One indirect method of prenatal diagnosis for these disorders begins with in vitro fertilization followed by removal of a single cell from several or all preimplantation embryos. Gender determination by PCR-based detection of male-specific sequences on the Y chromosome may be performed on all the embryos. In this way, male embryos, and the inherited X-linked disorder, may be avoided, and only female embryos are implanted. With respect to QC, it is advisable to involve only female laboratory workers in the PCR aspects of such work. Male workers who inadvertently contaminate samples with a single skin cell, for example, create the possibility of invalidating the assay's negative control. Worse, such contamination may lead to the artifactually incorrect laboratory finding that all the preimplantation embryos are male and therefore inappropriate for implantation.

2.5. Amplicon Carryover

PCR and/or other amplification technologies are exquisitely sensitive techniques. Poor attention to detail by technologists and/or sloppy conditions will eventually create a situation in which carryover amplified product (amplicons) contaminate some portion of the laboratory. Contaminating amplicons making their way into new PCR reactions act as suitable amplification substrates, thereby generating false-positive results. Laboratories must be constantly diligent to avoid the possibility of contamination.

The reagent preparation area for amplification technologies is the area that must be kept the most pristine, such that all possibility of amplicon contamination is avoided. Ideally, this is a separate room with positive air pressure (air flows out of and not into this room). What one is striving to avoid in this area is the introduction of amplified products from other areas of the lab. Patient specimens and extracted DNA should also never enter the reagent preparation area since their contamination of reagents can also lead to false-positive results, although on stochastic grounds, this is less likely to occur than contamination by the vast quantities of amplicons generated by a PCR reaction. A separate room for reagent preparation may be impractical or impossible, so one may use a hood or an enclosed benchtop box (a.k.a. "dead box") with a UV light source turned on when the area is not in use. Contaminating amplicons or DNA entering the reagent preparation area through a careless hand or an air current are sterilized by the UV light through the creation of thymine dimers that make the DNA unsuitable as a substrate in amplification reactions. The reagent preparation area should have dedicated equipment; nothing should be returned to this area once it has left.

Separate the specimen preparation area from the area where PCR reactions are constructed. Thus, aerosolized patient nucleic acid cannot contaminate subsequently constructed PCR reaction tubes, thereby generating false-positive results. Use dedicated equipment for each area. Before PCR reaction construction, wipe down lab benches and pipeters with 10% bleach and then 70% ethanol to do away with any contaminating DNA molecules that may be present.

When all reagents have been added, PCR reaction tubes should be capped before being brought to the thermal cycler. When PCR is completed, capped tubes should be brought to the area where the results of the reaction are analyzed. This "dirtiest" area of the laboratory is the one where sloppy technique will ultimately generate false-positive results in subsequent reactions. The opening of post-PCR tubes generates aerosols that may contain millions of copies of a specific amplicon *(9)*. Consider using gauze pads to open post-PCR reaction tubes gently so that aerosols are absorbed by the pads and may be discarded. It is best if this area is a separate room not vented back to other areas of the PCR laboratory. Again, equipment (including labcoats) in this area should be dedicated. In all areas, it is best to use positive-displacement pipeters, or air-displacement pipeters with specially plugged, and aerosol-resistant PCR tips, i.e., hydrophobic microporous filters where the filter is bonded onto the walls of the pipet tip. Frequent changing of gloves in the PCR analysis area is indicated, as are disposable gowns, masks, and caps. Sticky floor mats help reduce the possibility of amplicons moving into clean areas of the laboratory on the soles of shoes.

Chemical sterilization methods exist and should be employed when possible, but should not be thought of as a "crutch" that eliminates the need for cleanliness and scrupulous technique. Isopsoralens included in PCR reactions intercalate in double-stranded DNA, crosslinking the strands on activation with UV light. Such DNA is an unsuitable substrate in PCR, because strand dissociation via denaturation cannot occur; such denaturation is a necessary step in PCR. However, the presence of crosslinked amplicons can still be assessed by a number of methods, including agarose gel electro-phoresis, so the assay can be completed.

Inclusion of deoxyuridine in place of thymidine in the reaction mixture does not alter amplification, gel analysis, or product hybridization. However, it does serve as the basis of an effective amplicon sterilization technique. Prior to thermal cycling, uracil-N-glycoslyase (UNG) is added to PCR components and allowed to act on its substrate; the uracil residues in any contaminating carryover DNA that may be present. Simultaneously, UNG has no effect on patient DNA (or bacterial or viral DNA if one of these is the target of investigation) that contains no uracil, but only thymidine residues. Following this sterilization reaction, UNG is heat-inactivated and PCR may proceed with the threat of false positivity owing to contamination removed *(4,10)*.

3. CONCLUSION

Molecular pathology is the newest discipline in the hospital pathology laboratory. We are still on something of a "learning curve" with respect to implementation of molecular pathology tests. Indeed, these tests are in a state of flux as different tech-nologies vie to become the methodology of choice. Only a few years ago, Southern blotting and the related slot/dot-blot technology dominated the field. These are labori-ous, multistep tests that demand high levels of QC to generate accurate results. In the early part of this decade, PCR had already made strong inroads into the field and now in the middle of the decade has come to dominate it. PCR is faster, easier, and less expensive to perform than Southern blot technology, but is fraught with its own set of QC issues, ranging from reaction optimization to carryover contamination control. Now, as the new century approaches, new in vitro nucleic acid amplification tech-niques like transcription-mediated amplification, LCR, nucleic acid sequence-based amplification (NASBA®), and others, such as bDNA amplification, are poised to cap-ture market share from PCR-based techniques, not strictly because the companies mar-keting them are superior marketers, but to a large degree because of availability in kit form, ease of use, FDA approval, and so on *(11)*. Finally, many companies are working to bring the cost of sequencing to a point at which it is affordable in the routine clinical laboratory. Arguably, sequencing is the gold standard for most molecular based diagnostics and will be a great benefit in the diagnostics laboratorian's armamentarium. Issues specific to QC for sequencing will have to be addressed before this methodology takes hold in the laboratory. This is truly a developing field and may appropriately be considered a "work in progress."

REFERENCES

1. Farkas, D. H. Establishing a clinical molecular biology laboratory, in *Molecular Biology and Pathology: A Guidebook for Quality Control*, Farkas, D. H., ed., Academic, San Diego, CA, pp. 15–16, 1993.
2. Farkas, D. H. Quality control of the B/T cell gene rearrangement test, in *Molecular Biology and Pathology: A Guidebook for Quality Control*, Farkas, D. H., ed., Academic, San Diego, CA, pp. 77–101, 1993.
3. Farkas, D. H. Specimen procurement, processing, tracking, and testing by the Southern blot, in *Molecular Biology and Pathology: A Guidebook for Quality Control*, Farkas, D. H., ed., Academic, San Diego, CA, pp. 51–75, 1993.
4. Spadoro, J. P. and Dragon, E. A. Quality control of the polymerase chain reaction, in *Molecular Biology and Pathology: A Guidebook for Quality Control*, Farkas, D. H., ed., Academic, San Diego, CA, pp. 149–158, 1993.
5. Kwok, S. and Higuchi, R. Avoiding false positives with PCR. *Nature* **339**:237–238, 1989.
6. Tsongalis, G. J. and Silverman, L. M. Molecular pathology of the fragile X syndrome. *Arch. Pathol. Lab. Med.* **117**:1121–1125, 1993.
7. Liu, X.-Y, Nelson, D., Grant, C., Morthland, V., Goodnight, S. B., and Press, R. D. Molecular detection of a common mutation in coagulation factor V causing thrombosis via hereditary resistance to activated protein C. *Diagn. Mol. Pathol.* **4**:191–197, 1995.
8. Crisan, D. bcl-2 gene rearrangements in lymphoid malignancies. *Clin. Lab Med.* **16**:23–47, 1996.
9. McCreedy, B. J. Detection of viral pathogens using PCR amplification, in *Molecular Methods for Virus Detection*, Wiedbrauk, D. L. and Farkas, D. H., eds., Academic, San Diego, CA, pp. 175–191, 1995.
10. Wiedbrauk, D. L. and Stoerker, J. Quality assurance in the molecular virology laboratory, in *Molecular Methods for Virus Detection*, Wiedbrauk, D. L. and Farkas, D. H., eds., Academic, San Diego, CA, pp. 179–181, 1995.
11. Farkas, D. H. *DNA Simplified: The Hitchhiker's Guide to DNA*. American Association for Clinical Chemistry, Washington, DC, pp. 7–58, 1996.

Prospects for the Future Role
of the Clinical Laboratory

Lawrence M. Silverman

1. TRAINING, CERTIFICATION, AND QUALITY ASSURANCE

Over the past 15 years, medical sciences and, in particular, clinical laboratory sciences have witnessed a revolution in molecular diagnostics. As of October, 1995, molecular diagnostics could be categorized into:

1. Molecular genetics for inherited diseases;
2. DNA diagnostics, nucleic acid-based diagnostic tests other than molecular genetics (forensics, paternity testing, infectious diseases, transplantation, and so forth); and
3. Molecular pathology: tissue-based testing primarily involving oncology.

Certification for laboratory directors is currently provided for molecular genetics through the American Board of Medical Genetics, whereas the American Board of Pathology has proposed future certification in molecular pathology. However, the field of molecular diagnostics is evolving so rapidly that these techniques are becoming widely used tools that can be applied to virtually all areas of laboratory medicine, making certification categories less clearcut. Eventually, laboratory directors who are certified in traditional specialties (clinical chemistry, hematology, and so on) will probably be intimately involved with molecular techniques, with or without additional certification.

Training and quality assurance are much more acute issues than certification. Currently, training of laboratory personnel varies from laboratory to laboratory, creating uncertainty regarding quality assurance. External proficiency testing is in its infancy, with the College of American Pathologists and American College of Medical Genetics jointly initiating a pilot program in molecular genetics. The College of American Pathologists also includes a checklist on Molecular Pathology in their inspections of clinical laboratories. At the same time, certain commercial reference laboratories are providing molecular testing that runs counter to recommendations of scientific advisory groups. At the present time, consumers of molecular laboratory services are in a position of *caveat emptor*!

What does the future hold for molecular testing? Undoubtedly, the situation will be compounded by the increased availability of presymptomatic testing, i.e., detecting

From: Molecular Diagnostics: For the Clinical Laboratorian
Edited by: W. B. Coleman and G. J. Tsongalis Humana Press Inc., Totowa, NJ

molecular events that predispose individuals to disorders prior to the onset of symptoms (*see* Section 2.4.). Currently, an example of this type of disorder is Huntington's disease. The implications of testing for this disorder, before symptoms are present, have been the subject of numerous debates and pilot studies. This scenario will be replayed with many other disorders, such as BRCA1, associated with familial breast and ovarian cancer.

2. ETHICAL, SOCIAL, AND LEGAL ISSUES OF MOLECULAR GENETIC TESTING

DNA-based genetic testing can be applied to various clinical situations, each associated with different concerns for the clinical laboratorian. Some of these concerns are unique to the techniques being used, such as direct mutation detection vs indirect linkage analysis. Other concerns depend on the specific clinical question being addressed, such as diagnostic testing, carrier testing within families with affected probands, general population carrier testing, presymptomatic testing, and susceptibility testing.

1. DNA-based testing can be used to assist in making or confirming the diagnosis of specific disorders, such as sickle-cell anemia or cystic fibrosis (CF). In this regard, the data can be directly transmitted to the ordering physician or health care professional with the appropriate interpretive comments. A major concern is that diagnostic testing only be performed on individuals who have already met clinical criteria for the specific disorder. For example, testing for deletions associated with Duchenne or Becker muscular dystrophy would not be useful for fascioscapulohumeral or limb-girdle muscular dystrophy, and thus, should be confined to individuals whose pattern of muscle weakness and serum creatine kinase (CK) levels are consistent with these disorders. Diagnostic testing can be further complicated by disease with adult-onset symptoms (*see* item 4).

2. Carrier testing can be simplified if an affected individual within the family is available for diagnostic testing. When the causative mutation(s) is known, appropriate family members can be accurately and quickly tested. However, information within a family must be confined to those individuals who have requested testing. These data must be handled with extreme concern for confidentiality, regarding both family and nonfamily members (i.e., insurance companies or employers). When there are unknown family mutations, carrier testing can still be performed by indirect linkage analysis; however, certain limitations apply to linkage analysis, which can result in less accuracy than direct approaches.

3. The accuracy of general population carrier screening depends on the percentage of disease-causing mutations that can be detected. Furthermore, the information from such programs must be coupled with appropriate educational material and genetic counseling. A recent report by the Office of Technology Assessment (OTA) (CF Carrier Screening, OTA, US Congress, 1992) identifies factors that will affect carrier testing in the general population and should be mandatory reading for anyone engaging in this area of testing.

4. Presymptomatic testing refers to those adult-onset disorders in which testing can identify affected individuals prior to the onset of symptoms. As one can imagine, the impact of this information, particularly for fatal disorders or those that cause severe limitations, can have psychological, economic, and legal implications. Thus, it is imperative that DNA-based genetic testing be ordered appropriately, after educational, psychological, and genetic counseling. Similarly, data must be only transferred to the appropriate health care professional, **never** directly to the patient. An example of an adult-onset disorder in which presymptomatic testing is available is Huntington's disease.

5. A relatively new category of DNA-based testing pertains to detecting mutations that may give rise to certain disorders, particularly cancer, over a life-time. Breast and ovarian cancer, as well as certain types of colon cancer, can cluster within families, usually exhibiting an autosomal dominant form of inheritance. Risk estimates are associated both with individuals who test positively and those who test negatively for causative mutations. However, the implications of these risk estimates must be transmitted to patients by experienced health care professionals, not by laboratory personnel.

There are many other social, ethical, and legal issues that must be addressed before other DNA-based genetic tests are offered on a large scale. Currently, issues have arisen pertaining to the use of archived human tissue for research and development activities. Generally, this material remains after ordered tests have been performed. Most institutions provide a general informed consent, which allows excess tissues to be used for research. However, ethicists argue that these forms are not sufficient and that specific consent forms must be generated each time a new research project is initiated using archived samples. Naturally, this creates concern among scientists who are already following proscribed procedures to ensure patient anonymity. Ethicists argue that these safeguards are not sufficient. Many other specific issues pertain to DNA-based forensic and paternity tests, which are currently being addressed by appropriate specialty groups. Readers are directed to the series of position statements issued on genetic testing by the American Society for Human Genetics published periodically in the *American Journal of Human Genetics*.

3. AUTOMATION AND NEW TECHNOLOGIES

A major limitation on availability of molecular testing is the lack of affordable kits and/or automation. Several promising technologies have failed to make CF testing cost-effective for routine labs, although certain testing strategies are successfully used by commercial labs. Nevertheless, the dearth of high-quality kits and high-throughput instrumentation is the greatest hindrance to availability. A ray of hope comes from the recent FDA approval of Roche Molecular Systems Amplicor chlamydia and HLA kits, whereas hepatitis C kits are available in Europe. As more kits enter the marketplace, more labs will be able to justify high volume molecular tests. However, automation and kit development have been limited, to a large extent, by legal restraints associated with amplification technologies.

An attractive approach for mutations analysis and identity testing is the use of reverse dot blots or slot blots, also developed by Roche Molecular Systems (Alameda, CA). The key feature of this is a membrane-bound oligonucleotide, which is specific for sequence of the gene to be analyzed, for example, CFTR. After the sample is amplified by PCR, the product is hybridized to the membrane, with biotin attached to the PCR primers. Streptavidin-horseradish peroxidase then forms the basis on the color reaction that identifies specific sequences in the sample. Thus, through the use of multiplex PCR, multiple regions of a gene are analyzed for specific mutations. This approach is currently being tested for general use for CF mutations analysis, and is available for genotyping the HLA-DQA1 locus for identity testing.

A bright spot on the horizon is the continued development of exciting new technologies that expand the molecular testing armamentarium. I would like to highlight several of the most promising developments.

3.1. The Protein Truncation Assay

Although many new technologies are residues of basic research, very few become useful in clinical settings. An exception is the Protein Truncation Assay (PTA), which is now used for screening mutations that lead to premature truncation of proteins, especially those having tumor suppressor activity. The basis of this assay is a report by Sarkar and Sommer (1989, *Science* **244**:331–334) which describes the use of RNA sequence and its protein product to screen for mutations leading to premature truncation. In rapid succession, papers appeared using this technique to screen dystrophin, NF1, APC, and BRCA1 (the latter three code for tumor suppressors). The detection rates vary from gene to gene, but average between 70 and 80%, significantly better than any single molecular test. Until labs have more experience with this technique, positive results (i.e., the appearance of a truncated protein) should be confirmed, preferably by genomic DNA sequence. A major drawback to this technique is the use of RNA as starting material, since most laboratories tend to archive DNA rather than RNA. RNA is generally used since RT-PCR reverse-transcribes RNA to cDNA, which contains continuous coding regions (exons) without intervening sequence (introns). There are some genes that contain large exons, which can be screened using genomic DNA rather than RNA. An example of this is exon 11 of BRCA1, which contains approx 60% of the entire coding region. Moreover, transformed lymphoblastoid cell lines are convenient sources of both DNA and RNA. As more tumor suppressor genes are identified, this technique will become more popular. Efforts are under way to both automate the assay and formulate PTA kits.

The BRCA1 protein is thought to act as a tumor suppressor; yet germline mutations in this gene account for only ~5% of all cases of breast cancer that are limited to those families with multiple cases of breast and ovarian. The more common form of breast cancer is sporadic; however, the BRCA1 gene is rarely mutated in tumors removed from sporadic breast cancer patients. This disparity has led researchers to look for other genes that might be involved in sporadic breast cancer, or other abnormalities of BRCA1 structure or function. Evidence shows that at least one other gene is involved in familial breast cancer, named BRCA2, which is linked to chromosome 13 (BRCA1 is linked to chromosome 17). However, BRCA2 accounts for fewer cases of familial breast cancer than BRCA1, and virtually none of the sporadic cases. However, researchers now believe that the BRCA1 protein does not function normally in the majority of sporadic cases. Data show that the BRCA1 protein, which normally is transported to and functions in the nucleus, remains in the cytoplasm to a large extent in sporadic breast cancer.

3.2. Combination of Molecular Markers and Protein Assays

In the near future, patients with breast cancer will probably be assessed using a combination of molecular markers in a tiered-testing format. For example, BRCA1, as discussed above, will be important for individuals with a history of early onset breast and/or ovarian cancer in their families. BRCA1 mutations will be detected by a series of techniques, depending on several factors, including ethnicity. For example, two mutations (185 del AG and 188 del 11) account for ~33% of all familial breast/ovarian cancer in Ashkenazi Jews. For these mutations, simple, inexpensive direct mutation analysis can be performed. Similarly, other more expensive techniques, such as PTA (*see* Section 3.1.) can be reserved for families who are either negative for direct mutational analysis or are not part of an ethnic group with recognized, common mutations. In this fashion, testing can be performed efficiently and at the lowest cost.

Additionally, other markers associated with breast cancer include p53 and the ataxia telangectasia (AT) gene. In the latter case, individuals heterozygous for truncating mutations in the AT gene have been reported to be at a significantly increased risk for developing breast cancer. In the case of p53, those patients whose tumors are positive for p53 mutations have a significantly poorer prognosis than those without p53 mutations.

It is conceivable to picture the following scenario involving:

1. Genomic DNA and RNA screening for mutations in BRCA1 (and possibly BRCA2) for families with early onset breast/ovarian cancer;
2. RNA screening for truncating mutations in AT to detect individuals with increased susceptibility to environmental risk factors, i.e., radiation;
3. Tissue screening for p53 mutations to determine prognosis; and
4. Tissue screening for BRCA1 protein localization.

This type of tiered-testing pattern emphasizes the need to integrate molecular techniques involving DNA, RNA, protein analysis, and immunohistochemistry to maximize information at an affordable price.

3.3. Molecular Diagnosis of Blood Group Incompatibilities

Another exciting area is the use of molecular techniques to genotype various components of the Rh blood group (D, C, E, and so on). Approximately 1/1000 live births have some form of sensitization, which can be demonstrated prenatally by conventional serological testing if fetal blood is obtained by fetoscopy, which is associated with increased fetal risks. However, molecular determination of Rh genotypes can be performed by DNA amplification of cultured amniocytes. Caution must be taken, however, to avoid misidentification of the fetal genotype owing to maternal contamination. The possibility of misidentification is reduced by culturing since fetal cells, rather than maternal cells, are selected by special culturing conditions. Additionally, paternal genotyping can reduce the risk of misidentification.

3.4. "DNA on a Chip"

Several recent developments involve the use of silicon-glass chips to serve as a platform for either amplification (PCRChips) or nucleic acid hybridization. Both approaches use microsamples and exploit the miniaturization that results from micromachining developed for computer chip production. One scenario involves attaching oligonucleotides to a chip in a 1028 × 1028 array based on selected sequence variations, so that sample DNA will only hybridize, under specific conditions, to complementary oligonucleotides. Following a subsequent signal-generating step, this approach could make large-scale sequencing more efficient or detect mutations in specific disorders characterized by extreme allelic heterogeneity, such as CF.

4. CONCLUSION

In the preceding chapters, each author has addressed the latest developments in his/ her specific area of expertise. In addressing the future prospects for the clinical laboratory, I have also mentioned recent developments, some of which are already making an impact, and others that may do so in the near future. Unfortunately, by the time this book is published, most of these predictions (including mine) will be challenged by newer technological developments and increased understanding of disease mechanisms. That is the nature of this field—a never-ending saga of scientific breakthroughs, significant contributions from the biotechnology industry (and occasional hindrances), ethical dilemmas, and ultimately, promises of a brave, new world. What we have learned from the last 15 years, however, is that many of the promises, unfortunately, go unfulfilled.

Index

A

Abetalipoproteinemia, genetics, 278
Achondroplasia, genetics, 253
ACTH insensitivity, genetics, 257
Adeno-associated virus,
  genome, 205
  life cycle, 205
  mediation of gene transfer, 205, 206
Adenosine, structure, 17, 18
Adenosine deaminase, gene therapy of
    deficiency, 208
Adenovirus,
  gene therapy,
    E1A replacement in vector, 204,
      205
    gene size capacity, 205
    helper cells, 205
    longevity of vector, 205
  gene transfer by conjugation, 200
  genome, 203, 204
A DNA, structure, 17, 19
Agarose gel electrophoresis,
  DNA,
    extraction, 44
    quantitation, 44, 45
    resolution, 66
  factors affecting migration rate, 130
  matrix properties, 131, 132
  northern blotting, 76, 78
  pH, 131
  principle, 65, 66, 130, 131
  reverse-transcription polymerase
    chain reaction products, 112,
    113
  size standards, 67, 68, 134
  Southern blotting, 66–68
  staining, 68
Aldosterone synthetase deficiency,
    genetics, 258
Anatomy, history, 7
Androgen resistance, genetics, 259
Antibiotic resistance, detection,
  aminoglycosides, 353
  β-lactams, 352, 353

  rifampin, 353
  vancomycin, 353, 354
APC,
  multiplex polymerase chain reaction,
    153
  protein truncation test, 153–155
Apo A-I,
  deficiency, 280
  gene, 280
  polymorphism, 280
Apo B, gene, 277
Apo B-100, familial defective disorder,
    279
Apo C-II abnormality, genetics, 261, 276
Apo E,
  deficiency, 282
  polymorphism, 281, 282
Arterial thrombotic disease, risk factors,
    284–286
AT, *see* Ataxia telengiectasia
AT-III,
  deficiency, 287
  polymorphism, 286, 287
Ataxia telengiectasia (AT),
  clinical manifestations, 237
  diagnosis, 238
  genetics, 238, 303, 304
  incidence, 237, 303
  malignancy association, 237, 238
Autoradiography, blot interpretation,
    72, 73, 78, 79
Autosomal-dominant disorders,
    heredity, 222, 223

B

B-cell,
  arrest in neoplasia, 321
  clonality determination,
    polymerase chain reaction, 319,
      327–329, 337
    Southern blot, 319, 323–325, 327
  development,
    differentiation, 319, 321
    markers, 319, 320

immunoglobulin gene
      rearrangement, 322, 323
B DNA, structure, 17, 19
Birth defects, prevalence, 193, 219
Blood,
    blood group incompatibilty
          diagnosis, 377
    cancer, *see* Lymphoma
    history of diagnostic testing, 8–11
Bloom's syndrome, genetics, 303, 304
BRCA1, mutations and cancer, 301, 302,
    376
Breast cancer,
    clinical outcome prediction, 309
    heredity, 301, 302
    markers, 376, 377

C
Cancer, *see also specific cancers*; Tumor
    cell-cycle regulation, 297
    clinical outcome prediction, 307–309
    early detection,
          colorectal cancer, 305, 306
          genetic test design, 305
          importance, 293, 304, 305
          lung cancer, 306
          pancreas cancer, 307
    genes associated with cancer, 296–299
    multistep carcinogenesis, 293–298
    screening, 309, 310
Cardiovascular disease (CVD), *see also*
      specific diseases
    genetics, 271–274
    multifactorial etiology, 271, 272
    risk factors for coronary artery
          disease, 271, 272
CETP, *see* Cholesterol ester transfer
      protein
CF, *see* Cystic fibrosis
Charcot-Marie-Tooth disease (CMT),
    clinical manifestations, 238
    diagnosis, 239, 240
    genetics, 239
    types, 238
Chlamydia pneumoniae, diagnosis of
      infection, 346, 347
Chlamydia trachomatis, diagnosis of
      infection, 349, 350
Cholesterol ester transfer protein
      (CETP), deficiency, 281
Chromosome,

aberrations,
    detection, 30
    types, 29, 219
pathogen analysis, 354
Cloning,
    blunt ends, 53, 54
    cohesive ends, 53
    defined, 50
    DNA ligation, 51, 52
    libraries,
          applications, 55
          complementary DNA libraries, 54,
                55
          genomic libraries, 54
          screening, 54
    modification of DNA fragments, 52,
          53
    restriction enzymes, 51
Clostridium difficile, diagnosis of
      infection, 351, 352
CMT, *see* Charcot-Marie-Tooth disease
Coagulation pathway, 283, 284
Colorectal cancer,
    clinical outcome prediction, 308
    development and progression, 297, 298
    early detection, 305, 306
    hereditary cancers, 300, 301
Competitive oligonucleotide priming
      (COP),
    primers, 151, 152
    principle, 150, 151
COP, *see* Competitive oligonucleotide
      priming
CVD, *see* Cardiovascular disease
Cystic fibrosis (CF),
    allele-specific polymerase chain
          reaction, 150
    gene therapy, 209
    multiplex polymerase chain reaction
          analysis, 153
    mutation screening by reverse dot
          blotting, 129
    restriction fragment length
          polymorphism analysis, 144, 146
    symptomatic treatment, 193
Cytosine, structure, 17, 18

D
Denaturing gradient gel electrophoresis
      (DGGE),
    computer modeling, 139

GC clamp, 140
interpretation of gels, 139
principle, 137–139
sensitivity, 141
Dentatorubral-pallidoluysian atrophy
    (DRPLA),
    diagnosis, 233–235
    features, 231
    molecular mechanisms, 233
    parental transmission bias, 232, 233
    trinucleotide repeat instability, 231,
        232
DGGE, *see* Denaturing gradient gel
    electrophoresis
Diabetes insipidus,
    familial hypothalamic disease, 250
    familial nephrogenic disease, 250
Diabetes mellitus,
    glycogen synthetase deficiency, 262
    history of diagnostic testing, 8, 10, 11
    hypoglycemia of infancy, 263
    insulin,
        mutations, 263
        receptor abnormalities, 262
    maturity-onset diabetes of the young,
        262
    mitochondrial DNA abnormality, 262
    types, 262
Diagnostic laboratory,
    economics, 4, 5, 12
    genetic disease diagnosis, 227
    history of development, 7–11
    logistics, 4
    organization, 4
    staff, 3
    training and certification, 373
DM, *see* Myotonic dystrophy
DMD, *see* Duchenne muscular
    dystrophy
DNA, *see also* Southern blot
    base pairing, 17
    branched DNA detection,
        pathogens, 342
        polymerase chain reaction, 97, 99,
            100
    cloning, *see* Cloning
    damage and mutation, 29–31
    extraction,
        agarose gels, 44
        pathogen diagnosis, 345, 346
    genetic code, 20, 21

genomic organization,
    eukaryotes, 20, 36
    plasmids, 37, 42
    prokaryotes, 35, 36
    viruses, 36, 37
isolation,
    eukaryotic genomic DNA,
        automation, 40
        blood, 40
        cell lysis, 39
        considerations in protocol
            selection, 37
        cultured cells, 40
        forensic samples, 41
        guanidium isothiocyanate
            extraction, 39, 40
        organic extraction, 38, 39
        preserved tissue, 41
        proteinase K treatment, 37–39
        pulsed-field gel electrophoresis,
            41
        RNA degradation, 38, 39
        tissue, 40, 41
    plasmid DNA, 42–44
    viral DNA, 41
point mutations, 30, 31, 220
quantitation,
    absorption, 44
    dot blot, 45
    gel electrophoresis, 44, 45
recombination, 22
repair, 22, 29, 297, 303, 304
replication, 22
sequencing methods,
    automation, 58
    chain termination, 56, 57
    chemical cleavage, 55, 56
    clinical application, 123
silicon chip platforms, 377
structure, 16, 17, 19
DNA polymerase I, *see* Klenow
    fragment
Dot blot,
    DNA quantitation, 45
    reverse dot blot and mutation
        detection, 128–130, 375
Dropsy, history of diagnostic testing, 8
DRPLA, *see* Dentatorubral-
    pallidoluysian atrophy
Duchenne muscular dystrophy (DMD),
    clinical manifestations, 240

diagnosis, 240–242
genetics, 240
Dystrophin gene,
multiplex polymerase chain reaction
analysis, 152
protein truncation test, 153, 155

E
Electrophoresis, *see* Agarose gel
electrophoresis; Polyacrylamide
gel electrophoresis
Enhancer,
inducibility, 195
mechanism of action, 195
promoter matching, 194, 195
tissue specificity, 195, 196
Escherichia coli O157, H7, detection, 352
Estrogen resistance, genetics, 259
Ethics, molecular genetic testing, 374, 375
Ethidium bromide, DNA staining in
gels, 45

F
Factor V,
mutation in venous thrombosis, 289
quality control in assay, 366
Factor VII, polymorphism and arterial
thrombotic disease, 286
Familial adenomatus polyposis (FAP),
diagnosis, 306
genetics, 300, 301, 306
Familial combined hyperlipidemia
(FCH), genetics, 276, 277
Familial dyslipidemia, genetics, 261
Familial hyperapobetalipoproteinemia
(FHB), features, 278
Familial hypercholesterolemia (FH),
genetics, 260, 261, 278
Familial hypertriglyceridemia (FHTG),
genetics, 276, 277
Familial hypoalphalipoproteinemia,
features, 280, 281
Familial hypobetalipoproteinemia,
genetics, 279
Familial hypocalciuric hypercalcemia
(FHH), features, 255
Familial hypoparathyroidism, features,
255
FAP, *see* Familial adenomatus polyposis
FCH, *see* Familial combined
hyperlipidemia

FH, *see* Familial hypercholesterolemia
FHB, *see* Familial
hyperapobetalipoproteinemia
FHH, *see* Familial hypocalciuric
hypercalcemia
FHTG, *see* Familial
hypertriglyceridemia
Fibrinogen, polymorphism and arterial
thrombotic disease, 284, 285
FISH, *see* Fluorescence *in situ*
hybridization
Fluorescence *in situ* hybridization
(FISH),
chromosomal abnormalities,
cytogenetic analysis,
applications,
genetic disease diagnosis, 164,
171, 172
tumor pathology, 164, 170, 171
fluorescence microscopy and
imaging, 170
limitations, 172
probes,
hybridization, 168, 170
labeling, 167
types, 165
steps, 154–165
leukemia analysis, 170, 335
principle, 163, 164
Fragile X syndrome (FRAXA),
diagnosis, 233–235
features, 229
genotype and phenotype correlation,
232
molecular mechanisms, 233
parental transmission bias, 232, 233
quality control in assay, 366, 368
trinucleotide repeat instability, 231, 232
FRAXA, *see* Fragile X syndrome

G
Generalized thyroid hormone resistance
(GTHR),
clinical manifestations, 253
genetics, 254
Gene therapy,
cancer approaches, 209, 210
cystic fibrosis, 209
enhancers, 194–196
expression vector localization by *in
situ* hybridization, 178, 179

gene transfer,
adeno-associated virus-mediated gene transfer, 205, 206
adenovirus-mediated gene transfer, 203–205
assays, 196, 197
direct injection, 197, 198
ex vivo versus in vivo transfer, 197
hepatitis delta virus, 206, 207
herpesvirus, 206, 207
liposome-mediated gene transfer, 198
molecular conjugation, 199, 200
retrovirus-mediated gene transfer, 200–203
infectious disease, 210
promoters, 194–196
replacement therapy, 193, 194
severe combined immunodeficiency, 208
transgene expression,
assay, 196, 197
detection by *in situ* amplification, 185, 186
factors influencing, 196
vaccination, 211
Genome,
DNA libraries, 54
junk DNA, 218
organization,
eukaryotes, 20, 36
humans, 217, 218
plasmids, 37, 42
prokaryotes, 35, 36
viruses, 36, 37
Glucocorticoid,
resistance, 258
suppressible aldosteronism, 258
Growth hormone,
African Pigmy short stature, 252
familial isolated disease, 251
Pit-1 deficiency disorder, 251
pituitary tumor secretion, 252
resistance syndrome, 252
GTHR, *see* Generalized thyroid hormone resistance
Guanidium isothiocyanate, extraction of nucleic acids, 39, 40, 105
Guanosine, structure, 17, 18

H
HA, *see* Heteroduplex analysis
HD, *see* Huntington disease

Hepatic lipase, deficiency, 276
Hepatitis C virus, diagnosis of infection, 350, 351
Hepatitis D virus, mediation of gene transfer, 206, 207
Heredity,
autosomal-dominant disorders, 222, 223
autosomal-recessive disorders, 222, 223
genetic imprinting, 223, 224
Mendelian laws, 222, 223
uniparental disomy, 223
unstable mutations, 223
X-linked disorders, 224–226
Hereditary neuropathy with liability to pressure palsies (HNPP), genetics and diagnosis, 239, 240
Herpes simplex virus encephalitis (HSVE), diagnosis, 348
Herpesvirus, mediation of gene transfer, 206, 207
Heteroduplex analysis (HA),
gel electrophoresis, 136, 137
principle, 136
sensitivity, 137
HIV, *see* Human immunodeficiency virus
HNPP, *see* Hereditary neuropathy with liability to pressure palsies
Hodgkin's lymphoma, *see also* Lymphoma
diagnosis, 331, 332
minimal residue disease detection, 335, 336
treatment, 331
HPV, *see* Human papillomavirus
HSVE, *see* Herpes simplex virus encephalitis
Human immunodeficiency virus (HIV),
diagnosis of infection, 184, 350
gene therapy, 210
Human papillomavirus (HPV), infection detection by *in situ* amplification, 184, 185
Huntington disease (HD),
diagnosis, 233, 234
features, 231
genotype and phenotype correlation, 232
molecular mechanisms, 233

parental transmission bias, 232, 233
trinucleotide repeat instability, 231, 232
11β-Hydroxylase deficiency, genetics, 257
21-Hydroxylase deficiency, genetics, 257
Hypergonadotropic ovarian dysgenesis, genetics, 259
Hyperparathyroidism, causes, 254, 255

I
Imprinting, heredity, 223, 224
In situ hybridization (ISH), *see also* Fluorescence *in situ* hybridization
    applications,
        expression vector localization for gene therapy, 178, 179
        tumor gene expression, 177, 178
        viral DNA detection, 177, 179, 180
    controls, 176
    messenger RNA detection, 172
    principle, 163, 164
    probes,
        hybridization reaction, 175, 176
        labeling, 174, 175
        types, 174
    sensitivity, 179, 180
    steps, 172, 173
    tissue preparation,
        embedding, 173
        fixation, 173
        protease treatment, 173, 174
In situ polymerase chain reaction,
    applications,
        transgene detection in gene therapy, 185, 186
        tumor gene expression, 185
        viral infection detection, 184, 185
    controls, 183, 184
    limitations, 186
    messenger RNA detection and controls, 182, 183
    mispriming and hot starts, 181, 182
    polymerase chain reaction conditions and optimization, 180, 181
    principle, 94, 180
    product detection, 182
    sensitivity, 163, 180
    tissue preparation, 180
Insulin, *see* Diabetes mellitus
ISH, *see In situ* hybridization

J
Jansen-type metaphyseal chondrodysplasia, features, 255

K
Kallman's syndrome,
    diagnosis, 249
    genetics, 250
Klenow fragment,
    chain termination DNA sequencing, 57
    polymerase chain reaction, 90

L
Laboratory, *see* Diagnostic laboratory
Laron's syndrome, genetics, 252
LCAT, *see* Lecithin:cholesterol acyl transferase
LDL, *see* Low-density lipoprotein
Lecithin:cholesterol acyl transferase (LCAT), deficiency, 281
Legionella pneumophila, diagnosis of infection, 346
Leukemia,
    acute myelogenous leukemia, 332
    chronic myelogenous leukemia and diagnosis by Philadelphia chromosome, 333–335
    fluorescence *in situ* hybridization analysis, 170, 335
    minimal residue disease detection, 335, 336
Li-Fraumeni syndrome, genetics, 300
Library, *see* Cloning
Liddle's syndrome,
    clinical presentation, 258
    genetics, 258, 259
Ligase chain reaction, *see* Polymerase chain reaction
Linkage analysis, diagnostic testing, 226, 242
Lipoprotein, *see also specific lipoproteins*
    components, 274
    high-density lipoprotein, familial disorders of metabolism, 279–281
    lipid disorder classification, 275
    low-density lipoprotein,
        familial disorders of metabolism, 277–279
        heredity of particle size, 279
    types, 274

Lipoprotein(a), familial excess, 283
Lipoprotein lipase (LPL),
  genetics of deficiency, 276
  plasma inhibitor, 276
Liposome, mediation of gene transfer,
  198
Low-density lipoprotein (LDL),
  familial disorders of metabolism,
    277–279
  heredity of particle size, 279
LPL, *see* Lipoprotein lipase
Lung cancer, early detection, 306
Lyme disease, diagnosis, 348
Lymphoma, *see also* Hodgkin's
    lymphoma; Non-Hodgkin's
    lymphoma
  cell-surface antigens in diagnosis,
    317, 318
  classification, 317
  clonality determination,
    polymerase chain reaction, 319,
      327–329
    Southern blot, 319, 323–325, 327
  minimal residue disease detection,
    335, 336

M
Male familial precocious puberty,
  genetics, 259, 260
McCune-Albright syndrome, genetics, 260
Medicine, history of diagnostic
    medicine,
  ancient history, 5-6
  current developments, 11, 12, 375–378
  early modern period, 8–11
  Reformation, 6, 7
Melanoma, heredity, 302
MEN 1, *see* Multiple endocrine
    neoplasia type 1
MEN 2, *see* Multiple endocrine
    neoplasia type 2
Mendelian laws, 222, 223
Messenger RNA (mRNA),
  functions, 23
  in situ hybridization detection, 172,
    182, 183
  isolation by oligo-dT
    chromatography, 46, 47, 105
  northern blotting, 74
  processing,
    capping of 5'-end, 24, 25

  editing, 26
  polyadenylation of 3'-end, 24, 25
  splicing, 23, 24
  size variance, 73, 74
  structure, 24–26
Mineralocorticoid excess syndrome,
    genetics, 258
Molecular biology,
  central dogma, 15, 16
  history of advances, 11, 15
mRNA, *see* Messenger RNA
Multiple endocrine neoplasia type 1
    (MEN 1), genetics, 256
Multiple endocrine neoplasia type 2
    (MEN 2),
  diagnosis, 264, 265
  genetics, 264, 265, 304
  treatment, 265, 266
Mutational analysis polymerase chain
    reaction,
  allele-specific polymerase chain
      reaction,
    gel electrophoresis, 149, 150
    primers, 149, 150
    principle, 146, 149
  chemical cleavage of mismatches, 141
  competitive oligonucleotide priming,
    primers, 151, 152
    principle, 150, 151
  denaturing gradient gel
      electrophoresis,
    computer modeling, 139
    GC clamp, 140
    interpretation of gels, 139
    principle, 137–139
    sensitivity, 141
  heteroduplex analysis,
    gel electrophoresis, 136, 137
    principle, 136
    sensitivity, 137
  hybridization,
    allele-specific oligonucleotide
        hybridization, 127, 128
    factors affecting efficiency, 124,
      125
    mechanism, 124
    rate, 125
    reverse dot blotting, 128–130
    temperature, 125, 126
  multiplex polymerase chain reaction,
    applications, 152, 153

principle, 152
principle, 94, 124
protein truncation test,
    gel interpretation, 155, 156
    principle, 153, 154
    template synthesis, 155
restriction fragment length poly-
    morphism analysis, 143, 144
ribonuclease cleavage of mismatched
    RNA:DNA duplexes,
    efficiency of cleavage, 141–143
    gel electrophoresis, 143
    nonisotopic assay, 142, 143
    principle, 141
single-strand conformational
    polymorphism,
    gel electrophoresis, 136
    principle, 134
    sensitivity, 134–136
site-directed mutagenesis, 145, 146
Mycobacterium tuberculosis, diagnosis of
    infection, 347, 348
Mycoplasma pneumoniae, diagnosis of
    infection, 347
Myocardial infarction,
    etiology, 272
    outcomes, 272, 273
Myotonic dystrophy (DM),
    diagnosis, 233, 234
    features, 231
    genotype and phenotype correlation,
        232
    molecular mechanisms, 233
    parental transmission bias, 232, 233
    trinucleotide repeat instability, 231,
        232

N
NASBA, *see* Nucleic acid sequence
    based amplification
Neurofibromatosis 1 (NF 1),
    clinical manifestations, 236, 304
    diagnosis, 237
    genetics, 236, 237, 304
    incidence, 236, 304
NF 1, *see* Neurofibromatosis 1
NHL, *see* Non-Hodgkin's lymphoma
Nitrocellulose membrane,
    northern blotting, 78
    Southern blotting,
        capillary transfer, 70

electrotransfer, 70, 71
fixing of DNA, 71
vacuum transfer, 71
Non-Hodgkin's lymphoma (NHL), *see
    also* Lymphoma
chromosomal translocations, 329–331
diagnosis by clonality determination,
    336–338
minimal residue disease detection,
    335, 336
proto-oncogenes, 329–331
Northern blot,
    agarose gel electrophoresis, 76, 78
    applications, 73, 85, 86
    hybridization,
        factors influencing, 84
        probe removal from blots, 85
        washing of membranes, 84, 85
    interpretation, 78, 79
    membrane transfer, 78
    probes,
        complementary DNA probe
            construction, 81, 82
        nick translation, 80
        nonradioactive probes and
            detection, 83, 84
        random primer extension, 80, 81
        riboprobe construction, 82, 83
    protocol, 77
    ribonuclease inhibition, 74
    RNA preparation,
        isolation, 75
        quantitation, 75
    sensitivity, 103
    total RNA versus messenger RNA, 74
    troubleshooting, 79, 80
Nucleic acid sequence based
    amplification (NASBA), *see*
    Polymerase chain reaction
Nylon membrane,
    northern blotting, 78
    Southern blotting,
        capillary transfer, 70
        electrotransfer, 70, 71
        fixing of DNA, 71
        vacuum transfer, 71

O
Obesity, genetics, 263, 264
Oncogene, definition, 296
Ovarian cancer, heredity, 301, 302

P

p53, single-strand conformational
     polymorphism, 134
PAI-1, *see* Plasminogen activator
     inhibitor-1
Pancreas cancer, early detection, 307
PCR, *see* Polymerase chain reaction
Pepsin, tissue treatment for *in situ*
     hybridization, 173
PFGE, *see* Pulsed-field gel
     electrophoresis
Philadelphia chromosome, chronic
     myelogenous leukemia diagnosis,
     333–335
PHP, *see* Pseudohypoparathyroidism
Pit-1, deficiency disorder, 251
Plasmid,
     applications, 42
     copy number, 42
     isolation, 42–44
     organization, 37, 42
     pathogen analysis, 354
Plasminogen activator inhibitor-1 (PAI-
     1), polymorphism and arterial
     thrombotic disease, 286
Polyacrylamide gel electrophoresis,
     DNA sizing, 133, 134
     factors affecting migration rate, 130
     pH, 131
     polymerization of gel, 132
     pore size, 132, 133
     safety in handling acrylamide, 132
Polymerase chain reaction (PCR), *see
     also In situ* polymerase chain
     reaction; Mutational analysis
     polymerase chain reaction;
     Reverse-transcription polymerase
     chain reaction
     AmpErase system, 93
     antibiotic resistance detection, 352–354
     applications, 89, 94, 95, 123
     branched DNA detection, 97, 99, 100, 342
     buffer, 93
     clonality determination in
          lymphoma, 319, 327–329
     contamination prevention, 92, 93,
          369, 370
     deoxynucleotide triphosphates, 93
     Duchenne muscular dystrophy
          diagnosis, 241, 242
     genomic DNA target sequence
          analysis, protocol, 94

ligase chain reaction, 95
     long-range reactions, 92
     nucleic acid sequence based
          amplification, 95, 97
     pathogen diagnosis, 341, 345–352,
          355, 356
     polymerases,
          Klenow fragment, 90
          Taq polymerase, 90, 92, 93, 97, 123
     primer design, 93
     principle, 89, 90, 124
     quality control, 364–370
     sensitivity, 89, 90, 92
     trinucleotide repeat disorder
          diagnosis, 233–235
Polymorphism,
     definition, 220
     types, 220–222
Probe, oligonucleotide,
     complementary DNA probe
          construction, 81, 82
     fluorescence *in situ* hybridization,
          hybridization, 168, 170
          labeling, 167
          types, 165
     in situ hybridization,
          hybridization reaction, 175, 176
          labeling, 174, 175
          types, 174
     membrane attachment in reverse dot
          blots, 128
     nick translation, 80
     nonradioactive probes and detection,
          83, 84, 127, 128
     pathogen diagnosis by hybridization,
          341, 342
     random primer extension, 80, 81
     riboprobe construction, 82, 83, 141
Promoter,
     core elements, 195
     enhancer matching, 194, 195
     inducibility, 195
     tissue specificity, 195, 196
Protein C, abnormalities in venous
     thrombosis, 287
Protein S,
     deficiency, 288
     functions, 287
Protein truncation test (PrTT),
     applications, 237, 376
     gel interpretation, 155, 156

principle, 153, 154, 376
template synthesis, 155
Proteinase K,
cell treatment in DNA isolation, 37–39
tissue treatment for *in situ*
hybridization, 173
PrTT, *see* Protein truncation test
Pseudohypoparathyroidism (PHP),
features, 256
genetics, 256
Pulsed-field gel electrophoresis (PFGE),
DNA isolation, 41
pathogen analysis, 355
Purine nucleoside phosphorylase, gene
therapy of deficiency, 208

Q
QC, *see* Quality control
Quality control (QC),
amplicon carryover prevention, 369,
370
commercial kits, 370
importance, 363
instrumentation, 363–365
results reporting, 365
test controls, 365–367

R
RACE, *see* Rapid amplification of
complementary DNA ends
Rapid amplification of complementary
DNA ends (RACE), *see*
Reverse-transcription polymerase
chain reaction
Restriction enzyme,
classification, 51, 144
quality control of digestions, 366, 367
restriction fragment length
polymorphism analysis, 143,
144, 220, 221
site-directed mutagenesis,
polymerase chain reaction
mediation and mutation
analysis, 145, 146
Southern blot analysis, fragmentation
of DNA, 64, 65
Retinoblastoma, genetics, 299, 300
Retrovirus,
gene therapy,
efficiency, 201
helper cell lines, 201

insertional oncogenesis, 200, 201
targeting of genes, 201
vector types, 202, 203
life cycle, 200
translation units, 200
Reverse-transcription polymerase chain
reaction,
agarose gel electrophoresis of
products, 112, 113
complementary DNA amplification,
cycle parameters for polymerase
chain reaction, 112
overview, 110
primer design, 110–112
contamination prevention, 114, 115
controls, 115
differential display, 118, 119
patch-clamp recording, simultaneous
measurement, 115, 116
principle, 94, 103, 104
quantitative analysis standards, 114
messenger RNA, 115–117
rapid amplification of
complementary DNA ends, 117,
118
restriction mapping of products, 113,
114
reverse transcription,
overview, 106
primer design, 109
priming first-strand
complementary DNA
synthesis, 107–109
reaction parameters, 109, 110
reverse transcriptase selection, 106,
107
RNA preparation,
isolation, 104–106
quantitation, 105
storage, 106
sensitivity, 103
sequence-specific hybridization in
verification, 114
sequencing of products, 113
Ribonuclease,
inhibition in RNA purification, 44, 45,
74, 104, 105
mutation detection by cleavage of
mismatched RNA:DNA
duplexes,
efficiency of cleavage, 141–143

gel electrophoresis, 143
nonisotopic assay, 142, 143
principle, 141
Ribosomal RNA (rRNA),
function, 27
structure, 27
RNA, *see also* Messenger RNA; Northern
blot; Reverse-transcription
polymerase chain reaction;
Ribosomal RNA; Transfer RNA
functions, 23, 26, 27, 45
isolation,
cell lysis, 46, 105
messenger RNA, 46, 47
northern blot preparation, 75
ribonuclease inhibition, 44, 45, 74,
104, 105
mapping, 49, 103
nucleic acid sequence based
amplification, 95, 97
plasmid-directed synthesis, 47–49
quantitation, 49, 75, 115–117
structure, 22, 23, 26–29, 45
rRNA, *see* Ribosomal RNA

S
SBMA, *see* Spinal and bulbar muscular
atrophy
SCA 1, *see* Spinocerebellar ataxia type 1
SCID, *see* Severe combined
immunodeficiency
Severe combined immunodeficiency
(SCID), gene therapy, 208
Sex reversal, genetics, 260
Sickle cell anemia,
allele-specific polymerase chain
reaction, 146
symptomatic treatment, 193
Single-strand conformational
polymorphism (SSCP)
gel electrophoresis, 136
principle, 134
sensitivity, 134–136
spinal muscular atrophy diagnosis,
235, 236
Site-directed mutagenesis, polymerase
chain reaction mediation and
mutation analysis, 145, 146
SMA, *see* Spinal muscular atrophy
Southern blot,
applications, 63, 64, 85, 86

clonality determination in
lymphoma, 319, 323–325, 327
DNA preparation,
agarose gel electrophoresis, 65–68
restriction enzyme fragmentation,
64, 65
Duchenne muscular dystrophy
diagnosis, 241
hybridization,
factors influencing, 84
probe removal from blots, 85
washing of membranes, 84, 85
interpretation, 72, 73
membrane transfers,
capillary transfer, 70
election of membrane, 68
electrotransfer, 70, 71
fixing of DNA, 71
vacuum transfer, 71
pathogen analysis, 354, 355
principle, 63
probes,
complementary DNA probe
construction, 81, 82
nick translation, 80
nonradioactive probes and
detection, 83, 84
random primer extension, 80, 81
riboprobe construction, 82, 83
quality control, 365, 366
sensitivity, 64
trinucleotide repeat disorder
diagnosis, 233–235
troubleshooting, 73
Spectrophotometer, quality control, 364
Spinal and bulbar muscular atrophy
(SBMA),
diagnosis, 233, 234
features, 231
genotype and phenotype correlation,
232
molecular mechanisms, 233
parental transmission bias, 232, 233
trinucleotide repeat instability, 231, 232
Spinal muscular atrophy (SMA),
diagnosis, 235, 236
genes, 236
incidence, 235
types, 235
Spinocerebellar ataxia type 1 (SCA1),
diagnosis, 233–235

features, 231
genotype and phenotype correlation, 232
molecular mechanisms, 233
parental transmission bias, 232, 233
trinucleotide repeat instability, 231, 232
SSCP, *see* Single-strand conformational polymorphism

T
Tangier disease, features, 280
Taq polymerase, polymerase chain reaction, 90, 92, 93, 97, 123
T-cell,
    clonality determination,
        polymerase chain reaction, 319, 327–329
        Southern blot, 319, 323–325, 327
    development, 321, 322
    markers, 322
    receptor genes,
        rearrangements, 322, 323
        types, 321, 322
β-Thalassemia,
    competitive oligonucleotide priming and mutation detection, 151
    mutation screening by reverse dot blotting, 129
bcl-2, translocation defects in lymphoma, 330, 331, 367, 368
Thymidine, structure, 17, 18
Thyroid-stimulating hormone (TSH), *see also* Generalized thyroid hormone resistance
    elective pituitary resistance, 254
    receptor mutations,
        activating mutations, 253
        inhibiting mutations, 253
Transfer RNA (tRNA),
    function, 26, 27
    structure, 26

Triglyceride, familial metabolic disorders, 275–277
Trinucleotide repeat, neurological disorders, 229, 231–235
Trisomy, fluorescence *in situ* hybridization analysis, 171
tRNA, *see* Transfer RNA
TSH, *see* Thyroid-stimulating hormone
Tumor, *see also* Cancer
    fluorescence *in situ* hybridization analysis, 170, 171
    gene therapy, 209, 210
    growth hormone secretion, 252
    in situ amplification analysis of gene expression, 185
    in situ hybridization analysis of gene expression, 177, 178
    thyroid genetics, 254
Tumor suppressor gene, definition, 296, 297

U
Uniparental disomy, heredity, 223
Urinalysis,
    ancient history, 5, 6
    early modern developments, 8

V
Vaccination, gene therapy, 211
Venous thrombosis, risk factors, 286–289
Vitamin D resistance, genetics, 256

W
Williams syndrome, features, 255
Wilms' tumor, genetics, 304

X
X-linked disorders,
    heredity, 224–226
    quality control in assay, 368, 369

Z
Z DNA, structure, 17, 19